ANTHROPOLOGY AND

MW00356464

CULTURE, ILLNESS, AND HEALING

Editors:

MARGARET LOCK

*Departments of Anthropology and Humanities and Social Studies
in Medicine, McGill University, Montreal, Canada*

ALLAN YOUNG

*Department of Anthropology, Case Western Reserve University,
Cleveland, Ohio, U.S.A.*

Editorial Board:

ATWOOD D. GAINES

*Departments of Anthropology and Psychiatry, Case Western Reserve
University and Medical School, Cleveland, Ohio, U.S.A.*

GILBERT LEWIS

*Department of Anthropology, University of Cambridge,
England*

GANANATH OBEYESEKERE

*Department of Anthropology, Princeton University,
Princeton, New Jersey, U.S.A.*

ANTHROPOLOGY AND EPIDEMIOLOGY

Interdisciplinary Approaches to the Study of Health and Disease

Edited by

CRAIG R. JANES

Department of Anthropology, University of Colorado, Denver, Colorado

RON STALL

Department of Urban Studies, Rutgers University, New Brunswick, New Jersey, and The Alcohol Research Group, Berkeley, California

and

SANDRA M. GIFFORD

Division of Community Health, State Health Commission of Victoria, Australia

D. REIDEL PUBLISHING COMPANY

A MEMBER OF THE KLUWER 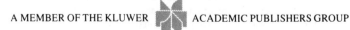 ACADEMIC PUBLISHERS GROUP

DORDRECHT / BOSTON / LANCASTER / TOKYO

Library of Congress Cataloging-in-Publication Data

Anthropology and epidemiology.

(Culture, illness, and healing)
Includes bibliographies and indexes.
1. Medical anthropology. 2. Anthropology,
Cultural. 3. Epidemiology. I. Janes, Craig R. (Craig
Robert), 1953– II. Stall, Ron, 1954– . III.
Gifford, Sandra M. IV. Series. [DNLM: 1. Anthro-
pology, Cultural. 2. Epidemiology. WA 105 A628]
GN296.A55 1986 306'.46 86–20434
ISBN 90–277–2248–X
ISBN 90–277–2249–8 (pbk.)

Published by D. Reidel Publishing Company,
P.O. Box 17, 3300 AA Dordrecht, Holland.

Sold and distributed in the U.S.A. and Canada
by Kluwer Academic Publishers,
101 Philip Drive, Assinippi Park, Norwell, MA 02061, U.S.A.

In all other countries, sold and distributed
by Kluwer Academic Publishers Group,
P.O. Box 322, 3300 AH Dordrecht, Holland.

All Rights Reserved
© 1986 by D. Reidel Publishing Company
and copyrightholders as specified on appropriate pages within.
No part of the material protected by this copyright notice may be reproduced or
utilized in any form or by any means, electronic or mechanical,
including photocopying, recording or by any information storage and
retrieval system, without written permission from the copyright owner

Printed in the Netherlands

TABLE OF CONTENTS

PREFACE

Over the past two decades increasing interest has emerged in the contributions that the social sciences might make to the epidemiological study of patterns of health and disease. Several reasons can be cited for this increasing interest. Primary among these has been the rise of the chronic, non-infectious diseases as important causes of morbidity and mortality within Western populations during the 20th century. Generally speaking, the chronic, non-infectious diseases are strongly influenced by lifestyle variables, which are themselves strongly influenced by social and cultural forces. The understanding of the effects of the behavioral factors in, say, hypertension, thus requires an understanding of the social and cultural factors which encourage obesity, a sedentary lifestyle, non-compliance with anti-hypertensive medications (or other prescribed regimens), and stress. Equally, there is a growing awareness that considerations of human behavior and its social and cultural determinants are important for understanding the distribution and control of infectious diseases. Related to this expansion of epidemiologic interest into the behavioral realm has been the development of etiological models which focus on the psychological, biological and socio-cultural characteristics of hosts, rather than exclusive concern with exposure to a particular agent or even behavioral risk. Also during this period advances in statistical and computing techniques have made accessible the ready testing of multivariate causal models, and so have encouraged the measurement of the effects of social and cultural factors on disease occurrence. Finally, (perhaps in partial response to the previous reasons) the disciplines of epidemiology and anthropology have undergone a parallel evolution. Epidemiologists have been forced to define and measure complex social processes hypothesized to impact on health and disease states. Anthropologists, on the other hand, have become increasingly interested in the potential contributions of their discipline to resolve the day-to-day problems of specific populations, and especially so within the realms of disease occurrence and medical care. These convergent interests have created the opportunity for mutually beneficial cross-disciplinary pollination.

The original idea behind this book can be said to have been formed, in large part, in conversations between epidemiologists and medical anthropologists interested in the effects of social and cultural variables on health. This volume has benefited most particularly from the experience of researchers in the Department of Epidemiology and International Health and Medical Anthropology Program of the University of California, San Francisco, and in the School of Public Health of the University of California,

vii

Craig R. Janes et al. (eds.), Anthropology and Epidemiology, vii—viii.
© *1986 by D. Reidel Publishing Company.*

Berkeley. Acting on a growing interest on these two campuses, particularly, among medical anthropologists either training or working in epidemiology, Sandra Gifford and Ron Stall organized a session for the 1983 meetings of the American Anthropological Association. Most of the contributors to the book presented papers at this session or acted as discussants. The interest attracted by the symposium and the lively discussion that followed the presentation of papers convinced us of the need for this book. It became clear that the idea of combining or integrating medical anthropology and epidemiology represented an area of recognized potential.

Anthropology and epidemiology are multifaceted disciplines that claim a diverse population of practitioners, teachers, and writers. There is thus no single integrative model that embodies the many strengths of the two fields. It is not simply a matter of applying anthropological techniques or theories to understanding disease and disorder; a wide range of possible research alternatives exists — from enlivening epidemiological data with ethnographic detail to direct involvement by anthropologists in epidemiological research. In this book we have endeavored to collect articles that represent several analytic approaches to the concurrent use of anthropology and epidemiology in the study of a variety of diseases and disorders. Other diseases, different approaches, and varying integrative models exist; we hope they are explored in subsequent publications. If the directions signaled by these diverse contributions illuminate paths for future research, and invite further discussion and debate in the disciplines touched by anthropology and epidemiology, we will feel our purpose in undertaking this project was achieved.

Following our basic agenda to provide a sampling of research that draws on various integrative models of anthropology and epidemiology, we have structured the book according to major disease categories, and within these broad categories case studies of particular places and peoples that range from indigenous cultures of the Third or Fourth Worlds, to contemporary, white, urban-American subcultures. We set the scene for these case studies in Section I with a series of theoretical and historical essays that examine the logic and historical underpinnings of interdisciplinary collaboration. Section II offers three case studies of anthropological contributions to the study of infectious disease. Section III presents two anthropological perspectives on the major non-infectious conditions of cardiovascular disease and breast cancer. Section IV considers the applicability of social science models and methods in the case of three classes of mental health "disorders" — suicide, alcohol problems, and hyperactivity in children.

Readers will note that the contributions of anthropology in this volume are predominantly social/cultural in nature. In addressing our many goals in constructing this book, we were unable to give to physical/biological anthropology the justice it is due for its many contributions to human paleoepidemiology, genetic epidemiology, and human ecology. In partial defense of this omission, we feel that because the integration of epidemiology and social/cultural anthropology has remained most problematic, one goal has been to encourage cross-disciplinary dialogue in this area. We hope that as interest in the potential for collaboration grows, future volumes will appear that contain contributions from other sub-fields of anthropology as well.

This volume was not conceived of as a primer in either epidemiology or anthropology. Many excellent introductory texts and collections exist. In the field of epidemiology we refer the reader to the introductory texts by Abraham and David Lilienfeld, *Foundations of Epidemiology*, 2nd ed., New York: Oxford University Press, 1980; and Judith Mausner and Anita Kramer, *Epidemiology — An Introductory Text*, Philadelphia: W. B. Saunders Company, 1985. For readers unfamiliar with epidemiologic concepts and terminology, we suggest a concise dictionary by John Last, *A Dictionary of Epidemiology*, New York: John Wiley and Sons, 1978. For readers unfamiliar with anthropology, specifically medical anthropology, we suggest perusal of the following texts: George Foster and Barbara Anderson, *Medical Anthropology*, New York: Wiley, 1978; Lorna G. Moore, et al., *The Biocultural Basis of Health: Expanding Views of Medical Anthropology*, St. Louis, Missouri: Mosby, 1980; and Ann McElroy and Patricia Townsend, *Medical Anthropology: An Ecological Perspective*, North Scituate, Massachusetts: Duxbury, 1979. For those interested in case studies of the relationship between anthropology and public health, the following remains a classic reference: Benjamin Paul (ed.), *Health, Culture, and Community*, New York: Russell Sage Foundation, 1955. For more advanced reading in medical anthropology, the series *Culture, Illness, and Healing*, edited by Arthur Kleinman and published by the D. Reidel Company, is recommended.

This volume is the result of much hard work by many people. We would first like to thank the contributors for faithfully sending us their drafts and coping with our particular brand of "committee" editorship. Second, we would like to thank the many organizations that provided us with the necessary support to attend to the duties of editing. These include the Medical Anthropology Program of the University of California, San Francisco; the Alcohol Research Group of the Medical Research Institute, San Francisco, California; the Prevention Research Center of Berkeley, California; and the World Health Organization Centre (Region 8) For Diabetes Education and Control, Caulfield, Australia. We gratefully acknowledge the diligent labors of Cathy Wasserman in indexing the volume, and we thank Martin Scrivener of D. Reidel and the former series editor, Arthur Kleinman, for their assistance in bringing this book to publication.

June 20, 1986   SANDRA M. GIFFORD
                                                     CRAIG R. JANES
                                                     RON STALL

SECTION I

HISTORICAL AND THEORETICAL
PERSPECTIVES

FREDERICK L. DUNN AND CRAIG R. JANES

INTRODUCTION: MEDICAL ANTHROPOLOGY AND EPIDEMIOLOGY

As epidemiology has expanded its concerns in this century to encompass the full range of human disease and disorder, researchers have been forced to grapple with complex assemblages of psychological, social, cultural, demographic, and genetic factors in their quest to identify etiologic relationships and improve health services. The recognition that causal assemblages often include such phenomena as acculturation, "anomie", ethnicity, and poverty has led epidemiologists to look to the social sciences for help in explaining the relationship of social and cultural processes to health. One consequence of this interdisciplinary work has been the evolution of general models of health and disease that include, as a central component, the many dimensions of human behavior.

It is now recognized that any human disease or disorder is the result of many factors within what may be described as a "causal web", a web of determinants.[1] These webs, their extent varying with population characteristics such as size and density, include exogenous factors, biotic and nonbiotic; endogenous (genetic) factors; demographic factors; and behavior as governed by psychological, social, and cultural factors (Audy 1971; Audy and Dunn 1974; Dunn 1976a). Within any such causal web, many of the determinants of disease and disorder are behavioral.

It is the goal of epidemiology to identify and measure the relative importance of factors within the causal web of a disease or disorder. Because all diseases are caused, at least in part, by the behavior of individuals, groups, or communities, epidemiology must be a behavioral science. The concern with health-related behavior is something that epidemiology shares with medical anthropology, and is the basis of the complementarity of the two disciplines. Whereas epidemiology may be concerned primarily with determining the relationship of behavior to disease, medical anthropology most often focuses on the social and cultural correlates of behavior, or on the contexts of such behavior. The point of greatest possible complementarity and practical collaboration thus lies in exploring the nexus between the health consequences of behavior and the social and cultural correlates of that behavior.

Although anthropologists have worked in epidemiology, and significant scholarly attention has been given to the relationship between the social sciences and epidemiology (e.g., Cassel 1964; Fleck and Ianni 1958), the nexus in the causal web described above is not well understood in the case of many diseases and disorders. At present the problem areas that have profited most from cross disciplinary collaboration are the cardiovascular diseases

3

Craig R. Janes et al. (eds.), Anthropology and Epidemiology, 3—34.
© *1986 by D. Reidel Publishing Company.*

and some psychiatric disorders (e.g., Scotch 1963; Leighton 1959; Leighton et al. 1963). There are many reasons for a lack of research in this area. Disciplinary boundaries often restrict cross-disciplinary communication. Funding patterns also tend to follow disciplinary lines, and restrict interdisciplinary research. And perhaps most importantly, of all the social sciences anthropology holds to a methodological tradition that diverges in significant ways conceptually as well as operationally from that of epidemiology.

Despite such differences and barriers, however, integration of the two traditions holds promise for both understanding and preventing disease. It is important for epidemiologists to understand the complex nature of the human behavior they try and capture through quantitative measurement. It is equally important for anthropologists to recognize the powerful models used in epidemiology to identify patterns of cause and effect. Complementary research would profit both disciplines.

The papers that follow are case studies that illustrate various facets of the relationship between medical anthropology and epidemiology. Although several articles have appeared that consider the relationship of "anthropology and epidemiology", especially in recent years (e.g., Rubinstein 1984), we are unaware of other wide-ranging attempts to explore these relationships. Despite the wide-ranging goals of this book, however, we must also point out two limitations: almost all of the case material relates to anthropological perspectives on epidemiology and epidemiological problems; and although anthropology is a composite discipline — physical or biological as well as social and cultural — this work is almost exclusively concerned with epidemiology in relationship to social and cultural anthropology. Concerning the first limitation, this book offers a distinctly anthropological view of epidemiology. This is not to say that it will appeal only to other anthropologists. There is much in this work to interest and to serve as an "invitation" to the epidemiologist. Concerning the second limitation, we recognize the importance of work in biological/physical anthropology that is epidemiological, or makes a significant contribution to epidemiology. Anthropologists have worked for some time in the areas of human paleontology, genetic epidemiology, and human ecology, making significant contributions to understanding the impact of disease on the human organism. Perhaps in due time another book may be assembled that emphasizes epidemiology in relationship to physical/biological anthropology.

In the following sections we examine the logical basis of the complementarity of medical anthropology and epidemiology. We divide this discussion into two parts. In part one we describe the kinds of collaborative relationships that have characterized the relationship of these two disciplines and discuss the conceptual basis of this collaboration. In part two we turn to a discussion of how anthropology may benefit the application of epidemiologic data through facilitating programs of disease prevention and control.

PART ONE: AREAS OF CONCEPTUAL AFFINITY

Different But Complementary Traditions

The relationship between anthropology and epidemiology has grown chiefly through the efforts of anthropologists working "in epidemiology". At least a few epidemiologists were aware, even many years ago, that anthropologists were potential contributors to epidemiological research (Fleck and Ianni 1958; Cassel 1964). Others such as Buck et al. (1970) recruited anthropologists to serve as members of teams engaged in epidemiological fieldwork. Although anthropologists today are involved in studies across the whole spectrum of epidemiological concern, it is clear that the earliest points of contact with the field were in two areas: psychiatric epidemiology, and epidemiological research in "traditional", non-Western societies, in developing countries, or in other settings where it was considered that anthropologists were likely to be particularly "useful" by virtue of their special knowledge.

It is understandable that the earliest common ground between the disciplines was found in the psychiatric area — in which the medical (and epidemiological) side was represented by persons with at least some exposure to the social and behavioral sciences. In addition, social scientists were involved in psychiatric epidemiology from its beginnings in the nineteenth century (Grob 1985). Among the earliest examples, then, of anthropological-epidemiological collaboration are studies such as those undertaken by the Leightons, Hughes, and others in Stirling County, Nova Scotia, and in the Yoruba country of Nigeria (A. Leighton 1959; D. Leighton et al. 1963; A. Leighton et al. 1969).

More recently, anthropologists have involved themselves in the field of communicable disease epidemiology. Infectious and parasitic disease investigators have seldom had much exposure to the social sciences in their training, and have therefore — unlike those in psychiatric research — been slow to appreciate the possibilities of collaboration with anthropologists or other behavioral scientists (Dunn 1979a, 1984). Very few anthropologists have as yet found opportunities for work similar to that described by Nations in her contribution to this volume on diarrheal disease research in Brazil (pp. 97—123), or by Gorman in his role as an anthropologist facilitating research on AIDS in the gay community of San Francisco (pp. 157—172).

Today, of course, it is in chronic non-infectious disease epidemiology — especially work on cancer, heart disease, and genetic disorders — that anthropology is most significantly represented. Anthropologists such as Scotch (1960) were drawn into epidemiologic studies in the chronic disease field from their beginnings in mid-century and their influence was evident in the writings of pioneering chronic disease epidemiologists such as Cassel (1964; and see Trostle, this volume, pp. 59—94).

The increasing involvement of social scientists in epidemiology parallels the historical development of epidemiology as a distinguishable discipline. Through the first half of this century epidemiologists were largely self-taught, or learned by example in doing research. Many were physicians; some were statisticians. The physicians came, of course, from professional schools; most, in their university years, were not exposed to research in any systematic fashion, that is, to the methods, traditions, principles, limitations, and ethical considerations that are now a normal part of research training. Those whose inclinations led them into epidemiological research became "epidemiologists", if they chose to identify themselves as such, largely by virtue of their research experience. A background of formal epidemiological training — beyond, perhaps, a course or two in a school of public health — was certainly the exception until the 1950s and 1960s. Thus the profession (discipline) of epidemiology in this country was established and long dominated by several generations of physician-scientists and statisticians whose sense of professional identity was not always very strong (see Stallones 1963). Things have changed dramatically since that time. During what Rothman (1980) calls the "boom period" (1950—1980) of epidemiology, textbooks appeared, theory flowered, the ranks increased, and epidemiologists were trained as such.

The epidemiology of today is very different to that of 1950 in terms of its practitioners; its professional identity; in its confidence, flexibility, and capacity for interdisciplinary collaboration — for incorporating new ideas and for taking advantage of research methods offered by other fields; and in its research emphases. Among other differences, for example, in 1950 the communicable diseases still dominated the concern of most epidemiologists; a few were interested in mental disorders; a very few in the chronic non-infectious diseases and disorders. Now epidemiologists are concerned to a much greater extent with chronic non-infectious diseases, and have expanded their interest to include events or disorders such as suicide, child abuse, accidents, and substance abuse.

The field of anthropology has undergone a similar kind of development within the same approximate time period. Although anthropologists have been trained as such for a significantly longer period than epidemiologists, it was not until the 1940s that they began to turn significant attention to applying anthropological expertise to the solution of human problems. Since this time there has been an enormous theoretical growth in the field of anthropology. In very broad terms, it can be said that sociocultural anthropology has moved from a field where the major research question is why and how cultures differ — explored by the early ethnological theorists — to understanding the dynamics of human behavior, the acquisition and use of beliefs by individuals, and the adaptive significance of patterns of behavior. In addition, there has been a significant increase in applied research, particularly in the past twenty-five years, that has led to the development of knowledge regarding specific classes of topics, or "problems"; e.g., economic development, education, aging, and health.

Although the two fields do have a long and productive historical relationship, a review of current textbooks of epidemiology and anthropology would suggest that the two disciplines are separated by serious analytic differences. Because of a focus in anthropology on the details of social, cultural and biological variability, the basic analytic focus in data collection has been on relatively small, and generally "bounded" groups of people: communities, villages, and cultures.[2] Furthermore, traditional descriptive anthropology, or ethnography, is primarily qualitative and "vertical" in nature. The field worker concentrates on the study of one or only a very few social units (households, groups, villages, etc.) of a particular society. Each unit is studied in great detail and in regard to many aspects of day-to-day life. Much is observed, much is recorded of values, attitudes, and behavior; and as the work proceeds many questions are posed and answered. The results of these vertical studies form the basis of analytic or theoretical anthropology (ethnology). In the study of illness and disease, anthropology has been primarily concerned with understanding the social and cultural contexts in which an illness event is embedded; e.g., the sick role, ethnomedicine, and the social structure of medical systems. More recently, many medical anthropologists have extended their research into the realm of medical ecology, a field that shares many research goals with epidemiology.

Although epidemiology is similar to anthropology in possessing descriptive and analytic components, the topical focus of these components, and the methods they entail, are unique. Epidemiology is usually defined as the study of the distribution and determinants of disease and disorder in human populations. The primary units of analysis are large population aggregates identified in terms of geographic, administrative, or demographic boundaries. There is no assumption in epidemiology that members of the groups under scrutiny are related to each other, or see themselves related to each other, in any way other than as defined by the epidemiologist (i.e., being a member of a specific ethnic, sex, age, or residential group). Unlike descriptive anthropology, which is based on in-depth ethnographic study, descriptive epidemiology is quantitative and closely related in its "horizontal" methods to those of social survey research. Population-based data, often archival or based on the analysis of morbidity or mortality records, are collected from many demographic units, and the range of questions is restricted and usually specified prior to the initiation of research. Analytic epidemiology differs from the descriptive component primarily in terms of its focus on the identification of cause and effect in the case of a specific disease or class of diseases. Although some analytic designs in epidemiology require working with relatively small groups of people — for example, retrospective case-control designs — sample sizes are generally much larger than in the case of anthropology, and sample selection is based on demographic characteristics and disease status rather than on social or cultural features of the subject population.

Despite these differences, as we have seen, medical anthropologists and epidemiologists share a history of cooperation and common concern. Although in some cases this cooperation is based primarily on the value of "special" anthropological knowledge of the subjects of epidemiologic investigation — e.g., non-Western peoples — there are more fundamental reasons for a natural affinity of the two disciplines. Specifically, this affinity is based on complementary approaches to answering the following three major research questions that are characteristic of nearly all epidemiologic research: (1) what are the social, behavioral, demographic, and biological characteristics of persons who develop a disease; (2) what is the relationship of the disease to geographic, ecological, and social locales; and (3) what is the relationship of disease onset to suspected risk factors (cf. Mausner and Bahn 1974)?

These three questions are often associated with descriptive epidemiology, which seeks primarily to identify the amount and distribution of disease within a population. In this context it is fairly routine to focus on the demographic characteristics of *person,* (question 1); *place* (question 2); and *time* (question 3). For example, typical categories of data gathered in descriptive studies include age, sex, ethnicity, occupation, marital status, place of residence, age cohort, and differences in disease rates occurring over time. Analytic epidemiology, a more focused study of the determinants of disease and causal relationships, also operationalizes the categories of person, place, and time, but in a more specific way that is dependent on the relationship between hypothesized risk factors and a disease. For example, social support and exposure to social and cultural contexts characterized by poverty and anomie are characteristics of person and place that have been analyzed in relationship to cardiovascular disease. The time dimension in analytic epidemiology involves methodological techniques for sorting out cause and effect.

In contemporary epidemiology, different aspects of person and place — for example things intrinsic or extrinsic to the person, and things in the social, physical, or biologic environment — have been combined into ecological models that stress the interrelations of causal factors. The idea of "causal web" we alluded to earlier in this introduction is one such model. The essence of this model, developed in response to the overly deterministic focus on a few agents during the germ-theory era of the early 20th century, is that effects never depend on single isolated causes, but occur as a consequence of "a complex genealogy of antecedents" (MacMahon and Pugh 1960). A simpler and more graphic representation of this idea, emphasizing man-environment relations, is that of the "wheel of causation". The wheel consists of a hub representing an individual or group of individuals, and includes genetic, psychological, and behavioral attributes. Surrounding this hub are the biological, physical, and social environments. The relative importance of the different components of the wheel depend upon the disease or disorder being studied. Like the idea of a causal web, the wheel model implies multiple and interrelated etiologic factors (Mausner and Bahn 1974: 35—36). Finally, all etiologic models include some conception of time, generally expressed as the "natural history" of a disease. Natural history is generally broken down into necessarily general and arbitrary stages which indicate an individual's susceptibility to disease, the point at which anatomic or functional changes occur, and the point where disability results if the deleterious anatomic or functional changes are not arrested (Mausner and Bahn 1974: 6—9). Factors whose presence appears to be associated with increasing susceptibility are termed risk factors. The importance of determining the natural history of any disease lies in identifying appropriate points for disease prevention or control. Usually this is best done at the stage of susceptibility, which is in turn recognized on the basis of risk factors — characteristics of person and place identified through analytic research.

Although this description of epidemiologic models and concepts is necessarily brief, it should be apparent to the medical anthropologist that there are several significant points at which anthropology and epidemiology share many concepts and where anthropology may offer some significant empirical input. In the following paragraphs we illustrate the complementarity of anthropology and epidemiology by citing the potential of social science contributions to answering research questions within the categories of person, place, and time. At the conclusion of this discussion we offer a model for organizing anthropological-epidemiological research on health-related behavior.

Characteristics of Persons

The first question commonly addressed in epidemiologic studies regards the relationship of characteristics of individuals or groups to disease. These characteristics may also include attributes that contribute to health, or what is commonly termed "host resistance". Many of the attributes of persons that affect health will be behavioral (e.g., food habits), will stem from social, psychological, or cultural processes (e.g., social integration or social support), or will be meaningful in the context of some group of people or beliefs (e.g., ethnicity or religion). The potential for interdisciplinary collaboration in identifying and understanding these attributes should be evident.

Consider, for example, how the study of the effects of social networks on health provides an opportunity for anthropological input. The concept of social networks was defined by pioneering anthropological researchers (e.g., Mitchell 1969), and later operationalized by epidemiologists to test an hypothesized relationship between social network formation and health status (e.g, Berkman and Syme 1976; Pilisuk and Froland 1978). The study of social networks and health represents an example of the diffusion of an anthropological concept to epidemiology. In its travels across disciplinary boundaries, however, the definition of the concept of social networks has been stripped of some of its original meaning. In health studies the interest is usually in measuring the size and integration of a network, or determining which relationships in a network are psychologically meaningful and supportive. In its original conceptualization, however, the idea of social network involved two qualitative dimensions, and within these, several sub-dimensions (Mitchell 1969). First, the structure and shape of a social network, termed its "morphology", represents the size, differentiation, and density of relationships. Second, the quality of relationships in a network, termed the interactional dimension, represents the content and meaning of each constituent relationship. There are, further, certain regular and systematic relationships between structures and meanings. There are many kinds of meanings, and each may represent a different dimension of social support, the aspect of presumed interest in most epidemiological studies. The importance of recognizing the many dimensions of social networks, and thus of social support in the context of health, cannot be underestimated. For example, which relationships, imbued with certain meanings, function to provide people under stress with the most fundamental kind of support? Or, what kind and how much social support derives from friendship ties; from kinship ties? Therefore, while epidemiologic analysis has demonstrated the relationship of some social network attributes to health, a significant unexplored area remains that would benefit from anthropological research.

Characteristics of Places

The second question epidemiologists commonly ask about a disease is "what is its relationship to geographic, ecological, and social locales"? This question is most often directed at identifying the existence of environmental pathogens, or of unhealthful environmental processes. Remember that in the epidemiological classification, this notion includes the social, physical, and biologic environments. Anthropological input to answering this question has often been made through applying the special knowledge gained in the course of ethnographic case studies of particular communities, cultures, or ecological settings. For example, Page et al. (1974) used the published results of ethnographic research to rank Solomon Islands societies on the basis of acculturation to Western culture. These societies were then compared in an effort to isolate the relationship of characteristics of lifestyle (e.g., nutrition and exercise) to blood pressure levels. Anthropologists have also been involved in identifying the socio-ecological changes that occur when people migrate from one environment to another (e.g., Beaglehole et al. 1977; Baker et al. in press; Graves et al. 1983; Janes this volume: pp. 175—211; Prior et al.

1974; Scotch 1963), or are exposed to the particular social and cultural upheavals of post-colonial modernization (e.g., Dressler 1982, 1985).

Characteristics of Time

A third question of importance to epidemiologists is "what is the relationship of disease onset to suspected risk factors?" This is a methodological question related to the assessment of cause and effect relationships. This issue is central to analytic epidemiology, where the discipline of epidemiology is the strongest conceptually, and where anthropology may stand to gain the most in terms of design and methodology. As we have described, analytic epidemiology most often tries to explain the occurrence of an event based on a wide range of individual, group, and environmental "facts". A number of research models rather unique to epidemiology have been developed to evaluate the relationship of these facts to each other and to the event of interest over time; e.g., retrospective and prospective case-control designs and methods for determining the risks attributable to individual causal factors. Given these methodological traits, would not it be of anthropological interest to apply epidemiological models to occurrences of witchcraft, or of political succession, or of spirit possession? Although to date few anthropologists have explicitly attempted such applications of epidemiological methods to anthropological problems, the contributions of those who have are significant (e.g., Rubel et al. 1984).

Another dimension of time that is of interest to anthropologists is that of the natural history of a disease or disorder. Every disease, particularly chronic disease that may last a lifetime, has a distinctive historical pattern. A natural history can be conceived of as a continuum of anatomical or behavioral changes, but is of necessity broken into several stages. In epidemiology it is important to know the differences between the "stage of susceptibility", where a disease has yet to develop but the predisposing conditions (risk factors) are present; the "stage of presymptomatic disease", where pathogenic changes have started to occur but cannot be (or are not) clinically recognized; and the "stage of clinical disease" where pathogenic changes are noted (Mausner and Bahn 1980). The staging of a disease is important in epidemiology for permitting uniform diagnoses across clinical institutions and national boundaries, identifying stages where prevention or control efforts might be effectively aimed, and identifying the point at which behavioral or anatomical changes can be seen to constitute a clinical disease.

Natural history has been of interest to anthropologists in cases where nosology is poorly developed, for example in the case of behavioral disorders such as alcohol or drug abuse, and in the area of psychiatry. In these cases it is often difficult to separate deviant behavior from a clinically identifiable disorder. There is often a great difference between how the epidemiologist might choose to define the clinical stage of a disease (the "etic" view), or how the individuals or groups to which they belong define it (the "emic" view). This distinction, which corresponds roughly to that between "illness" and "disease" in medical anthropology (see Chrisman 1985), carries some interesting implications for the practice of epidemiology. In the case of alcohol use, for example, an epidemiologist must often make an *a priori*; decision about the point at which consumption becomes problematic. Anthropological input could be usefully made in defining, from an "emic" point of view, the differences between the "stage of susceptibility" (i.e., heavy consumption); and the "stage of clinical disease" (i.e., alcoholism) for a particular community or ethnic group (see Stall this volume: pp. 275—301; Bennett and Ames 1985). In this volume the paper by Rubinstein and Perloff (pp. 303—332) addresses the issue of how anthropological input may contribute to understanding the natural history of attention deficit disorder in children.

When the rates or distribution of a disease change over time, epidemiologists often seek to analyze the data by grouping individuals according to date and sometimes place of birth. These groupings are termed *cohorts*, and it is generally assumed, by virtue of the age-homogeneity within groups, that members' life experiences, including exposure to disease risks, are similar, and that these life experiences are unique in comparision with other cohorts. The epidemiologic interest in cohorts is in defining the particulars of socio-environmental contexts that characterize the life experiences of cohort members, thereby isolating elements deleterious to health. Anthropological input into isolating the particular life changes age groups experience, though presently limited to a few topics (e.g., aging), appears to be of particular value to the epidemiological analysis of cohort effects. In this volume, the paper by O'Neil (pp. 249—274) examines coping behavior in the context of specific age-cohorts, suggests why these cohorts developed distinct coping styles, and demonstrates how these styles moderate the social-change and stress process. Further research into defining specific cohort-groups in contexts of rapid social change and/or migration would be of particular benefit to elucidating the modernization and chronic desease link (see Janes 1984 for a discussion of the importance of migrant cohorts).

A Model of Health-Related Behavior

The distinctions between person, place, and time noted above are, of course, artificial ones, drawn here to illustrate the kinds of information epidemiologists seek in studying disease distribution and occurrence, and where medical anthropology may contribute to the epidemiologic enterprise. It should be clear, however, that significant to identifying the health-related characteristics of person and place is the understanding of psychological, social, and cultural correlates of individuals' behavior, as well as the determinants of the behavior of outsiders that may in turn affect the group or population at risk (for example, cigarette advertisers or public health officials). In order to point out the many areas where medical anthropological research can benefit the study of disease and disorder in communities, it is possible to construct a causal model that emphasizes the behavioral dimensions of the concepts of person and place (and in some cases, time) discussed above. It should be remembered throughout this discussion, however, that behavioral factors represent only a portion, although often a significant one, of the causal web.

Health-related behavior can be distinguished along three axes. First, behavior may be examined in relation to its deliberateness or purposefulness in effecting some health-related outcome. Many acts, though health-related in fact may not be so perceived by those engaged in the actions. Deliberate behavior, on the other hand, comprises all those actions which individuals or groups undertake with an awareness (or assumption) that they may have some impact, favorable or unfavorable, on human health. Second, it is also possible to distinguish between those behaviors, deliberate or non-deliberate, that serve to promote or maintain health, or which contribute to ill-health or mortality. Third, important in this scheme is the behavior of, and as defined by, outsiders, including those concerned with control, prevention, health promotion, and treatment who are not themselves members of the community at risk. It is thus possible to distinguish eight areas of behavioral research, each of which requires attention for a comprehensive understanding of behavior relevant to the epidemiology of any disease or disorder.

To demonstrate the usefulness of this model of community-based health behavior, we have summarized the behavioral dimensions of two important chronic conditions, one infectious in origin and characteristic of developing countries, and the other of non-infectious etiology which is the greatest cause of death in the developed world. The behaviors implicated in these two diseases, filariasis and cardiovascular disease are summarized in Tables I and II, respectively. Tables IA and IIA outline the influence of intra-community behaviors of groups or individuals on disease. Tables IB and IIB indicate known or hypothesized relationships between the extracommunity behavior of groups and disease. We believe that the behavioral model described here is a useful heuristic for conceptualizing appropriate avenues for health research, as well as for organizing what is known about the behavioral dimensions of any disease or disorder.

Methodological Issues

Up to this point we have focussed on areas of common interest to anthropology and epidemiology. However, there are, as noted previously, significant differences in both the typical scope of research and the kinds of methods that each discipline emphasizes. The major difference is one of measurement. Anthropology developed primarily as a qualitative enterprise, while epidemiology, with its close ties to statistics, has remained a quantitative science. We do not wish to enter into the qualitative/quantitative debate here, nor

TABLE IA

Cardiovascular disease-related behavior in the community

DELIBERATE BEHAVIOR	NONDELIBERATE BEHAVIOR
Part 1: Health-enhancing behavior (of the individual, the group, or the entire population in the community)	
1. Cultural values that prescribe regular visits to medical practitioners.	1. Engagement in economic or leisure activities that are health enhancing — e.g., high levels of exercise, no obesity, no cigarette smoking — or general cultural values that emphasize lifestyles that are health enhancing.
2. Exercise.	2. Traditional dietary practices that lead to a diet low in saturated fats.
3. Food practices initiated or sustained for purpose of reducing serum cholesterol.	3. Belonging to a well-integrated group that subscribes to a coherent value system; i.e., social integration and stability.
4. Reducing weight; avoiding obesity.	4. Existence of social support through normal kin or peer relationships, or special rituals including religious involvement.
5. Stopping or avoiding smoking.	5. Exposure to little externally-stimulated social and cultural change; little potential for socially or culturally "incongruous" situations.
6. Ritual or therapeutic activities designed to improve health that comfort the individual, and have significant psychological and social impact that lowers stress through providing a sense of belonging, social support, and enhanced coping.	6. Strong individual coping capacities for dealing with potentially stressful situations.
Part 2: Health-lowering (ill-health provoking) behavior (of the individual, the group, or the entire population in the community)	
1. Avoidance of routine medical care or treatment, especially when high-risk conditions, such as hypertension, are present.	1. Adoption of activity patterns and lifestyles that are unhealthy (but not known to be); e.g., little exercise, poor diet, smoking, high saturated fat diet.
2. Eating a diet high in saturated fats.	2. Cultural values that tolerate or favor a dangerously obese body type.
3. Avoidance of exercise.	3. Exposure to stressful life situations with few social supports and/or poor coping abilities.
4. Avoidance of weight reduction.	4. Migration to an environment very different from that in which one was raised; particularly an urban environment.
5. Smoking.	5. Exposure to rapid social change, and/or socially or culturally incongruous situations.
	6. Behavior that results, either individually or collectively, in poverty, social alienation, or "anomie".

TABLE 1B

Extracommunity cardiovascular disease-related human behavior

DELIBERATE BEHAVIOR	NONDELIBERATE BEHAVIOR
Part 1: Health-enhancing behavior (affecting individuals, groups, or the entire population in the community)	1. Characteristics of the social and cultural environment in which the community is embedded that are benign in causing individuals stress: e.g., absence of political and structural characteristics such as racism and economic discrimination that might lead to poverty, social disorganization, and rapid social and cultural change.
1. Provision of adequate medical care to members of the community.	
2. Primary prevention activities: health education through mass-media or other channels to increase awareness of cardiovascular risk factors; general planned "cultural change" encouraging the adoption of healthy lifestyles.	
3. Secondary prevention activities: screening for high-risk cases; treatment of high-risk conditions such as hypercholesteremia and hypertension; and general risk-factor intervention activities, e.g., helping individuals lose weight, increase exercise, change diet, and stop smoking.	2. Provision of social and economic services to the community that helps prevent stress-producing conditions or helps buffer the effects of social and cultural change: e.g., social welfare programs for low-income families; bilingual education and vocational training programs for new migrants; and community development projects (facilitated by extracommunity representatives, funds, or agencies) leading to community self-determination.
Part 2: Health-lowering (ill-health provoking) behavior (affecting individuals, groups or the entire population in the community)	1. Failure to provide adequate medical care and screening services to community members due to shortages of skilled practitioners, lack of funds, or local underdevelopment.
1. Deliberate failure to provide, or take measures to provide, adequate medical care to at-risk community members.	
2. Promotion of activities that are known to be unhealthy; e.g., advertising tobacco or foods high in saturated fats.	2. Introduction of rapid social and cultural change through resettlement or urban-renewal programs, resulting in geographic displacement of community, or disrupting change to the community environment.
	3. Social, economic, or political alienation of community, or portions thereof, that results in social disintegration, significant poverty, and a loss of community control and capacity for self-determination.

TABLE IIA[a]

Filariasis-related human behavior in the community

DELIBERATE BEHAVIOR	NONDELIBERATE BEHAVIOR
Part 1: Health-enhancing behavior (of the individual, the group, or the entire population in the community)	
Greater Psychological (or Social) Significance:	1. Human cyclical activity patterns (circadian, monthly, seasonal, annual) that serve to minimize contact with biting vectors.
1. Ritual behavior stemming from theories of cause, prevention, control, and cure and performed by the overtly diseased, or by other members of the community on their behalf.	2. Water and refuse management practices that tend to minimize vector breeding and vector density relative to humans.
2. Traditional therapy (herbal, manipulative, surgical) which is often closely linked to ritual behavior.	3. Encouragement of domestic animals that divert biting vectors from humans.
Greater Biological Significance:	4. House construction preferences (e.g., tall house posts) or other arrangements to deter pest mosquito biting, that also serve to minimize contact with biting vectors.
1. Some forms of traditional therapy (?).	5. Migration to and settlement in an area of lesser filarial endemicity.
2. Behavior of the overtly diseased (and still microfilaremic) person that serves to lessen his/her contact with biting vectors. Such behavior may result from personal choice or community sanction.	6. Factors contributing to low human population density (especially in rural areas); marked geographical dispersal of small communities.
3. Voluntary and intentional migration to an area of lesser filarial endemicity.	7. Urbanization (in some circumstances, such as in parts of the South Pacific).
	8. High mobility (if primarily emigration): dispersal of infected persons to other communities; lowered or stabilized community population density.
	9. Strong adherence to "tradition", i.e. low sociocultural change (= greater potential for successful health education and community-based filariasis control).

Table IIA (*Continued*)

DELIBERATE BEHAVIOR	NONDELIBERATE BEHAVIOR
Part 2: Health-lowering (ill-health provoking) behavior (of the individual, the group, or the entire population in the community)	
1. Voluntary migration to and settlement in an area known to be hazardous because of endemic filariasis (acceptance of the known hazard, for example, because of pressing need for land that can be opened to agriculture).	1. Human activity patterns that maximize contact with biting vectors, e.g., daily or seasonal agricultural activities that coincide with mosquito biting peaks or with seasonal population maxima.
	2. Water and refuse management practices that maximize vector breeding and density.
	3. Concealment and immobilization, voluntary or enforced, of overtly diseased (and still micro-filaremic) persons under conditions that allow for increased contact with vectors.
	4. House style preferences that favor contact with biting vectors; squatter type housing (in some circumstances).
	5. Migration to and settlement in an area of greater filarial endemicity without awareness of the increased hazard.
	6. Factors contributing to high human population density, especially in rural areas.
	7. Urbanization (in some circumstances).
	8. Low mobility (little emigration): infected persons remain in the community; openness to immigration, on the other hand, may add infected persons to the population.
	9. Rapid sociocultural change: behavior stemming from changing attitudes due to modernization, increased education, etc. (may = decreased responsiveness to traditional community leadership, and thus lower potential for success in community-based filariasis control).

[a] Source: Dunn (1976b)

TABLE IIB[a]

Extracommunity Filariasis-related human behavior

DELIBERATE BEHAVIOR	NONDELIBERATE BEHAVIOR
Part 1: Health-enhancing behavior (affecting individuals, groups, or the entire population in the community)	1. Changes introduced and encouraged for reasons having nothing directly to do with filariasis and having the indirect effect of decreasing vector density relative to humans, vector breeding, biting, etc. *Examples:* Fortuitous location of a new school building outside of the area of transmission; changes in house style, water supply, sanitary arrangements, agricultural activity patterns, transport, economic activities, etc.
1. Prophylactic or definitve chemical or other therapy serving to eliminated source of micro-filariae.	
2. Preventing infected outsiders from entering the community.	2. Mandatory and fortuitous resettlement of groups or the entire population in an area of low, or no, filarial transmission.
3. Regional or local vector control activities.	
4. Introducing and encouraging use of screening, bednetting, changes in house construction, domestic animals that will attract vector mosquitos, etc.	
5. Encouraging changes in water, refuse, and vegetation management to deter vector breeding and alter vector resting behavior.	
6. Encouraging changes in human activity patterns (e.g., agricultural) to minimize contact with biting vectors.	
7. Mandatory and deliberate resettlement of the population in an area of lesser, or no, filarial endemicity.	

Table IIB (Continued)

DELIBERATE BEHAVIOR	NONDELIBERATE BEHAVIOR
Part 2: Health-lowering (ill-health provoking) behavior (affecting individuals, groups, or the entire population in the community)	1. Deficiencies in a mass chemoprophylaxis program that lead to grudging participation or to outright rejection of the program by the population at risk. The outcome may be a lowering of community health or, at best, no improvement in the level of health as a result of the program. (In these situations failures in communication and education are often critical, but these may be underlain by problems of control team morale, e.g., poor working conditions, inadequate salaries, transport problems, and personality conflicts within the team.)
1. Regional changes in water distribution (irrigation schemes, dams, etc.) carried out with the recognition that the side effects may include increased filarial vector densities in some communities or community subsistence zones but these effects were considered to be outweighed by other considerations such as opening up of new land to agriculture and hydroelectric power gains.	2. Deficient vector control program, for reasons ranging from poor control team morale to community resistance because of problems secondary to the use of insecticides.
2. Mandatory resettlement of a population in an area of known filarial transmission, but this disadvantage is considered to be outweighed by other advantages (as 1 above).	3. Mandatory resettlement in an area of unrecognized filarial endemicity.
	4. Introduced change that has the unforeseen consequence of increasing vector contact with humans, e.g., a change in agricultural activity patterns, a conversion from domestic animals to tractors for plowing, and poor siting of new housing.

[a] Source: Dunn (1976b).

suggest avenues for integrating the two styles of research; ample writing on this subject already exists. We suggest, however, that measurement differences are easily bridged by realizing that in most cases they complement one another nicely. Qualitative research is powerful in achieving results of great validity (accuracy). Quantitative research, on the other hand, accompanied by sound sampling methods and procedures for limiting observer bias, is generally credited for its reliability (replicability) (see Babbie 1983: chapter 10 for a balanced discussion of qualitative and quantitative research). Although one kind of measurement is very difficult to combine with the other in a single step, qualitative and quantitative measurement may inform the other at different stages of the research process.

Many of the papers that follow in this book illustrate how the two styles of measurement may be used to explore an epidemiologic problem, or an anthropological problem identified by epidemiologic data. In Janes's study of hypertension in Samoan migrants (pp. 175—211), an initial period of qualitative research was used as a data base for designing the quantitative portion of the study, and aided analysis of the quantitative results. The comparative design of Kunstadter's (pp. 125—156) study of health in several ethnic groups in northeastern Thailand was based, in part, on knowledge of the ethnographic differences between the groups and the implications these had for understanding variance in mortality and morbidity rates. Rubinstein and Perloff (pp. 303—332) discuss how qualitative research might aid in defining attention deficit disorder among children in epidemiological studies. Nations (pp. 97—123) illustrates how qualitative research on local ethnomedical beliefs yields diagnostic categories of diarrheal disease that are grounded in cultural reality, and are thus useful for descriptive-level epidemiological studies of incidence, mortality, and attack rates.

On the other hand, the results of quantitative research may suggest further avenues for qualitative inquiry, or may suggest problems that require analysis that demands the strength of a qualitative approach. Gifford's analysis (pp. 213—246) of how clinicians and patients interpret attributions of risk for breast cancer — attributes based on quantitative analysis — is one such example. O'Neil's study (pp. 249—274) of stress among Inuit adolescents in the Canadian arctic was suggested in part by previous epidemiological research on acculturation that indicated the relationship of social and cultural processes to stress-related diseases and/or disorders.

As these and other examples in the book show, anthropological input into epidemiological research is important for developing appropriate measurement techniques, designing culturally-sensitive questionnaires or interview instruments, and for facilitating entree into subject communities. It is here that the concomitant employment of qualitative and quantitative methods is of great utility. Qualitative methods add meaning and a deeper social and cultural dimension to quantitative measures. On the other hand, quantitative measures may direct qualitative research by pointing to patterned relationships between variables that require further in-depth analysis.

In the latter case, anthropological analysis of causal factors may hold promise not only for illuminating an epidemiologic issue, as in the examples described above, but may contribute to development of anthropological theory. In the next section we discuss this kind of cross-disciplinary collaboration.

Epidemiology in Anthropology

With its central interest in identifying determinants of disease and disorder, the maturation of epidemiology has been accompanied by a gradual increase in the size and complexity of causal assemblages — those arrays of determinants that are scrutinized in virtually every investigation. It is ironic that the technology that has permitted this expansion — developments in the handling of large quantities of data, and refinements in statistical techniques — has now brought epidemiology to a point where it is generally appreciated that the "solutions" to some problems can only be approached but never reached. This complexity of determinants and the acknowledgement of the existence of "subjective" factors has forced some of the epidemiological pioneers into the realm of medical ecology, beyond the simple, uncomplicated world of "old-fashioned" epidemiology. It is these causal assemblages — these complexes of environmental, host-biological, and host-behavioral factors — that offer possibilities for anthropologists, for those aware that they are available in the epidemiological literature. Consider the following examples.

Cultural anthropologists have joined epidemiologists, geographers, and nutrition scientists in many-faceted studies of lactose intolerance in populations around the world. It was the ideas of a cultural geographer, Simoons (1966, 1970), that stimulated much of the recent work on this problem. Publication of his cultural historical hypothesis based on a survey of the epidemiological and nutritional literature was followed by a variety of studies and reviews (e.g., McCracken 1971; Kretchmer 1972) of a complex that includes: deficiency of the enzyme lactase and consequent lactose intolerance in adults and older children in some populations, gastrointestinal disorders associated with milk consumption in the face of incapacity to digest milk sugar, processing of dairy products, animal husbandry, and traditional dairying.

In this example, epidemiological data were available for lactose intolerance and for a few of the determinants that seemed to have influenced its distribution in human populations. In this case, however, epidemiologists had not developed a "causal assemblage" in the sense described above. Indeed, the complexity of causes — the complex or assemblage — came to be recognized largely through the efforts of a cultural geographer and several anthropologists and nutrition scienctists.

For other diseases and disorders, however, assemblages — clusters of causes, or causal data — of considerable scope and complexity have already been defined by epidemiologists. It now appears that some of these may be of interest to anthropology; with few exceptions this potential has not yet been investigated or exploited. We do not refer primarily to those causal factors (with which epidemiologists have often been concerned) that are of obvious interest to social scientists, e.g., social class and mobility, or migration and spatial mobility, or ethnicity. Nor, indeed, do we refer to the potential interest of any single determinant or category of determinants. It is the web of causes, and the complex causal relationships within the network — that hold promise. Quite apart from their epidemiologic significance these associations may have value in anthropological research. These assemblages, described by epidemiologists for their own purposes, can also be inspected by others whose points of view and research interests may have little or nothing to do with disease, health, or ill-health.

The well-known story of malaria, the sickle-cell trait, and agriculture in Africa is an example of such work. The beginnings of this research, by Allison (1954, 1961), were essentially epidemiological and analytic. Livingstone (1958, 1964), although an anthropologist, extended the work in the same vein as Allison while also opening up some leads for anthropologists to follow. It was Weisenfeld (1967) who finally drew the strands together in a fundamentally anthropological interpretation of an assemblage that included the malaria parasite, *Plasmodium falciparum,* the *Anopheles gambiae* complex of mosquito species, the sickle-cell trait and disease, forest clearing for agriculture, African cereal crop cultivation, African root and tree crop cultivation, the westward dispersal of many Malayo-Polynesian traits in Africa, climatic variation, and time. The biocultural evolutionary synthesis that has emerged from these studies has probably been of greater fundamental importance in anthropology than in any of the other disciplines that the work has touched, including human genetics.

Consider also the case of coronary heart disease. Epidemiological attention has for many years been directed to the study of such risk factors as excess body weight, cigarette smoking, sedentary occupations, limited physical exercise, high blood pressure, certain diets, certain personality types, and conditions contributing to sociocultural or psychological stress. Interest has centered on the correlation between each factor and the disease — or mortality due to the disease. The relative strengths of most of these associations are now well established, at least for some populations in industrialized countries. Little attention, however, has been given to the types and strengths of associations within groups or clusters of these determinants; and few epidemiologists have any incentive to explore how these determinants may be linked to other factors that appear to be quite outside the field of concern of a heart disease researcher (e.g., social structure, social networks ethnic identity, community organization). It is here that opportunities are open for investigations that may be rewarding for anthropology. We suggest that anthropologists look into these associations not as further contributions to coronary disease epidemiology, but for their own sake, exploring links and relationships no more improbable that those between African agriculture practices, the sickle-cell trait, and *Anopheles gambiae* mosquito behavior would have seemed thirty years ago.

One example of the theoretical potential of epidemiological findings for anthropology is the recent increase in research on "stress" and disease. For the most part, stress has been measured, usually indirectly, as arising from some social condition (usually change). The resulting measure has then been examined in relationship to a variety of disorders, for example, hypertension, symptoms of mental illness, and general level of health (e.g., Antonovsky 1979; Dohrenwend and Dohrenwend 1981; James and Kleinbaum 1976; Jenkins 1976; Marmot and Syme 1976; Syme et al. 1964, 1966; Tyroler and Cassel 1964). Anthropologists such as Dressler (1982), however, have established the causal linkages between specific stress-producing conditions and the broader social and cultural processes stemming from poverty, colonialism, and social change. In this volume, the paper by O'Neil (pp. 249—274), though ostensibly written as a critique of epidemiological under-standings of the stress-disorder relationship, holds great potential for enrich-ing anthropological understandings regarding the relationship of changing "Fourth World" communities to the colonial units in which they must function, and in illuminating the fundamentals of change — particularly the role of cohorts. In examining the negative aspects of such social and cultural processes, anthropology stands to gain new insight into the particulars of acculturation — long an elusive and poorly understood phenomenon.

For a final example, consider what might be gained — of anthropological significance — from an investigation of the associations among unemploy-ment, strength and integrity of traditional medical beliefs and practices, and urbanization. Each of these has been tied into the assemblage of deter-minants of suicide mortality in various parts of the world — along with bereavement, depression, family integrity, life threatening illness, and numer-ous other factors. What kinds of links exist between the supposed causal factors that underlie successful suicide? How are the links maintained, reinforced, weakened? What can inspection of these links tell us about the psychosocial condition of a society? Would a study of this assemblage ultimately contribute more to anthropological theory than to medical sci-ence? O'Neil's paper, referred to above, provides a few partial answers to these questions, but more importantly, points the way for further — and primarily anthropological — research.

Although the direct application of epidemiological data or findings to anthropological theory has not been attempted beyond the few examples cited above, it is important to recognize that epidemiology has had a considerable, if indirect, influence on the field of medical anthropology. Anthropologists have undertaken to use epidemiological data in the interest of furthering understanding of mankind's past (e.g., Stearn and Stearn 1945;

Dobyns 1963), and in understanding the impact of disease on contemporary social structure and culture (e.g., Lindenbaum 1979; Krech 1978).

Is there really such a thing, however, as "epidemiology in anthropology" any more than there is (or is not) a "statistics in anthropology"? In practice, it is not "epidemiology" *per se,* but "the epidemiology of ____" that has the potential to influence or expand anthropological theory. Thus, in the examples that we have noted, it is the determinants, "causes", and risk factors in, for example, suicide and malaria — as they are revealed, described, and analyzed by epidemiological (and other) techniques — that may or may not affect the anthropological discipline. Perhaps it is more nearly correct to speak of, e.g., "the anthropology of malaria" or "the anthropology of heart disease", just as we commonly consider religious institutions or political systems in anthropology. We must leave this question open.

PART TWO: MEDICAL ANTHROPOLOGY IN DISEASE
PREVENTION AND CONTROL

Concepts of Prevention

One of the goals of epidemiological research is to provide data upon which sound prevention programs can be built, and to inform the clinical identification and treatment of specific disease or disorders. As such, it is critical that epidemiological knowledge include some understanding of how the social and cultural environment affects the health-related behavior of individuals. The process of applying epidemiological data to prevention represents a small but developing area in medical anthropology that holds great promise.

Prevention is a broad term that includes several strategies for reducing or treating ill-health. *Primary* prevention encompasses all measures that prevent the outbreak of a disease. This includes the reduction of individuals' exposure to causal agents or environmental processes that lead to mental or physical ill-health, as well as the alteration of individual susceptibility to risk. *Secondary* prevention involves strategies for the detection and diagnosis of disease at an early stage, usually through screening and identification of "high-risk" groups. Health efforts tend to consist of remedial efforts to reduce risk or treat disease in its early stages. *Tertiary* prevention consists of the amelioration, treatment, or cure of clinical disease (Mausner and Bahn 1980; Ratcliffe et al. 1984).

Public health educators base health promotion and prevention programs on knowledge provided by epidemiologic studies of specific diseases.[3] Such knowledge generally consists of a clearly identified set of risk factors plus some measurement of the relative strength of each risk in predicting an unhealthy outcome. Risk factors of most interest to public health workers are those that stem from the behavior of individuals or alterable aspects of the natural environment — the success of any prevention program depends on either convincing individuals to change their behavior or changing the environment to remove factors that place individuals at risk for disease.

Because the vast majority of health-related behaviors, both deliberate and non-deliberate, are strongly influenced by — if not fully determined — by social and cultural factors, public health educators must be aware of the socio-environmental contexts of risk as well as the nature of individual risk characteristics. Furthermore, because the focus in prevention is on behavior change, successful prevention programs depend on a detailed and sound theoretical understanding of human behavior. Without significant input from the social sciences in terms of analyzing the contexts and determinants of individual risk-taking behavior, epidemiologic data provide a generally weak basis for the design of sound prevention strategies. For example, although a large body of epidemiologic research concerns the health effects of smoking, far too little addresses the causes of smoking itself, and thus how individuals can be prevented from smoking.

Medical Anthropology and Prevention

Although the relevance of medical anthropology for facilitating the application of epidemiologic knowledge might appear from the preceding discussion to be clear, in practice this relevance remains largely theoretical. Currently, the most promising areas for involvement are in international health, mental health prevention among culturally unique communities, and prevention of disorders that develop as a direct result of social interaction, such as alcohol and drug abuse.

In much of the developing world the major infectious and parasitic diseases and nutritional disorders remain profoundly important, although increasing attention is being directed towards non-infectious diseases such as heart disease and diabetes (Basch 1978). Also important in many developing countries are those general health education efforts relating to family planning, maternal and child health, improving community sanitation, and nutritional counseling. Much of this effort is, however, undertaken without the support of behavioral research and adequate sociomedical consultation and advisory services. It is critical that research priority be given to topics that are directly related to disease prevention and control and that aim at enhancing community responsibility and control over the planning and implementation of prevention activities. This includes enhancing community understanding of psychological and social factors affecting prevention, participation in case finding and treatment; input into overcoming the constraints in mass drug administration or vaccination; and overcoming cultural constraints on programs of health education.

The importance of anthropological research in conjunction with infectious disease epidemiology pertains not only to "traditional" non-Western settings. Gorman's paper in this volume (pp. 157—172) demonstrates the relevance of anthropological insight into the gay community for understanding the epidemiology of Acquired Immune Deficiency Syndrome (AIDS). In particular, his paper seeks to understand the structure and content of the gay sociocultural system as it relates to individual behavior implicated in the transmission of AIDS. As he points out, such information is necessary for developing prevention measures that can be integrated into the various lifestyles of the gay community.

The epidemiology and prevention of mental illness is another area in which medical anthropologists have had substantial input, and yet is one that would benefit from additional research. In particular, anthropologists have played important roles in isolating the social and cultural factors that lead to mental disorders (e.g., Leighton 1959; Leighton et al. 1963). The extension of these findings to the prevention of mental illness in different communities and population groups remains in a nascent stage, but one that holds promise. For example, the National Institute of Mental Health sponsored a conference in May, 1984 in which several medical anthropologists, psychologists, and psychiatrists gathered to discuss the relevance of medical anthropological input into preventive programming. Several long-term projects designed and implemented by medical anthropologists are currently underway, and their success will show whether anthropological expertise increases the success of such programs (cf. Manson, forthcoming).

Of interest in the area of mental health, and a topic that has not benefited from much anthropological interest, is the epidemiology and prevention of violence: suicide, family violence, accidents, and physical assault. Because such phenomena appear related to socio-environmental factors, and directly affect the nature of social relationships within communities and families, anthropological research would be both relevant and productive.

Related to the field of mental illness epidemiology and prevention is that of substance abuse. Anthropologists have had a long-standing interest in this area (e.g., Bennett 1984; Everett et al. 1976; Heath et al. 1981). Much of the interest has been in comparing alcohol and drug use cross-culturally, but a growing number of investigators are turning their attention to studying the determinants, distribution, prevention, and treatment of substance abuse problems within developed countries (e.g., Ablon 1974; Heath et al. 1981; Stall this volume: pp. 275—301; Wolin and Bennett 1983).

Prevention programs may include other than health promotion or primary prevention activities. For many diseases, particularly those where etiology and natural history are poorly understood, secondary prevention is extremely important. In secondary prevention, the goal is to identify either high-risk individuals and give them a more intense level of medical care, or to identify early stages of these diseases that are, presumably, more amenable to clinical amelioration. Often, secondary prevention is aimed at preventing short and long-term complications due to the disease. Screening criteria for early disease identification are frequently based on epidemiological data. For example, in the case of breast cancer, discussed in the paper by Gifford (pp. 213—246), women with certain characteristics — e.g., increasing age, history of bilateral pre-menopausal breast cancer in a first degree relative, late age at birth of the first child, and a history of fibrocystic breast disease — are given "risk profiles" based on what is known through epidemiological research to be the relative risk of each of these factors. Women considered "high risk" are subject to closer medical scrutiny and sometimes surgical intervention. Although such scrutiny may permit earlier detection of the disease, the meaning of epidemiological risk factors is often poorly understood by clinicians. This has serious implications for patient management. Often, as Gifford points out, doctors diagnose women as being "at risk" in the same sense that they diagnose a disease. The result is that women's lives become medicalized, and they come to think of themselves as being in a "pre-disease" state. Being diagnosed "at risk" creates a state between health and illness. Such a diagnosis can result in a great deal of pain and doubt, and can compromise the ability of women to live reasonably normal lives. The role of the medical anthropologist in facilitating the translation of epidemiological knowledge into clinical practice, is in such cases, first to convey to clinicians both epidemiological and lay concepts of risk, and second, to suggest strategies for both clinicians and patients to make decisions about risk management that are based on sound epidemiological principles. Although this is an area of activity usually thought of as "clinical anthropology", it is of relevance to our discussion here because it addresses the application of epidemiological data to prevention.

DISCUSSION

As the previous sections illustrate, the interfaces between epidemiology and anthropology are complex, involving many varieties of collaboration. To summarize, we note two broad areas of research collaboration between anthropology and epidemiology. The first involves direct collaboration between the two disciplines. The second involves more indirect contributions to epidemiology, and to public health planning, policy, and implementation; or, conversely, contributions to anthropological theory from epidemiologic research.

Direct collaboration represents the involvement of anthropologists in more traditional epidemiological research — developing research designs, defining variables, testing specific hypotheses that have a social or cultural basis, and facilitating case-finding and case-definition issues. This kind of collaboration corresponds partly with what we might call "anthropology in epidemiology" (as in "anthropology in medicine"), but represents primarily the actual association and active cooperation of epidemiologists and anthropologists.

Indirect collaboration involves three types of activities, each entailing only loose or tangential cooperation between anthropologists and epidemiologists. First, anthropologists may explore in depth the socio-cultural correlates of causal assemblages that have already been identified in epidemiology. For example, a researcher may investigate the determinants of behavior that results in the transmission of a specific disease such as filariasis or schisto-somiasis. The collaboration is indirect because the specific etiological agent of these diseases may already be identified; what the anthropologist does is amplify the behavioral dimensions of a causal assemblage. The importance of this kind of research lies in providing data vital to the successful imple-mentation of disease control and prevention programs. Second, anthropolo-gists may look to epidemiological data as providing clues for anthropological theory and hypotheses. We have defined this as representing "epidemiology in anthropology". Here the collaboration of anthropologists and epidemiolo-gists may take the form of communication through professional journals. Third, anthropologists involved in prevention-oriented research may consult with epidemiologists, though this will vary depending on the nature of the disorder being studied. Where the epidemiological relationships between behavioral factors and disease have been identified, as in the case of many infectious diseases, the role of the anthropologist may be in designing culturally-appropriate control measures in collaboration with public health educators. However, where a disorder or class of disorders is poorly understood, such as in the case of alcohol problems or mental illness, anthropologists may be much more directly involved in the interaction of basic epidemiological work and applied prevention efforts. Thus, collabora-tion at this level demands eclectic use of an array of anthropological and epidemiological skills.

Within these categories of collaboration — direct and indirect — the research expertise required of the anthropologist, the potential for indepen-dent or "traditional" research, and the range of methodological tools avail-able to the anthropologist will differ. For example, in contexts of direct and close collaboration, anthropologists may find themselves working primarily as epidemiologists. The papers by Kunstadter (pp. 125—156), Gorman (pp. 157—172), Stall (pp. 275—301), and Rubinstein and Perloff (pp. 303—332) reflect such a role. In these cases anthropologists must be conversant in epidemiological research techniques, including the design and execution of structured and quantitative research projects. Anthropological expertise is provided in the context of designing research instruments, evaluating known epidemiological relationships that are related to complex social and cultural processes, or facilitating acceptance of the research team by the community being studied.

Where collaborative relationships are less direct, anthropologists have much more flexibility in designing research and developing alternate strate-gies for data collection and analysis. At one end of a continuum, anthropolo-gists may take a traditional anthropological approach to an epidemiological problem. The papers by O'Neil (pp. 249—274) and Janes (pp. 175—211) represent, in essence, ethnographic analyses of stress, an identified risk factor for a number of chronic, non-infectious diseases or disorders. At the other end of this continuum, anthropologists may employ anthropological theory and method to understand how epidemiological knowledge can be applied. Anthropological approaches can also help illuminate and deepen understandings of causal assemblages. Finally, such an approach can feed back into the development of anthropological theory. At this level, the research design as well as the primary research questions remain primarily anthropological. For example, Gifford's paper shows how basic anthropological research methods are used to understand the relationship of clinical uncertainty about risk, and epidemiological, clinical and lay beliefs surrounding the natural history of breast cancer to the clinical management of patients at risk. The importance of research at this end of the continuum lies not so much in elucidating etiological relationships between behavioral factors and disease, as in illuminating the application of epidemiological knowledge.

Regardless of the level of collaboration, it is essential that anthropologists intending to work in some relationship with epidemiology develop an understanding of the methods and theories of the discipline. The opposite, of course, is also true — epidemiologists who have an interest in social and cultural factors must also develop some knowledge of method and theory in anthropology. Many graduate training programs in medical anthropology are beginning to train students in the basics of epidemiology, selected topics in biomedicine, statistics, demography, and medical geography (Dunn 1979b). Because health is a phenomenon not restricted to the purview of any one discipline, it is critical that health researchers, including behavioral scientists, be trained — or at least exposed to — a wide variety of fields and methods.

Although we have spoken throughout this Introduction of "anthropology and epidemiology" — due to the demands of simplicity as well as some allegiance to the fields in which we were trained — such specific phrasing may be overly parochial. Anthropology shares much with sociology as well as with some branches of psychology, demography, and geography. Epidemiology, as we have pointed out, is a rather new discipline related to a number of basic and applied health sciences, including immunology, physiology, pathology, microbiology, parasitology, environmental toxicology, public health education, and statistics. Thus, we believe it may be equally valid to speak of this book as presenting case studies in multidisciplinary health research.

Although the articles to follow stand in and of themselves as significant contributions to medical anthropology and epidemiology, we would like to look forward to a time when collections such as this one become unnecessary. This is not to suggest that the topic of cross-disciplinary collaboration is or will become unimportant, but that we hope it will become an institutionalized aspect of health research and health care; not a phenomenon that is unique enough to cause remark in scholarly publications. The articles presented herein represent first, albeit seemingly small steps, toward such interdisciplinary development.

NOTES

1. Health can be defined as *the capacity of the individual or group (or society) to profit from experience and to respond to insults — physical, biological, social, and psychological.* These coping and learning capacities vary constantly throughout the life span of the individual or group. Fine variations may occur, e.g., on a circadian or monthly basis; other differences in these capacities occur in relation to age. Still others reflect previous experience — immunological, physiological, psychosocial, and so forth. Health of the individual — as coping and learning capacity — therefore reflects endogenous, genetically governed personal characteristics blended with all that has been learned (even immunologically) through accumulated experience. In this sense, then, health can never be "complete" but it can certainly be optimal, for time, place, and circumstances. Thus any degree of ill-health reflects some limitation of the person's ability to respond and/or learn. This limitation may be primarily social or psychological, but not necessarily so (Dunn 1984).

2. Although we use the terms society and culture (and the adjectives social and cultural, or sociocultural) frequently and generally in unison, these refer to quite distinct classes of phenomena. Following Kluckhohn (1949: 21—24), we define a "society" as a group of people who interact more with each other than they do with other individuals, and in a patterned way that can be generalized to constitute a social structure. The adjective "social", then, refers to these patterned interactions. "Culture", on the other hand, is an abstraction that encompasses a peoples' way of thinking, feeling, and believing. Culture constitutes a storehouse of the pooled learning of the group, and as such defines and guides much of the patterned interaction we call "social". However, not all social behaviors are culturally governed; new situations arise for which there are no precedents, and thus no cultural solutions. The term "cultural" thus refers to beliefs, values, attitudes, and cognitions; the very basis of overt behavior such as speech, tools, housing styles, and so forth.

3. Epidemiology and public health, particularly public health policy, were at one time more closely integrated than they are today (see Trostle, this volume, pp. 35—57). Since the development of epidemiology into a "full-grown" discipline, however, "there has been a general tendency for epidemiology to ignore its natural and historical relationship with public health, and much health policy has tended to ignore the need for epidemiological consideration (Lilienfeld 1984: 241)". However tenuous the interrelationship of public health and epidemiology today, one still nourishes the other to a greater extent than perhaps the practitioners of each would recognize.

REFERENCES

Ablon, Joan
    1974 Al-Anon Family Groups: Impetus for Learning and Change Through the Presentation of Alternatives. American Journal of Psychotherapy 28: 30—45.
Alland, Alexander
    1970 Adaptation in Cultural Evolution: An Approach to Medical Anthropology. New York: Columbia University Press.
Allison, A. C.
    1954 Protection Afforded by Sickle-Cell Trait Against Subtertian Malarial Infection. British Medical Journal 1: 290—294.

1961 Genetic Factors in Resistance to Malaria. Annals of the New York Academy of Sciences 91: 710—729.

Antonovsky, Aaron
1967 Social Class and the Major Cardiovascular Diseases. Journal of Chronic Diseases 21: 65—106.

Audy, Ralph
1971 Measurement and Diagnosis of Health. In P. Shepard and D. McKinley (eds.), Essays on the Planet as a Home. New York: Houghton-Mifflin.

Audy, Ralph and Frederick L. Dunn
1974 Health and Disease, and, Community Health. In F. Sargent II (ed.), Human Ecology. Amsterdam,New York: American Elsevier.

Babbie, Earl R.
1983 Practicing Social Research. 3rd ed. Belmont, CA: Wadsworth.

Baker, Paul T., Joel M. Hanna and Thelma S. Baker (eds.)
In Press The Changing Samoans: Health and Behavior in Transition. New York: Oxford University Press.

Basch, Paul F.
1978 International Health. New York: Oxford University Press.

Beaglehole, R. C. et al.
1977 Blood Pressure and Social Interaction in Tokelau Migrants in New Zealand. Journal qf Chronic Diseases 29: 371—380.

Bennett, Linda A. (ed.)
1984 Contributions from Anthropology to the Study of Alcoholism. In M. Galantner (ed.), Recent Developments in Alcoholism, Vol. 2. New York: Plenum Press.

Bennett, Linda A. and Genevieve M. Ames (eds.)
1985 The American Experience with Alcohol: Contrasting Cultural Perspectives. New York: Plenum Press.

Berkman, Lisa and S. Leonard Syme
1979 Social Networks, Host Resistance, and Mortality: A Nine-Year Follow-up Study of Alameda County Residents. American Journal of Epidemiology 109: 186—204.

Buck, A. A., R. I. Anderson, T. T. Sasaki et al.
1970 Health and Disease in Chad: Epidemiology, Culture and Environment in Five Villages. Baltimore: Johns Hopkins University Press.

Cassel, John
1964 Social Science Theory as a Source of Hypotheses in Epidemiological Research. American Journal of Public Health 54: 1488—1494.
1976 The Contribution of the Social Environment to Host Resistance. American Journal of Epidemiology 104: 107—123.

Caudill, William
1953 Applied Anthropology in Medicine. In A. L. Kroeber (ed.), Anthropology Today. Chicago: University of Chicago Press.

Chrisman, Noel J.
1985 Alcoholism: Illness or Disease? In Linda A. Bennett and Genevieve M. Ames (eds.), The American Experience With Alcohol. New York: Plenum Press.

Dobyns, H. F.
1963 An Outline of Andean Epidemic History to 1720. Bulletin of the History of Medicine 37: 493—515.

Dohrenwend, B. and B. Dohrenwend (eds.)
1981 Stressful Life Events and Their Contexts. New York: Prodist.

Dressler, William W.
1982 Hypertension and Culture Change: Acculturation and Disease in the West Indies. South Salem, NY: Redgrave.
1985 Psychosomatic Symptoms, Stress, and Modernization: A Model. Culture, Medicine, and Psychiatry 9: 257—286.

Dunn, Frederick L.
  1976a Traditional Asian Medicine and Cosmopolitan Medicine as Adaptive Systems. *In* C. Leslie (ed.), Asian Medical Systems: A Comparative Study. Berkeley, CA: University of California Press.
  1976b Human Behavioural Factors in the Epidemiology and Control of *Wuchereria* and *Brugia* Infections. Bulletin of the Public Health Society, Malaysia 10: 34—44.
  1979a Behavioural Aspects of the Control of Parasitic Diseases. Bulletin of the World Health Organization 57: 499—512.
  1979b Biomedical Anthropology: An Introductory Course for Graduate Students. *In* Harry F. Todd and Julio L. Ruffini (eds.), Teaching Medical Anthropology: Model Courses for Graduate and Undergraduate Instruction. Washington, D.C.: Society for Medical Anthropology.
  1984 Social Determinants in Tropical Disease. *In* K. S. Warren and A. A. F. Mahmoud (eds.), Tropical and Geographical Medicine. New York: McGraw-Hill.
Everett, M. W. et al.(eds.)
  1976 Cross-Cultural Approaches to the Study of Alcohol: An Interdisciplinary Perspective. The Hague: Mouton.
Fleck, A. C. and F. A. J. Ianni
  1958 Epidemiology and Anthropology: Some Suggested Affinities in Theory and Method. Human Organization 16: 38—40.
Graves, Theodore, D., Nancy B. Graves, Vineta Semu et al.
  1983 The Price of Ethnic Identity: Maintaining Kin Ties Among Pacific Islands Immigrants to New Zealand. Paper presented at the XV Pacific Sciences Congress, Dunedin, New Zealand, 1983. Forthcoming, Journal of Behavioral Medicine.
Grob, G. N.
  1985 The Origins of American Psychiatric Epidemiology. American Journal of Public Health 75: 229—236.
Heath, Dwight B. et al. (eds.)
  1981 Cultural Factors in Alcohol Research and Treatment of Drinking Problems. Journal of Studies on Alcohol (supplement) 9.
James, S. A. and Kleinbaum D. G.
  1976 Socioecologic Stress and Hypertension Related Mortality Rates in North Carolina. American Journal of Public Health 67: 634—639.
Janes, Craig R.
  1984 Migration and Hypertension: An Ethnography of Disease Risk in an Urban Samoan Community. Ph.D. Dissertation in Medical Anthropology, University of California, Berkeley and San Francisco.
Janes, Craig R. and Ivan G. Pawson
  1986 Migration and Biocultural Adaptation: Samoans in California. Social Science and Medicine 22: 821—834.
Jenkins, C. David
  1976 Recent Evidence Supporting Psychologic and Social Risk Factors for Coronary Disease. New England Journal of Medicine 294: 987—994; 1033—1038.
Kluckhohn, Clyde
  1949 Mirror for Man. New York: McGraw-Hill.
Krech, Stephen III
  1978 Disease, Starvation, and Northern Athapaskan Social Organization. American Ethnologist 1: 103—127.
Kretchmer, Norman
  1972 Lactose and Lactase. Scientific American 227(4): 70—78.
Leighton, Alexander H.
  1959 My Name is Legion: Foundations for a Theory of Man in Relation to Culture. New York: Basic Books.

Leighton, Alexander H., Adeoye T. Lambo, Charles C. Hughes et al.
   1969 Psychiatric Disorder Among the Yoruba. Ithaca, NY: Cornell University Press.
Leighton, Dorothea, John S. Harding, David B. Macklin et al.
   1963 The Character of Danger: Psychiatric Symptoms in Selected Communities. New York: Basic Books.
Lieban, Richard
   1973 Medical Anthropology. In J. J. Honigmann, ed., Handbook of Social and Cultural Anthropology. Chicago: Rand-McNally.
Lilienfeld, Abraham M.
   1984 Epidemiology and Health Policy: Some Historical Highlights. Public Health Reports 99: 237—241.
Lindenbaum, Shirley
   1979 Kuru Sorcery. Palo Alto: Mayfield.
Lindheim, Roslyn and S. Leonard Syme
   1983 Environments, People, and Health. Annual Reviews of Public Health 4: 335—359.
Livingstone, F. B.
   1958 Anthropological Implications of Sickle-Cell Gene Distribution in West Africa. American Anthropologist 60: 533—562.
   1964 Aspects of the Population Dynamics of the Abnormal Hemoglobin and Glucose-6-Phosphate Dehydrogenase Definciency Genes. American Journal of Human Genetics 16: 435—450.
Manson, Spero (ed.)
   In Press Medical Anthropology: Implications for Stress Prevention Across Cultures. Primary Prevention Publication Series, National Institute of Mental Health, Government Printing Office.
MacMahon, B. and T. F. Pugh
   1960 Epidemiologic Methods. Boston: Little, Brown, and Co.
Marmot, Michael and S. Leonard Syme
   1976 Acculturation and Coronary Heart Disease in Japanese-Americans. American Journal of Epidemiology 104: 225—247.
Mausner, Judith S. and Anita K. Bahn
   1974 Epidemiology — An Introductory Text. Philadelphia: W. B. Saunders.
McCracken, R. D.
   1971 Lactase Deficiency: An Example of Dietary Evolution. Current Anthropology 12: 479—517.
Mitchell, J. Clyde
   1969 The Concept and Use of Social Networks. In J. C. Mitchell (ed.), Social Networks in Urban Situations: Analyses of Personal Relationships in Central African Towns. England: Manchester University Press.
Montgomery, Edward
   1973 Ecological Aspects of Health and Disease in Local Populations. Annual Review of Anthropology 2:30—35.
Page, L. B., A. Damon, and R. C. Moellering
   1974 Antecedents of Cardiovascular Disease in Six Solomon Islands Societies. Circulation 49: 1132—1146.
Paul, Benjamin D.
   1963 Anthropological Perspectives on Medicine and Public Health. Annals of the American Academy of Political and Social Sciences 346: 34—43.
Pilisuk, Marc, and Charles Froland
   1978 Kinship, Social Networks, Social Support, and Health. Social Science and Medicine 12B: 273—280.
Prior, I. A. M. et al.
   1974 The Tokelau Island Migrant Study. International Journal of Epidemiology 3: 225—232.

Ratcliffe, John, Lawrence Wallack, Francis Fagnani et al.
  1984 Perspectives on Prevention: Health Promotion vs. Health Protection. *In* J. de
        Kervasdoue, J. R. Kimberly, and V. G. Rodwin (eds.), The End of An Illusion: The
        Future of Health Policy in Western Industrialized Nations. Berkeley: University of
        California Press.
Rothman, K. J.
  1981 The Rise and Fall of Epidemiology, 1950—2000 A.D. New England Journal of
        Medicine 304: 600—602.
Rubel, Arthur J., Carl W. O'Nell, and Rolando Collado-Ardau
  1984 Susto, A Folk Illness. Berkeley, CA: University of California Press.
Rubinstein, Robert A.
  1984 Epidemiology and Anthropology: Notes on Science and Scientism. Communication
        and Cognition 17: 163—185.
Scotch, Norman A.
  1960 A Preliminary Report on the Relation of Sociocultural Factors to Hypertension
        Among the Zulu. Annals of the New York Academy of Sciences 84: 1000—1009.
  1963 Sociocultural Factors in the Epidemiology of Zulu Hypertension. American Journal
        of Public Health 53: 1205—1213.
Simoons, F. J.
  1969 Primary Adult Lactose Intolerance and the Milking Habit: A Problem in Biological
        and Cultural Interrelations. I. Review of the Medical Research. American Journal of
        Digestive Diseases 14: 819—836.
  1970 Primary Adult Lactose Intolerance and the Milking Habit: A Problem in Biological
        and Cultural Interrelations. II. A Cultural Historical Hypothesis. American Journal
        of Digestive Diseases 15: 695—710.
Stallones, R. A.
  1963 Epidemi(olog)²y*. American Journal of Public Health 53: 695—710.
Stearn, E. W, and A. E. Stearn
  1945 The Effect of Smallpox on the Destiny of the Amerindian. Boston: Bruce Hum-
        phries.
Syme, S. Leonard et al.
  1964 Some Social and Cultural Factors Associated with the Occurrence of Coronary
        Heart Disease. Journal of Chronic Diseases 16: 277—289.
  1966 Cultural Mobility and Coronary Heart Disease in an Urban Area. American Journal
        of Epidemiology 82: 334—345.
Syme, S. Leonard and Lisa Berkman
  1976 Social Class, Susceptibility and Sickness. American Journal of Epidemiology 104:
        1—8.
Tyroler, Herman A. and John Cassel
  1964 Health Consequences of Culture Change. II. The Effect of Urbanization on Coro-
        nary Heart Disease in Rural Residents. Journal of Chronic Diseases 17: 167—177.
Weisenfeld, S. L.
  1967 Sickle-Cell Trait in Human Biological and Cultural Evolution. Science 157: 1134—
        1140.
Wolin, S. J. and L. A. Bennett
  1983 Heritage Continuity Among the Children of Alcoholics. *In* E. Gottheil et al. (eds.),
        Etiologic Aspects of Alcohol and Drug Abuse. Springfield, IL: Charles Thomas.

JAMES TROSTLE

EARLY WORK IN ANTHROPOLOGY AND EPIDEMIOLOGY: FROM SOCIAL MEDICINE TO THE GERM THEORY, 1840 TO 1920

INTRODUCTION

Epidemiologists and social scientists are collaborating today on research topics ranging from the epidemiology of violence to the behavioral patterns associated with coronary heart disease, lung cancer, or Acquired Immune Deficiency Syndrome (AIDS). They are uncovering significant etiological links between the social environment and health status, employing social categories such as bereavement (Jacobs and Ostfeld 1977), marital status (Gove 1973), social class (Antonovsky 1967; Syme and Berkman 1976), and social dislocation (Neser et al. 1971). Moreover, social scientists in general, and medical anthropologists in particular, are making independent contributions to epidemiological knowledge through their research on lactose intolerance (McCracken 1971), the relationship between malaria and sickle cell anemia (Wiesenfeld 1967), and the etiology of the slow virus *kuru* (Farquhar and Gajdusek 1981; Fischer and Fischer 1961; Gajdusek 1977; Lindenbaum 1982).

But contemporary researchers studying the health effects of the social environment are repeating many themes that were well developed more than a century ago. These include emphasizing the impact of economies and politics on health status, stressing the preventive aspects of medicine, ascertaining the effects of migration and social change on the health of populations, and hypothesizing that diseases are transmitted and maintained by means of social as well as biological forces.

These themes were clearly voiced at the beginning of this century, as shown by the following quotation:

Man has learned to make himself independent of the direct influence of nature. Between man and nature there is culture, which is linked to the social structures between which alone, man can be truly man .... Hygiene must therefore also study intensively the effects of these social conditions in which men are born, live, work, enjoy themselves, procreate and die. It thus becomes *social* hygiene, which takes its place beside physical-biological hygiene as a necessary supplement. (Alfred Grotjahn, *Was ist und wozu treiben wir Soziale Hygiene?*, 1904. Translated and quoted by Rosen 1947: 711—712, emphasis in the original.)

Although contemporary research linking society and culture to health thus has venerable roots, the relationship between epidemiology[1] and anthropology[2] remains largely unexplored: the joint history of these disciplines might generously be characterized as a history of benign neglect. Yet many anthropologists and epidemiologists have collaborated on studies of health services delivery and disease etiology, and their literatures contain theories

35

Craig R. Janes et al. (eds.), Anthropology and Epidemiology, 35—57.
© 1986 *by D. Reidel Publishing Company.*

and data of mutual interest. This article will review the history of some of these collaborative projects and important theories, and will explore what they have contributed to contemporary studies in the two fields.[3] I will show that the relationship between epidemiology and anthropology dates to the founding of these disciplines; that the earlier collaborative projects produced important results; and that the theories and methods used in previous projects can profitably be used by contemporary researchers.

This article will slight pre-19th century history, since digging too far into the past will uncover only distant ancestors. Instead it examines 19th century statistical and non-statistical analyses of health-related observations, as well as "epidemiological" work which manifested social or behavioral concerns. Following Ackerknecht (1948a: 592—593), I distinguish three broad groups of researchers in the 19th century: those who worked on a *historical* or *geographical* epidemiology, concentrated on the temporal and spatial factors involved in disease transmission; those who developed a *sociological* epidemiology, concerned with the host, and with the ways in which the social environment itself influenced morbidity and mortality; and those who developed a *biological/parasitological* epidemiology, directed toward discovering specific agents of disease. These categories are not mutually exclusive divisions, since for example a biological epidemiologist might use a geographical approach in studying disease etiology; they are meant rather to emphasize different "modal" approaches to the study of disease. Some emphasized place or time, while others concentrated on person or agent. We must examine each approach if we want to understand the many disparate components of 19th century epidemiological work.

This essay is designed to lend some sense of historical context to today's interdisciplinary concerns. Its motivation is therefore "presentist": its purpose is to interpret the past in order to understand the present (see Stocking 1968c: 4).[4] But despite having a presentist motivation I do not mean to imply that the events recounted in these pages followed some inevitable or even cumulative progression. The analytic categories of the past may appear to be similar, or even identical, to ones we use today, but they were employed to answer questions which were developed within other social and theoretical contexts. Some of these categories, such as host, agent, and environment, have sufficient general importance that they transcend the boundaries of one particular historical moment; these will be used as linking themes in this essay. Others, such as telluric and miasmatic theories[5] of disease causation, have more circumscribed historical significance; these mark the discontinuities between past and present.

I. EARLY AUTHORS AND INFLUENCES

Epidemiologists interested in history commonly trace the concerns of their discipline back 2400 years to Hippocratic texts, particularly *Airs Waters Places* (Gordon 1953, 1958; Greenwood 1932; Lilienfeld and Lilienfeld 1980; Susser 1973).[6] According to these analysts, the Hippocratic contribution is valuable for its stress on the environment as a factor in disease causation. In *Airs Waters Places* physicians are urged to examine the seasons, winds, water, position, and soil of unfamiliar towns in order to understand the epidemic diseases of their inhabitants. More important for our purpose, diseases are discussed as attributes of populations, and particular causal emphasis is placed on the "mode of life" of a town's populace: "whether they are heavy drinkers, taking lunch, and inactive; or athletic, industrious, eating much and drinking little" (Hippocrates 1957: 73).

The environmental and analytical emphases of the Hippocratic approach were soon supplanted by a focus on divine causation, and on knowledge as something to be received rather than created. Medieval medicine had comparatively little to do with populational attributes, quantification, or careful observation. Not until the end of the Renaissance and during the Enlightenment did scholars shed the inherited mysticisms of the past, and begin to develop what some call the early ideas of modern epidemiology. Commonly cited from this period is the descriptive work of Europeans such as Girolamo Fracastorius (1484—1553) on contagion, John Graunt (1620—1674) on vital statistics, Thomas Sydenham (1624—1689) on malaria and clinical observation, and Bernardino Ramazzini (1633—1714) on occupational diseases. In the 18th century important etiological work was done by James Lind (1716—1794) on scurvy, Percival Pott (1714—1788) on scrotal cancer, and George Baker (1722—1809) on the "Devonshire Colic" (lead poisoning). Johann Peter Frank published the first volume of his *System of a Complete Medical Police* in 1779, which was an important early work in public health (Frank 1976). Less well known is the epidemiological work of the Reverend Cotton Mather of Boston, who in 1721 used mortality statistics to prove that those with smallpox inoculations fared better than those without. The medical historian Richard Shryock reports that Mather's work on inoculation may be seen as the chief medical contribution of 18th century America (1960: 58).

Mather was a vigorous opponent of witchcraft, but he was almost as vigorous (and colorful) a proponent of the significance of living patterns for health:

Some Sins there are that Naturally do Quicken the pace of Death. By intemperance men shorten their Lives. The Lewd Livers themselves do call it Living Apace. The Intemperate and Immoderate are but Short-lived; a Short-Age their Portion! In Excessive Eating, Men dig their own Graves with their Teeth. In Excessive Drinking, men Drown their Despised Lamp. Intoxications are Suffocations. By unchaste Excesses, men extinguish their Brightness in a Premature Snuff of Rottenness. Excesses of Grief and Care, and Labour, do work Death. (Cotton Mather 1712, *A Sermon Occasioned by the Raging of a Mortal Sickness in the Colony of Connecticut and the Many Deaths of our Brethren There*, excerpted in Winslow 1952: 15).

Mather's proscriptions for a healthy life formed part of a religious campaign against "unchaste Excesses"; such religious tenets provided an important rationale for health-enhancing behavior in the 18th century. Many individuals who emphasized the importance of social factors to health in the 19th century did so motivated by moral, political, and economic beliefs as dogmatic as those held by Mather.

Yet change is not driven only by the words and deeds of great individuals; we must note that theoretical, technological, and bureaucratic developments have significantly changed the course of epidemiology. For example, in the early 19th century the focus of medical research changed from a generalized pathology concerned with bodily humors, to a localized pathology concerned with bodily structures; only then did most research come to focus on specific diseases (Shryock 1961: 94). Accurate quantitative descriptions of specific diseases could occur only after these diseases could be identified with some certainty and consistency (Susser 1973); thus epidemiologic measures such as disease incidence or prevalence also depended on diagnostic sophistication.

One bureaucratic change was crucial to diagnostic sophistication: the development of the hospital. Physicians in hospitals could see for the first time beyond the particularities of their own practices; they could examine many patients with the same disease, be that disease rare or epidemic. Consistent and general diagnostic portraits of a disease could thus be built out of many individual cases,[7] and could be used in turn to improve the accuracy of case ascertainment.

But epidemiologic measures depend on numerators *and* denominators, that is, they require finding and diagnosing cases, *and* completely measuring the population at risk. Diagnostic sophistication alone, which would only affect a numerator, was not a sufficient cause of improvements in epidemiologic measures. Methods of record keeping which would reveal accurate population denominators were also important. At about the same time that diagnostic methods were changing, so too were some states developing these systems of record keeping, advancing beyond the early British Bills of Mortality upon which John Graunt based his pioneering studies (Graunt 1939 [1662]).

In some instances the development of epidemiologic research is said to have been dependent on governmental administrative procedures. While French epidemiology was dominant in the early 1800s, it declined by the mid-19th century, and the center of epidemiological development shifted to England. This shift has been traced to the presence in England of a well-developed system of vital statistics, and the absence of such a system in France (Lilienfeld and Lilienfeld 1980, Rosen 1955: 40). Within the first 40 years of the 19th century four general censuses were carried out in England, and civil registration of vital statistics was established (Rosen 1955: 39).

Finally, progress in research was dependent upon, and caused increasing interest in, new technological developments. The stethoscope appeared in 1819; compound microscope in the 1830s; ophthalmoscope and laryngoscope in the 1850s; microtome in the 1860s; and tissue staining in the 1870s. Each of these tools of measurement created new classes of knowledge, and allowed epidemiological inquiry to focus on more carefully defined categories of disease and agent. As we shall see, these new tools of measurement also restricted the depth of field of the scientific lens: a broad concern with the social environment narrowed toward the end of the century to a concern with particular aspects of the biological environment. Analysis of poverty largely gave way to analysis of pathogens.

The next four sections present selected 19th century contributions to epidemiology and anthropology. The first three of these sections distinguish among biological, geographical, and sociological epidemiologies. The work of a few individuals is highlighted within each section in order to present detailed examples of these different research traditions. The final section contains a brief account of the period from 1870 to 1920, during which the biological tradition in epidemiology expanded into bacteriological investigations.

II. THE RISE OF FIELD EPIDEMIOLOGY: BEHAVIORAL RESEARCH BY BIOLOGICAL/PARASITOLOGICAL EPIDEMIOLOGISTS

A new kind of epidemiological research began in the mid-19th century, in which investigators resorted to fieldwork (so-called "shoe-leather epidemiology") to trace the origin and course of illness through populations. Fieldwork was used to collect data to ascertain how the environment caused disease: a struggle was in full swing in the mid to late 19th century between *miasmatists* (who believed that epidemics were caused by decaying matter circulating in the atmosphere), and *contagionists* (who believed that epidemics were caused by infectious organisms spread by contact, vapor, or via contaminated articles). With each group continuing to marshal evidence in support of its theories, the latter half of the 19th century saw many investigations of the health effects of the environment (Ackerknecht 1948a, Terris 1985). Peter Panum and John Snow, who fit most easily into our category of biological epidemiologists, are good examples of the type of fieldwork done by 19th century biological epidemiologists. William Farr, another epidemiologist/statistician of the same period, deserves mention for his emphasis on the social environment. The work of each of these men will be described in turn, and used to exemplify similar work being done by many others.

Peter Panum (1820—1885)

In 1846, Peter Ludwig Panum investigated a measles epidemic on the Faroe

Islands, a Danish possession lying northwest of Scotland. This is the first work which might qualify today as combining anthropological and epidemiological methods, and took place just as these disciplines became established.[8]

In accordance with the prevailing emphasis on broad environmental factors leading to disease, Panum defined his research problem as the need "to study the hygienic factors which affect the state of health of the inhabitants" (1940: 3). Panum devoted numerous pages of his report to an ethnographic account of his five month stay on the islands, including descriptions of geography, topography, climate, vegetation, clothing, occupations, food, and social conditions. Through collecting individual measles case reports from 52 villages, Panum was able to define both the length of the incubation period of the disease and the duration of its infectivity. Since no one was attacked a second time, and since isolating cases through quarantine successfully restricted transmission of the disease, he concluded that measles had a contagious rather than a miasmatic origin. In fact he pointed to the practical advantages of establishing such an origin:

For if people believe that the causes of the disease are *generally dispersed in the atmosphere*, they can have no hope of protecting themselves against it, and will not be disposed to take precautions in this respect, since such measures must be regarded as vain; but if it is considered as settled that measles is transmitted only to such individuals as are susceptible to the infectious material which every measles patient carries, whether the infectious matter is suspended in the air *most nearly surrounding the patient*, or is entangled in clothes and the like, there may be hope of setting limits to the spread of the disease, and the necessary provisions in this direction will be instituted with reasonable hope of a successful result (1940 [1847]: 72, emphasis in the original).

For our purpose Panum's work is most notable for his use of observational methods. He did not emphasize social conditions to the extent that either Snow or Farr did; rather he included them as some of the many potentially relevant aspects of the external environment. Thus he mentioned that "the wealthier and more enlightened" seemed exempt from the gastric irritation that sometimes followed infection by measles; that there were occupational hazards from accidents and exposure to the severe climate, compensated by the benefits of physical exercise; and that the social life of the islands seemed to include qualities of simplicity, calmness, helpfulness, and little debauchery. Although he speculated that these last four factors might contribute to the relatively low Faroese mortality rate, he concluded that the major factor causing the favorable rates was the absence on the Islands of many of the infectious diseases then common in Europe.

Panum's approach suggests that some 19th century studies of disease transmission resulted in a cataloguing of social factors without explicit theoretical justification. Intervention strategies were similarly broad: as one analyst has put it, the scope of 19th century public health measures was "breathtaking" (Starr 1982: 180). Interventions to rid the environment of filth and foul odors had salutary effects on public health, but often not for the reasons put forth by those responsible. For example, the public health engineering of Max von Pettenkofer is famous for dramatically improving sanitation and health in Munich.[9] Pettenkofer fought to improve the systems of food inspections, water supply, and sewage disposal, and to reduce the level of overcrowding in dwelling units. Yet Pettenkofer was a leading opponent of the theory of contagion, and is almost as well known today for his dramatic demonstration of his contempt for Robert Koch's work on the path of infectivity of cholera: in 1892 he drank a culture of cholera bacilli, and startled the contagionists by not contracting the disease.

John Snow (1813—1858)

John Snow, probably the most celebrated 19th century epidemiologist, began his active research on cholera two years after Panum's measles investigation. Snow has been called the prototypical field epidemiologist because much of his data were gathered through personal observations and neighborhood surveys. His 1855 book, *On the Mode of Communication of Cholera*, is a methodical, well-documented argument for a contagious and water-borne transmission of cholera — this some 30 years before Robert Koch isolated the cholera vibrio. Snow examined the pathology of cholera as a clue to the manner of its communication. For example, he noted that cholera infections commenced in the alimentary canal, and he reasoned that such a focus of first infection suggested that some substance had been ingested. He then presented examples of the spread of the disease in mines, row houses, and entire neighborhoods, and in this process isolated important factors in the transmission of the disease, and contradicted arguments in favor of a miasmatic cause. Snow mapped the topography of a cholera outbreak near Cambridge and Broad Streets in London by means of a painstaking door to door survey, and isolated the probable source of the epidemic to a particular well. His subsequent removal of the Broad Street pump handle as a preventive measure has taken on great historical and symbolic significance.

Another of Snow's innovations occurred in what he called a "grandest scale experiment" (1936 [1855]: 75), one of a series of comparisons by which he implicated sewage polluted water in cholera mortality. Two different water supply companies had separate but interwoven systems of pipes in the Southwark area of London. They drew water from the Thames at two different sites, one of which was heavily polluted with sewage. Some blocks in the district had pipes from both suppliers, therefore Snow could compare exposed (case) and unexposed (control) groups. Since there were no important differences in pricing or service from the water companies, and since pipes once laid by one company were not replaced by those of another, the two groups appear to have been randomly assigned to their water source. Snow realized the significance of this for his research, noting that the population was "divided into two groups without their choice" (1936: 75).

Snow distinguished the water source by sodium chloride levels, and showed that those who used the badly polluted water had a higher incidence of cholera than did those who used the less polluted water. The death rate among residents of houses that used polluted water was about nine times higher than among residents of those that used less-polluted water.

In his ensuing discussion of the relevant causal factors in the epidemic, Snow analyzed seasonal factors, the sex differential and associated behavioral differences in exposure to water, and occupational factors. The study stands out as an early example of behavioral research and of quasi-experimental design in epidemiology. Nonetheless, as in the work of Panum and other biological epidemiologists, few explicitly social theories guided the social and behavioral aspects of this research. The procedural synthesis of ethnographic and epidemiologic methods preceded the synthesis of social theory and epidemiologic theory.

William Farr (1807—1883)

A third figure important to any discussion of mid-19th century epidemiology is William Farr. Farr was head of the statistical department in the English Registrar-General's office, and for almost 40 years was responsible for the vital statistics issued by that office. Along with researchers such as Florence Nightingale and John Simon, Farr was a prototypical British 19th century liberal, committed to social reforms, and committed to statistics as a means to advance these reforms.[10] Although not a field researcher in the fashion of Panum and Snow, Farr nonetheless was one of the most forcible 19th century proponents of an epidemiological focus on social factors, and thus provides a bridge to a more sociological (and radical) type of epidemiological research. The following quotation illustrates the depth of his understanding and commitment:

Different classes of the population experience very different rates of mortality, and suffer different kinds of diseases. The principal causes of these differences, besides the sex, age, and hereditary organization, must be sought in three sources — exercise in the ordinary occupations of life — the adequate or inadequate supply of warmth and of food — and the differennt (sic) degrees of exposure to poisonous effluvia and to noxious agents (1975 [1885]: 166).

Farr assisted Snow in his cholera investigations by providing Snow with the addresses of persons who had died from the disease. Although he was eventually convinced by Snow's research that cholera was a water-borne disease, Farr in the meantime championed the importance of elevation as the primary risk factor for contracting the disease. He explained an inverse effect of altitude on cholera mortality by referring to such "noxious agents" as "chemical modifications of organic matter", or "aqueous vapours impregnated with the products of chemical action" (Farr 1975: 347—351). Like

Pettenkofer, Simon, and others, Farr was an anticontagionist and a social reformer, whose work manifests the conflicting etiological theories of late 19th century medical research.[11]

III. GEOGRAPHICAL EPIDEMIOLOGY

Studies in geographical epidemiology emerged from an intellectual tradition distinct from that of the biological epidemiologists. The field of medical geography, as geographical epidemiology was sometimes known, expanded in the late 18th century, as European colonialist expansion brought a need for information about health conditions in foreign lands. Government-sponsored health surveys, or "medical topographies" appeared, written by Germans such as Johann Peter Frank (1976 [1779]) and Leonhard L. Finke (1792), and North Americans such as Daniel Drake (1850) and Noah Webster (1799). These focused on European, American, and foreign regions, and served both to catalogue dangers and explore the possible etiological importance of geography.

August Hirsch (1817—1894)

Perhaps the most important medical geographer of the 19th century was August Hirsch. Hirsch was a colleague of Rudolf Virchow, whose work we shall next discuss under the heading 'Sociological Epidemiology'. From 1866 to 1893 Hirsch co-edited with Virchow the *Jahresbericht ueber die Leistungen und Fortschritte der Gesamten Medizin* [*Yearbook of Accomplishments and Progress of Medicine*]. It is said that Virchow encouraged Hirsch to write his three volume *Handbook of Geographical and Historical Pathology*, the work for which Hirsch is best known (Ackerknecht 1953: 147). Hirsch is claimed as a father figure by modern medical geographers (e.g. May 1978 and Sigerist 1933), but his work is also important in epidemiology and in medical anthropology — in fact Hirsch may have been the first to have used the term "Medical Anthropology" (1883: vii).

Hirsch's work was a compendium of mid-19th century knowledge about diseases of organs, infectious, parasitic, and so-called 'constitutional' diseases. He used epidemiological categories of person, place, and time, though he emphasized place and time. His vision of the goal of historico-pathological and geographico-pathological inquiry was the following:

to exhibit the particular circumstances under which diseases have occurred within the several periods of time and at various parts of the globe; to show whether they have been subject to any differences, and of what kind, according to the time and place; what causal relations exist between the factors of disease acting at particular times and in particular places, on the one hand, and the character of the diseases that have actually occurred, on the other; and finally to show how those diseases are related to one another in their prevalence through time and through place (1883: 5).

Hirsch's first volume, on acute infectious diseases, included chapters on influenza, dengue, sweating sickness and military fever, smallpox, measles, scarlet fever, malaria, yellow fever, cholera, plague, typhus, relapsing fever, bilious typhoid, and typhoid. A tremendous amount of detail was furnished about the worldwide occurrence of these diseases: the chapter on yellow fever, for example, contained 20 pages of charts describing epidemics both by chronology and by latitude. Without knowing about the significance of the *Aedes aegypti* mosquito as a vector, Hirsch discussed the geographic distribution of the disease, and detailed the effects (or irrelevance) of such factors as temperature, moisture, wind, altitude, soil, population size, hygiene, poverty, and migration.

Geographical epidemiology thus represents an epidemiology concerned with broad temporal and geographical comparisons. This approach manifests the same concern for, and attention to, the study of "natural experiments" that can be seen in Snow's cholera work. It is an example of the comparative use of regional aggregate data for epidemiological analyses.

IV. THE SOCIAL THEORISTS: SOCIAL MEDICINE AND SOCIOLOGICAL EPIDEMIOLOGY

Much of what Ackerknecht called "sociological epidemiology" overlaps work in 19th century social medicine. Rosen has distilled three early principles of this field: health is a social concern; social and economic conditions have an important effect on health and disease; and social and individual measures must be taken to promote health and prevent disease (1947: 678—682). The social medicine movement began in France, where physicians such as Jules Guérin (1801—1886) and Louis René Villermé (1782—1863) documented the poor physical health of factory workers, and the effects of society on disease.[12] The work of the Belgian mathematician Adolphe Quetelet (1796—1874) was also important, through his systematic contributions to the developing field of statistics. Quetelet used the term *"statistique morale"* (translated as "moral statistics") for the study of non-physical human characteristics (Lazarsfeld 1961: 168). At a time when there were no experimental or laboratory methods to assess the public health (except for the kind of natural experiment capitalized upon by Snow), the use of statistical techniques to analyze observational data rapidly became important and popular. Adherents of social medicine saw moral statistics as providing objective and irrefutable proof of their contentions.

In the 1840s the center of development of social medicine moved to Germany. It expanded forcefully into the realm of politics around the time of the unsuccessful German revolution of 1848. This can be seen in the work of Rudolf Virchow, Solomon Neumann, and Rudolf Leubuscher, each of whom proposed specific measures for government action in support of health. These measures included providing medical care to the poor, regulating

working conditions in factories, and establishing the rights to work; education; food; and housing. Friedrich Engels also made an important contribution to social medicine concerning these issues, with the 1845 publication of
The Condition of the Working-Class in England (1973).[13]

Among the English, Farr and Snow were only a few of those who argued
for better working conditions: Edwin Chadwick, an anticontagionist like
Pettenkofer, also described the diseased state of the working class in his
1842 *Report on an Inquiry into the Sanitary Condition of the Labouring
Population of Great Britain.* Chadwick's report was emulated in the United
States by John Griscom in his 1845 report titled *The Sanitary Condition of
the Laboring Population of New York with Suggestions for its Improvement,*
and by Lemuel Shattuck in his 1850 *Report of a General Plan for the
Promotion of Public and Personal Health . . . relating to a Sanitary Survey of
the State.* But these British and North American studies did not extend their
criticisms of conditions in the workplace into more general criticisms of
society or theoretical analyses of social structure.

Two 19th century scientists merit extended discussion as major contributors to the literature on social factors in disease causation: Rudolf Virchow,
who exemplified the political involvement of mid-19th century proponents of
social medicine, and Emile Durkheim, who composed what is perhaps the
first work in social epidemiology.

Rudolf Virchow (1821—1902)

Virchow was a polymath with illustrious careers in medicine, politics, and
anthropology. His fame and influence were widespread in the 19th century
academic world; thus it is no coincidence that Panum studied pathological
anatomy with him in 1847 and 1851, and that the pre-eminent anthropologist Franz Boas came under Virchow's influence when Boas was
affiliated with the Berlin Ethnological Museum in 1883—1886 (Ackerknecht
1953: 235).[14]

Virchow was sent by the government in 1848 to investigate a typhus
epidemic in the famine-ridden Prussian province of Upper Silesia. According
to Ackerknecht's (1953) biography of Virchow, his experiences during this
three week study were to form and consolidate many of the later themes of
his career. Ackerknecht writes that Virchow's report to the government is
"an unusual and original document. Its fine clinical and pathological findings
are embedded into an amazingly competent 'anthropological' (sociological)
and epidemiological analysis" (1953: 15). Not only did Virchow blame the
government for the epidemic and famine, but as lasting solutions to the
problems he prescribed education, freedom, and prosperity rather than the
short term palliatives of food aid or new drugs.

Virchow's often-quoted dictum that "Medicine is a social science, and
politics nothing but medicine on a grand scale" dates from this time, as does

his idea that "the physicians are the natural attorneys of the poor, and the social problems should largely be solved by them" (1953: 243n.). Solomon Neumann, a colleague of Virchow's, had said much the same thing a year earlier:

> No special proof is required to see that the majority of the diseases which either prevent the full enjoyment of life or kill a considerable number of people prematurely are not due to natural physical, but to artificially produced social conditions . . . . Medical science is by its very nature a social science, but until this is actually recognized and conceded to medicine, we shall be unable to enjoy its benefits and shall have to be satisfied with an empty shell (Neumann 1847, excerpted in Rosen 1941: 14—15).

Ackerknecht points out that these ideas are not equivalent to the modern notion that medicine itself is a social science. Virchow, Neumann, and other activist physicians of the time meant rather that social science was contained in medicine, and that physicians were therefore justified in being active in politics.[15]

The mid-19th century was a time of many interchanges between the social sciences and medicine/hygiene; Neumann's words show that the boundaries of these disciplines were not yet fixed. Each field provided theories and even metaphors for the other: the early French sociologist Saint-Simon called his new science "social physiology" (Harris 1968); while Virchow and Neumann called medicine a social science. The use of an organic analogy for society can be traced back to Thomas Malthus, in his 1803 *Essay on the Principle of Population*. Later in the 19th century it was again employed by Darwin, Wallace, Spencer, and other proponents of the theory of evolution.[16]

The work of Virchow and his colleagues is important today not only because they emphasized the need to study and intervene upon the social causes of disease. Virchow also was a (largely unacknowledged) forerunner of modern studies of the health effects of social change: he "developed a theory of epidemic disease as a manifestation of social and cultural maladjustment" (Rosen 1947: 679), and stated that epidemic diseases were markers of cultural change:

> Epidemic diseases exhibiting an hitherto unknown character appear and disappear, after new culture periods have begun often without leaving any trace . . . . The history of artificial epidemics is therefore the history of disturbances which the culture of mankind has experienced. Its changes show us with powerful strokes the turning points at which culture moves off in new directions. Every true cultural revolution is followed by epidemics, because a large part of the people only gradually enter into the new cultural movement and begin to enjoy its blessings (translated and quoted in Rosen 1947: 681).

While this idea is fundamentally similar to contemporary theories of the health effects of culture change, it differs in two important respects: it implies that diseases occur among those not yet included in culture change; and it provides few testable propositions that might explain the connection between social or cultural change and health. Contemporary cultural change has brought mixed blessings; "diseases of development" are a phenomenon of change not accounted for by Virchow's theory. Nonetheless, Virchow's statement here is a qualitatively different approach to the study of social factors from that of Snow, Panum, Farr, Chadwick, or other 19th century advocates of sanitary reforms.

Emile Durkheim (1858—1917)

The last 19th century work which I describe is transitional not only in time but also in topic, for it is with Durkheim that epidemiology began to develop strong theoretical arguments for focusing on the social causes of disease. Emile Durkheim, the French sociologist, published *Le Suicide* in 1897; this work stands as the ultimate expression of the moral statistics movement which had manifested itself earlier in the work of Farr, Quetelet, and Virchow. Durkheim took for his subject what most see as the ultimate individual act, and then demonstrated that there were specific, stable, and quantifiable aspects of suicide when it was viewed as a collective social phenomenon (1951: 41—57, 297—309). Durkheim's research strategy in *Suicide* followed the theory of sociological investigation he presented in his 1895 work *The Rules of Sociological Method*. In *Rules* Durkheim stated his well-known principle that "The determining cause of a social fact should be sought among the social facts preceding it and not among the states of the individual consciousness" (1964: 110). In *Suicide* this was stated as "the social suicide-rate can be explained only sociologically".

In a careful and logical progression Durkheim examined a succession of explanations for suicide, such as pathology, race, heredity, climate, temperature, and imitation, and in each case found no strong favorable statistical support. An impressive number of techniques were used in this process, including examinations of common variations in rates, common levels of changes in rates, geographical distributions, and rates in migrants versus residents.[17] In analyzing his data, Durkheim used rates adjusted for age, sex, marital status, and other variables which might otherwise have confounded his results. He also adopted measures of relative risk (what he called a "coefficient of preservation or of aggravation") in describing general susceptibility: "if we represent the suicidal tendency of married persons by unity, that of unmarried persons of the same average age must be estimated as 1.6" (1951: 73). Durkheim's work is thus not only well-grounded in theory, but also sophisticated in method.

In its forceful emphasis on collective and social forces affecting individuals, Durkheim's work presaged most of contemporary social epidemiology. He pointed out in *Suicide* that the power of social forces was indicated by the fact that "The individuals making up a society change from year to year, yet the number of suicides is the same so long as the society itself does not change" (*Ibid.*: 307).

Durkheim also questioned why some particular individuals commit suicide, while other apparently similar ones do not — a question which could be subsumed under the contemporary topic of "host susceptibility", referring to factors influencing whether or not potential hosts acquire diseases. Durkheim's finding that the number of suicides was constant from year to year caused him to reason that the "suicidogenetic current" of society did not touch all susceptible persons at once. But how was it that persons who committed suicide one year had been "provisionally spared" the year before from the influence of collective life (*Ibid.*: 324)? Durkheim answered that the collective forces impelling individuals towards suicide increased with time; these probably combined with repeated negative life experiences to take their toll on successive cohorts.

Durkheim stated that his ideas about social forces should only be added to the prevailing categories of physical, chemical, biological, and psychological forces (*Ibid.*: 325n.). Though his work is not commonly heralded as noteworthy in the history of epidemiology, those with a particular concern for social factors should view Durkheim as an innovator and major contributor. At a time when the germ theory dominated epidemiological research, and reinforced the ideas that each condition had a single specific cause and each cause a single specific condition, Durkheim's writings foretold the reemergence of an alternative model. During the bacteriological era sociological epidemiologists such as Durkheim and Virchow helped to preserve the theory that social factors also played a causal etiological role.

V. THE BACTERIOLOGICAL ERA: A FOCUS ON THE AGENT

For some 50 years between the 1870s and the 1920s the bacteriological paradigm was dominant, and was joined in the early 20th century by an appreciation for the importance of arthropod-borne diseases, nutrition, and disease transmission by healthy carriers. The dominance of the paradigm was ensured by its impressive research findings: the decade of the 1870s saw isolation of agents responsible for causing leprosy and anthrax; the 1880s found agents for typhoid, tuberculosis, cholera, diphtheria, and meningococcal meningitis; the 1890s, plague and malaria; and by 1910 pertussis, syphilis, and epidemic typhus. By 1920 vitamins had been discovered, and pellagra had been proven to be associated with nutritional deficiency.[18]

These many impressive research findings increased interest in their underlying assumption, namely that each disease has but one cause. This popular model of disease causation was contained in what has been called the Henle–Koch postulates. Jacob Henle in the 1840s, and his student Robert Koch in the 1880s and 1890s, developed much of the theory and evidence for the involvement of specific micro-organisms in specific diseases. As outlined by Koch, the necessary criteria for demonstrating organismic causation were the occurrence of an organism in every case of a particular disease, accompanied by an explanation of a plausible pathological course; the occurrence of the organism in no other diseases; and the isolability, culturability, and potential reinfectivity of the organism. Dubos has labelled this the "doctrine of specific etiology" (1959: 10).[19]

Despite the many advances of the bacteriological era, the doctrine of specific etiology did not resolve the important question of why some individuals were more susceptible to a given illness than others, nor did it provide testable hypotheses about the morbidity and mortality from starvation, nutritional deficiencies, and the occupational diseases of the new industrial era. The health profile of the industrialized world was changing by the middle of the 19th century, and had started to change even before the pathways of causation and transmission were established for many infectious diseases. This can be seen in the rates of decline for such diseases as yellow fever, smallpox, typhoid, malaria, and tuberculosis (Rosen 1958; McKeown 1979). The advocates of social medicine were concerned with the ways these new occupational conditions affected health, but they presented a minority view.

Studying the pernicious effects of the social environment also was not a mainstream effort in the social science of the day. Late 19th and early 20th century social science was more concerned with the social repercussions of Darwin's theory of evolution (the *Origin of Species* was first published in 1859), particularly the implications of the Malthusian "struggle for survival", coupled with Spencer's concept of the "survival of the fittest". Spencer's harsh version of this struggle was popular between the 1850s and 1890s, as was the social philosophy known as "Social Darwinism"; the adherents of these social movements believed in *laissez faire* capitalism, and felt that the new industrialism served as a valuable selective force.[20] Late 19th century anthropology also reflected this topic: in addition to employing their cross-cultural comparative method to understand the evolution of social structure, anthropologists like L. H. Morgan and E. B. Tylor were both at least partly interested in establishing the supremacy and higher evolutionary development of the white "race". The eugenics movement popular in the early 20th century (which involved statisticians like Francis Galton and Karl Pearson) revived some aspects of this social philosophy.

VI. SUMMARY

In tracing the theoretical affinities and collaborative efforts of two disciplines through time, one immediately faces the narrow temporal constraints given by the use of the word "discipline": anthropology and epidemiology as specific fields date back only some 200 years. The label "discipline" is fully appropriate for these fields only for the past 130 years, or since the founding of professional societies and the creation of academic departments. Much of the pre-20th century work that today we call epidemiological was known in its time as geographical pathology, social medicine, hygiene, historical pathology, or vital statistics. The constraints in defining a unified 19th century epidemiology also apply to defining a unified 19th century anthropology, which was variously practiced as ethnology, sociology, culture history, or comparative sociology. Anthropology and sociology, the two social science disciplines most relevant to this presentation, became separated only after many of the themes of social medicine had already been developed. This chapter emphasized anthropology, but by necessity it examined a broad range of 19th century disciplines.

Three broad categories can encompass 19th century epidemiological work: the biological; the historical/geographical; and the sociological. So-called "shoe-leather epidemiology", or field epidemiology, begins within biological epidemiology, and provides an example of the participant observation and interview techniques employed by many 19th century epidemiological researchers. This use of what anthropologists call ethnographic methods was due largely to the nature of the etiological theories guiding research at the time: a broad conception of the relevance of the environment motivated correspondingly broad surveys that included many different social factors.[21]

In geographical epidemiology one can see the beginnings of population comparisons on an international scale. Geographical epidemiology also established the utility of a focus on the analytic categories of place and time. We shall see in the next chapter how this focus has been employed by contemporary medical geographers.

In sociological epidemiology one can see the continuation and advancement of a concern for assessing the social environment. The analytic categories employed here were those of the person, or of the host and the environment. Nineteenth century sociological epidemiologists frequently articulated a political agenda as part of their recommendations for improvements in health. Some of the important themes stressed by these researchers were that changes in social and cultural patterns were accompanied by changes in health status; that poverty itself was an important etiological agent; and that it was not only more effective but also cheaper for governments to direct their efforts toward preventive medicine rather than curative medicine.

With the advent of bacteriology came an increased focus on the agent, which dominated the epidemiological literature for almost 50 years. Geographical and sociological epidemiology continued to survive while the bacteriological paradigm dominated research. However, under the influence of the doctrine of specific etiology and the philosophy of social Darwinism, the social and the geographical approaches lost some of their momentum in the period between 1870 and 1920. In the 20th century we can follow the resurgence of these categories in contemporary research.

ACKNOWLEDGEMENTS

My thanks to the following for comments on earlier drafts of this paper: Frederick Dunn, Linnea Klee, Lynn Morgan, S. Leonard Syme, Frank Zimmerman, the editors, and an anonymous reviewer.

I gratefully acknowledge the financial support received from the following sources: NIMH research fellowship number F31 MH09039, the Wenner-Gren Foundation for Anthropological Research, the Rennie Endowment at the University of California, Berkeley, and the Schepp Foundation.

NOTES

1. I will call *epidemiological* those investigations that focus on the distribution and determinants of diseases in human populations (MacMahon and Pugh 1970), and that commonly use the analytic categories of person, place, and time, as well as host, agent, and environment.

2. The hallmark of anthropological investigations in the United States is a focus on the concept of culture, defined in many ways (see Kroeber and Kluckhohn 1952), but generally referring to "learned modes of behavior that are socially transmitted from one generation to the next and from one society or individual to another" (Steward 1955: 44). The discipline contains four subfields: cultural or social anthropology (which I shall refer to most frequently here); physical anthropology; archaeology; and linguistics.

3. There is as yet no historical survey of the relationship between sociology and epidemiology. Wilson (1970) presents a full contemporary account of sociology and epidemiology, but includes little history.

4. See also Stocking's chapter " 'Cultural Darwinism' and 'Philosophical Idealism' in E.B. Tylor" (1968a) for an example and discussion of the differences between presentist and historicist approaches; for related examples of this distinction in the history of medicine see Figlio (1977) and Shortt (1981).

5. Telluric theories were popular 18th and 19th century explanations of disease causation based on exudations from the soil. Miasmatic theory held that epidemic diseases were caused by atmospheric conditions including noxious odors. Telluric and miasmatic theories competed with contagionist theories to the end of the 19th century (Ackerknecht 1948a; Rosen 1958). (See also Terris 1985, a paper recently brought to my attention by Fred Dunn which makes many points similar to those made in this paper.)

6. For an argument specifically rejecting Hippocratic origins, and arguing instead for roots in Bentham, Bacon, and Hume, see Roth (1976: 53—56).

7. See e.g. Ackerknecht (1967), Foucault (1973), Figlio (1977).

8. The first epidemiological society started in 1850 (The Epidemiological Society of London), and the first enduring anthropological society started in 1843 (the Ethnological Society of Great Britain, later the Royal Anthropological Institute). The *Societe des Observateurs de l'Homme*, an early French anthropological society, was founded in Paris in 1800, but disbanded in 1804. (See Stocking 1968b, 'French Anthropology in 1800'.)

9. See Pettenkofer's 1873 lectures on 'The Value of Health to a City' (1941).

10. See Eyler (1979), Chapter 2: 'Statistics: A Science of Social Reform', pp. 13—36.

11. See Ackerknecht (1948a): 'Anticontagionism between 1821 and 1867'.

12. See Ackerknecht (1948b: 117—157), 'Hygiene in France, 1815—1848', and Rosen (1947), 'What Is Social Medicine?'.
13. See also Marcus (1974); Waitzkin (1981).
14. Boas was soon to become the founder and chief spokesman for anthropology in the United States. See Boas, 'Rudolf Virchow's Anthropological Work' *Science* (1902), reprinted in G. Stocking (ed.), *The Shaping of American Anthropology, 1883—1911: A Franz Boas Reader*. New York: Basic Books, 1974, pp. 36—41. Kluckhohn and Prufer (1959: 21—24) state that Virchow was one of four influential men in Boas' thought.
15. Galdston adopts the same position (1951: 13—14), but compare Waitzkin (1981: 83—89).
16. In fact, in viewing social science as a physiological examination of the proper and harmonious workings of society, and in writing of the "functional unity" of society, 20th century functionalist theories in the social sciences continue to employ such an organic analogy.
17. See, e.g., Faris (1951), a review of *Suicide*, and Selvin (1958), which is an assessment of Durkheim's multivariate analyses in *Suicide*. For a contemporary report of a project combining epidemiological and case study analyses of suicide, see Sainsbury (1972).
18. These discoveries are detailed and placed in their historical context in Foster (1970); Rosen (1958); and Starr (1982).
19. Modern epidemiologists have repeatedly criticized the narrowness of the Henle—Koch postulates, and their lack of relevance to behavioral factors, but have also pointed out that the postulates never were recommended by their authors as rigid criteria of causation (see e.g. Cassel 1964; Evans 1976; Kark 1974: 154; and Susser 1973: 22—24).
20. See Hofstadter (1955): *Social Darwinism in American Thought*, and Stocking (1968a).
21. There are parallels to this in the development of ethnological theory: late 19th and early 20th century anthropological investigations commonly included a broad range of descriptive categories. The "historical particularism" advocated by the anthropologist Franz Boas caused his students to devote many years and pages to broad ethnographic observations. In fact, much of the medical anthropological work done at this time was undertaken because a broad inventory approach was fashionable in ethnography — a justification similar to that which motivated 19th century epidemiologists to collect information on social factors.

REFERENCES

Ackerknecht, E. H.
   1948a Anticontagionism between 1821 and 1867. Bulletin of the History of Medicine 22: 562—593.
   1948b Hygiene in France, 1815—1848. Bulletin of the History of Medicine 22: 117—155.
   1953 Rudolf Virchow: Doctor, Statesman, Anthropologist. Madison, WI: University of Wisconsin Press.
   1967 Medicine at the Paris Hospital, 1794—1848. Baltimore: Johns Hopkins University Press.
Antonovsky, A.
   1967 Social Class, Life Expectancy and Overall Mortality. Milbank Memorial Fund Quarterly 45: 31—73.
Boas, F.
   1902 Rudolf Virchow's Anthropological Work. Science 16(403): 441—445.
Cassel, J. C.
   1964 Social Science Theory as a Source of Hypotheses in Epidemiological Research. American Journal of Public Health 54: 1482—1488.

Chadwick, E.
    1965 Report on an Inquiry into the Sanitary Condition of the Labouring Population of Great Britain. Reprint of the 1842 edition. Edinburgh: Edinburgh University Press.
Darwin, C.
    1859 The Origin of Species. (A Variorum Text, 1959.) M. Peckham (ed.). Philadelphia: University of Pennsylvania Press.
Drake, D.
    1850 A Systematic Treatise, Historical, Etiological, and Practical, on the Principal Diseases of the Interior Valley of North America, as They Appear in the Caucasian, African, Indian, and Esquimaux Varieties of its Population. Cincinnati: Winthrop B. Smith and Company.
Dubos, R.
    1959 Mirage of Health: Utopias, Progress and Biological Change. New York: Harper and Row.
Durkheim, E.
    1951 Suicide: A Study in Sociology. (1st French ed., 1897.) J. A. Spaulding and G. Simpson, transl. Glencoe, IL: Free Press.
    1964 The Rules of Sociological Method. (1st French ed., 1895.) S. A. Solovay and J. H. Mueller, transl., G.E.G. Catlin (ed.), Glencoe, IL: Free Press.
Engels, F.
    1973 The Condition of the Working-Class in England. (1st German ed., 1845.) Moscow: Progress Publishers.
Evans, A. S.
    1976 Causation and Disease: The Henle—Koch Postulates Revisited. Yale Journal of Biology and Medicine 49: 175—195.
Eyler, J. M.
    1979 Victorian Social Medicine: The Ideas and Methods of William Farr. Baltimore: Johns Hopkins University Press.
Faris, R. E. L.
    1951 Review of Suicide, by Emile Durkheim. American Journal of Sociology 57(1): 100—101.
Farquhar, J. and D. C. Gajdusek (eds.)
    1981 Early Letters and Fieldnotes from the Collection of D. Carlton Gajdusek. New York: Raven Press.
Farr, W.
    1975 Vital Statistics. A Memorial Volume of Selections from the Reports and Writings of William Farr. Reprint of the 1885 edition. History of Medicine Series No. 46. New York: New York Academy of Medicine.
Figlio, K.
    1977 The Historiography of Scientific Medicine: An Invitation to the Human Sciences. Comparative Studies in Society and History 19: 262—286.
Finke, L. L.
    1946 On the Different Kinds of Geographies, but Chiefly on Medical Topographies, and How to Compose Them. (Translated from the German, with an Introduction by George Rosen.) Bulletin of the History of Medicine 20: 527—528.
Fischer, A. and J. L. Fischer
    1961 Culture and Epidemiology: A Theoretical Investigation of Kuru. Journal of Health and Human Behavior 2: 16—25.
Foster, W. D.
    1970 A History of Medical Bacteriology and Immunology. London: Heinemann Medical.
Foucault, M.
    1973 The Birth of the Clinic. An Archaeology of Medical Perception. (A. M. Sheridan Smith, transl.) New York: Vintage Books.

Frank, J. P.
    1976 A System of Complete Medical Police: Selections from Johann Peter Frank. (E.
          Vilim, translator of the 1799 edition, edited with an introduction by E. Lesky).
          Baltimore: Johns Hopkins University Press.
Gajdusek, D. C.
    1977 Unconventional Viruses and the Origin and Disappearance of Kuru. Science 197:
          946—960.
Galdston, I.
    1951 Social Medicine and the Epidemic Constitution. Bulletin of the History of Medicine
          25(1): 8—21.
Gordon, J. E.
    1953 Evolution of an Epidemiology of Health, Parts I, II, and III. In The Epidemiology of
          Health. I. Galdston, (ed.), pp. 24—73. New York: New York Academy of Medicine.
    1958 Medical Ecology and the Public Health. American Journal of the Medical Sciences
          235(3): 336—359.
Gove, W. R.
    1973 Sex, Marital Status, and Mortality. American Journal of Sociology 79: 45—67.
Graunt, J.
    1662 Natural and Political Observations Mentioned in a Following Index, and Made
          Upon the Bills of Mortality. London. Reprinted 1939. Baltimore: Johns Hopkins
          University Press.
Greenwood, M.
    1932 Epidemiology — Historical and Experimental. (The Herter Lectures for 1931.)
          Baltimore: Johns Hopkins University Press.
Griscom, J. H.
    1845 The Sanitary Condition of the Laboring Population of New York with Suggestions
          for its Improvement. New York: Harper and Brothers.
Harris, M.
    1968 The Rise of Anthropological Theory. New York: Thomas Crowell.
Hippocrates
    1957 Airs Waters Places. (W. H. S. Jones, transl.) In Hippocrates, with an English
          Translation. pp. 71—137. Cambridge, MA: Harvard University Press.
Hirsch, A.
    1883 Handbook of Geographical and Historical Pathology. Three Volumes. (C.
          Creighton, transl., from the 2nd German ed.) London: The New Sydenham Society.
Hofstadter, D.
    1955 Social Darwinism in American Thought (Revised Edition). Boston: Beacon Press.
Jacobs, S. and A. Ostfeld
    1977 An Epidemiological Review of the Mortality of Bereavement. Psychosomatic
          Medicine 39: 344—357.
Kark, S. L.
    1974 Epidemiology and Community Medicine. New York: Appleton-Century-Crofts.
Kluckhohn, C. and O. Prufer
    1959 Influences During the Formative Years. In The Anthropology of Franz Boas. W.
          Goldschmidt (ed.), American Anthropological Association Memoir 89. pp. 4—28.
Kroeber, A. L. and C. Kluckhohn
    1952 Culture: A Critical Review of Concepts and Definitions. Peabody Museum Papers
          47, 1. Cambridge, MA: Harvard University Press.
Lazarsfeld, P. A.
    1961 Notes on the History of Quantification in Sociology — Trends, Sources and
          Problems. In Quantification: A History of the Meaning of Measurement in the
          Natural and Social Sciences. H. Woolf (ed.), pp. 147—203. Indianapolis: Bobbs-
          Merrill.

Lilienfeld, A. M. and D. E. Lilienfeld
    1980 Foundations of Epidemiology (2nd ed.). New York: Oxford University Press.
Lindenbaum, S.
    1982 Review of Kuru: Early Letters and Fieldnotes from the Collection of D. Carlton
          Gajdusek, by J. Farquhar and D. C. Gajdusek. Journal of the Polynesian Society
          91(1): 150—152.
MacMahon, B. and T. F. Pugh
    1970 Epidemiology: Principles and Methods. Boston: Little, Brown and Company.
Malthus, T. R.
    1803 An Essay on the Principle of Population, or a View of Its Past and Present Effects
          on Human Happiness, with an Inquiry Into Our Prospects Respecting the Future
          Removal or Mitigation of the Evils which it Occasions. London.
Marcus, S.
    1974 Engels, Manchester, and the Working Class. New York: Vintage Books.
May, J. M.
    1978 History, Definition, and Problems of Medical Geography: A General Review.
          (Report to the Commission on Medical Geography of the International Geograph-
          ical Union, 1952.) Social Science and Medicine 12D: 211—219.
McCracken, R. D.
    1971 Lactase Deficiency: An Example of Dietary Evolution. Current Anthropology 12:
          479—517.
McKeown, T.
    1979 The Role of Medicine. Dream, Mirage or Nemesis? Princeton: Princeton University
          Press.
Neser, W. B., H. A. Tyroler, and J. C. Cassel
    1971 Social Disorganization and Stroke Mortality in the Black Population of North
          Carolina. American Journal of Epidemiology 93: 166—175.
Panum, P. L.
    1940 Observations Made During the Epidemic of Measles on the Faroe Islands in the
          Year 1846. New York: Delta Omega Society.
Pettenkofer, M.
    1941 The Value of Health to a City, Two Lectures, Delivered in 1873. (Translated from
          the German, with an Introduction by H. E. Sigerist.) Bulletin of the History of
          Medicine 10: 487—503, 593—613.
Rosen, G.
    1941 Disease and Social Criticism. A Contribution to a Theory of Medical History.
          Bulletin of the History of Medicine 10: 5—15.
    1947 What is Social Medicine? A Genetic Analysis of the Concept. Bulletin of the
          History of Medicine 21: 674—733.
    1955 Problems in the Application of Statistical Analysis to Questions of Health: 1700—
          1880. Bulletin of the History of Medicine 29: 27—45.
    1958 A History of Public Health. New York: MD Publications.
Roth, D.
    1976 The Scientific Basis of Epidemiology: An Historical and Philosophical Enquiry.
          Ph.D. Dissertation, Epidemiology Program, University of California, Berkeley.
Sainsbury, P.
    1972 The Social Relations of Suicide: The Value of a Combined Epidemiological and
          Case Study Approach. Social Science and Medicine 6: 189—198.
Selvin, H. C.
    1958 Durkheim's Suicide and the Problems of Empirical Research. American Journal of
          Sociology 63: 607—619.
Shattuck, L.
    1948 Report of a General Plan for the Promotion of Public and Personal Health ...

Relating to a Sanitary Survey of the State. (Reprint of the 1850 Boston edition.) Cambridge, MA: Harvard University Press.

Shortt, S. E.
  1981 Clinical Practice and the Social History of Medicine: A Theoretical Accord. Bulletin of the History of Medicine 55: 533—542.

Shryock, R. H.
  1960 Medicine and Society in America: 1660—1860. Ithaca, New York: Cornell University Press.
  1961 The History of Quantification in Medical Science. *In* Quantification: A History of the Meaning of Measurement in the Natural and Social Sciences. H. Woolf (ed.), pp. 85—107. Indianapolis: Bobbs-Merrill.

Sigerist, H. E.
  1933 Problems of Historical-Geographical Pathology. Bulletin of the History of Medicine 1: 10—18.

Snow, J.
  1936 Snow on Cholera; Being a Reprint of Two Papers by John Snow. (2nd ed. 1855.) New York: Commonwealth Fund.

Starr, P.
  1982 The Social Transformation of American Medicine. New York: Basic Books.

Steward, J. H.
  1955 Theory of Culture Change. The Methodology of Multilinear Evolution. Urbana, IL: University of Illinois Press.

Stocking Jr., G. W.
  1968a 'Cultural Darwinism' and 'Philosophical Idealism' in E. B. Tylor. *In* Race, Culture and Evolution: Essays in the History of Anthropology. G. W. Stocking Jr. (ed.), pp. 91—109. New York: Free Press.
  1968b French Anthropology in 1800. *In* Race, Culture and Evolution. G. W. Stocking Jr. (ed.), pp. 13—41. New York: Free Press.
  1968c On the Limits of "Presentism" and "Historicism" in the Historiography of the Behavioral Sciences. *In* Race, Culture, and Evolution. G. W. Stocking Jr. (ed.), pp. 1—12. New York: Free Press.

Susser, M.
  1973 Causal Thinking in the Health Sciences: Concepts and Strategies of Epidemiology. London: Oxford University Press.

Syme, S. L. and L. Berkman
  1976 Social Class, Susceptibility and Sickness. American Journal of Epidemiology 104: 1—8.

Terris, M.
  1985 The Changing Relationships of Epidemiology and Society: The Robert Cruickshank Lecture. Journal of Public Health Policy 6: 15—36.

Waitzkin, H.
  1981 The Social Origins of Illness: A Neglected Story. International Journal of Health Services 11: 77—103.

Webster, N.
  1799 A Brief History of Epidemic and Pestilential Diseases; with the Principal Phenomena of the Physical World which Precede and Accompany Them. (2 volumes) Hartford, CT: Hudson and Goodwin.

Wiesenfeld, S. L.
  1967 Sickle-Cell Trait in Human Biological and Cultural Evolution. Science 157: 1134—1140.

Wilson, R. N.
  1970 The Sociology of Health: An Introduction. New York: Random House.

Winslow, C. E. A.
    1952 The Colonial Era and the First Years of the Republic (1607—1709) — The
        Pestilence that Walketh in Darkness. *In* The History of American Epidemiology. F.
        H. Top (ed.), pp. 11—51. St. Louis: C. V. Mosby.

JAMES TROSTLE

ANTHROPOLOGY AND EPIDEMIOLOGY IN THE TWENTIETH CENTURY: A SELECTIVE HISTORY OF COLLABORATIVE PROJECTS AND THEORETICAL AFFINITIES, 1920 TO 1970

Whether you primarily enjoy the progress in scientific method and knowledge made during the last hundred years, or whether you prefer to ponder those epidemiological problems, unsolved by both parties [contagionists and anticontagionists] at the time and unsolved in our own day, all your conclusions will be right and good except for the one, so common in man, but so foreign to the spirit of history: that our not committing the same errors today might be due to an intellectual or moral superiority of ours. (Ackerknecht 1948: 593)

The preceding chapter traced biological, geographical, and sociological schools of epidemiological inquiry in the 19th century, and gave examples of how each contributed to the shape and themes of modern epidemiology. It also explored the rise and subsequent decline of 19th century interest in the etiologic significance of social factors. This chapter will trace the growing involvement of the social sciences in the 20th century history of social epidemiology,[1] concentrating especially on anthropology,[2] and parallels to the 19th century work.

The broad inclusion of social factors[3] in 19th century epidemiological studies was waning by the end of the century, as research shifted to attempts to find single causes for specific diseases. A concern for social factors was reborn in the second and third decades of the 20th century, when it became important to conceptualize and measure the etiological effects of the social environment. Diseases such as cancer, heart disease, and diabetes were coming to dominate the industrialized world's disease profile, and single-cause models were not sufficient to explain their etiology. At the same time national governments faced increasing pressure to provide adequate health services; the need for research on design, efficacy, and provision of these services became as pressing as research on etiology. Community medicine and chronic disease epidemiology thus helped to revitalize research on the health effects of society and culture.

In order to describe these two different areas in the development of social epidemiology and public health in the 20th century this chapter covers two topics in depth: research on community health care and community diagnosis developed at the Institute of Family and Community Health in South Africa; and research on social change and social disorganization developed largely at the Epidemiology Department of the University of North Carolina, Chapel Hill. These two centers have been selected for extensive descriptions because they sponsored fundamental 20th century work in social epidemiology.

Largely omitted here because of space constraints are the work of physical

59

Craig R. Janes et al. (eds.), Anthropology and Epidemiology, 59—94.
© 1986 *by D. Reidel Publishing Company.*

anthropologists in epidemiological research,[4] that of psychological anthropologists in the development of psychiatric epidemiology,[5] and the role of anthropology and epidemiology in the search for the etiology of specific diseases, such as *kuru*.[6] Projects and ideas involving social and cultural anthropologists will be emphasized instead.

I. THE REVIVAL OF INTEREST IN THE HOST AND THE ENVIRONMENT

Many authors have suggested that the high mortality from the influenza pandemic of 1918—1919 helped to rekindle research interest in the host and environment (e.g. Douall 1952: 75; Galdston 1951: 16; Gordon 1953: 61; Hamer 1929: 129). Influenza killed approximately 20 million people worldwide in those two years, or twice the number of soldiers who had been killed in the Great War that had just ended. One epidemic probably did not launch a half century of research, but it did harshly remind investigators that their knowledge of microbes was not sufficient to explain the natural history of epidemics.

Including the host and the environment in the natural history of epidemics accompanied a broader definition of epidemiology. As new categories of diseases were developed and the industrialized world's disease profile began to change, researchers began to apply their epidemiological methods not just to the acute infectious diseases such as influenza, but also to parasitic and nutritional diseases (Chapin 1928); chronic infectious diseases (Frost 1941 [1927]); chronic non-infectious diseases (Greenwood 1932); and even to mental illness (Elkind 1938).

The renewed interest in the social environment in the 1920s and 1930s did not include the political overtones and sweeping environmental and political changes that had been advocated by Engels and Virchow in the mid-19th century. This was partly because the successes of bacteriology provided more specific measures of intervention than earlier had been available. Moreover, at this time national health insurance and/or national health services were the focus of increasing interest in Great Britain, the European continent, the U.S.S.R., the U.S., and South Africa. Bismarck had introduced the first national compulsory health insurance system in Germany in 1883, and other Western countries were following suit. Reform efforts in the tradition of Chadwick and Farr predominated over revolutionary efforts in the tradition of Virchow or Engels; researchers developed new health programs and argued for new legislation rather than for dramatic structural changes.

One important experiment in constructing a national health service began in South Africa in the late 1930s. This culminated in the founding of the Polela (also spelled *Pho*lela) Health Unit in 1940, and the subsequent founding of the Institute of Family and Community Health (IFCH) in 1945.

The innovative research methods used at Polela and at the IFCH, the high quality of the investigators trained there, and the subsequent emigration of those researchers to other sites throughout the world combine to make these institutions the birthplace of the most important collective research effort in social epidemiology to date.

The significance of the Polela project was that it assessed the health status of a community using social science and epidemiologic methods, and drew on those assessments to develop and evaluate a comprehensive multi-disciplinary approach to improving community health. Many of the research topics explored at Polela were similar to those explored by 19th century proponents of social medicine: poverty and social class are important determinants of health; social and cultural change affect the transmission of illness; and group as well as individual interventions promote health and prevent disease. The authors of the major book about the project acknowledged these similarities, entitling their book *A Practice of Social Medicine* (Kark and Steuart 1962).

Reflecting on the Polela project a decade after its inception, the first medical director, Sidney Kark, commented on the gains made after the first year of the experiment. He described the increasing level of staff knowledge about the culture and social structure of the local inhabitants, stressed the importance of careful observations, and added:

The whole process of the health centre's development was one which reflected an increasing understanding of the individual in terms of his family situation, of the family in its life situation within the local community and finally the way of life of the community itself in relation to the social structure of South Africa. By this detailed study the centre had moved from the plane of vague generalization about the importance of various social forces to an increasing understanding of those forces in relation to health and disease as manifested in individuals.

It was not so much that the experiment had led to the discovery of the connection between social relationships and health. This has been a well-established thesis and has for many years been an accepted fact. Nor was it that the centre had been able to establish such a correlation. Sociologists and epidemiologists have developed methods for such studies and many have been the reports during the past century indicating the importance of such correlations. The significant feature of this year of experimental study was rather the fact that it had been possible to evolve a technique which included such concepts as an integral part of its daily practice. (S. Kark 1951: 677)

The most significant figures in the Polela account are Sidney and Emily Kark and John Cassel. The Karks and their colleagues used epidemiology, and especially a socially oriented epidemiology, to develop and evaluate a practice of community-oriented primary health care (COPC). Their practice focused on the social and cultural factors in the growth and development of children; the social pathology of veneral disease; nutrition and adjustment in health; and the evaluation of COPC's effect on health status. Somewhat later Cassel and his colleagues studied the health effects of social and cultural change, concentrating on the processes involved and possible ways of mediating the effects of socially stressful life experience, such as social support. The IFCH and the Epidemiology Department at North Carolina are not commonly known to anthropologists, and their anthropological emphases are not commonly recognized by epidemiologists, so they merit detailed consideration here.

II. THE EPIDEMIOLOGY OF COMMUNITY HEALTH: THE WORK OF SIDNEY AND EMILY KARK

The Kark's biographies help to explain the origins of the anthropological aspects of their research. Emily and Sidney Kark were medical students together at the University of the Witwatersrand in the early 1930s, and were strongly influenced by their association with the South African Institute of Race Relations, which included Winifred Hoernle, a leading anthropologist at the University (S. and E. Kark: personal communication). In 1934 the Karks began a 'Society for the Study of Medical Conditions Among the Bantu', and in 1938—1939 Sidney Kark was appointed as the physician of a national Bantu Nutrition Survey, conducted by the Ministry of Health. In 1939 S. Kark was selected by the Ministry of Health to head a new health unit in Polela, a small rural African community in the province of Natal.

The Polela Health Center was a pilot project designed to deliver effective and appropriate health services to rural South African communities.[7] The Polela staff consisted of the Karks as physicians, a medical aide and nurse, and five health assistants. Apart from the Karks all were Zulus and thus of the same nation as the people of Polela, but initially none came from the local community. Additional health workers and nursing assistants were recruited early on from the local community (S. Kark: personal communication; Kark and Kark 1981b). The shared experiences and exchanges among the medical aide, health assistants, nurse, doctors, and representatives of the community helped to bridge the gap between traditional Zulu health beliefs and practices and biomedical beliefs and practices;[8] these exchanges also reinforced the interest of the staff in social science methods.

From its inception the Polela Health Center was concerned with the social and cultural life of the surrounding community. The first activities of the Health Center included meetings with tribal chiefs and elders to discuss the program. The staff consulted other groups active in the community: women's groups; local missionaries; school teachers; and parents of schoolchildren. The community health educators made multi-purpose home visits to educate the community, learn about local health beliefs and practices, and identify those people most responsible for the dissemination of news and new ideas. Health center staff created an innovative gardening program, wherein people were provided with seeds, taught how to grow new varieties of vegetables, and shown how to prepare a variety of nutritious dishes that conformed with local preferences; in addition they created a cooperative seed-buying project and community market. Early clinical work included examining school-children, initiating a general medical clinic, and establishing a maternal and child health program. An important epidemiological project initiated by the center in 1942 and expanded in following years was a house-to-house survey to ascertain the health status of the community. The combination of survey work and action programs led the Karks to develop the concept of community health diagnosis, which includes monitoring a community's health as well as identifying targets for intervention (S. and E. Kark: personal communication; Kark and Kark 1981a).

The Polela Health Center was successful: in 1944 the South African National Health Services Commission issued a report (known as the Gluckman Report, after its Chairman) which recommended that a large number of new health centers throughout South Africa be constructed, organized and administered according to the Polela model. The Chief Health Officer of the Ministry of Health of South Africa predicted that by the end of 1949, 44 Health Centers would be established (Gale 1949: 634).

The Institute of Family and Community Health (IFCH) was created (Sidney Kark, Director) to train staff for the new Health Centers, conduct research through a special research unit, and practice family and community medicine. The Institute included seven Health Centers; the one at Polela was its rural community health center, and six new centers were established by the Institute in and around the city of Durban to serve communities of various incomes and ethnicities.[9] Each of these centers provided primary health care, and served as a source of information for cross-cultural comparative research on such topics as child rearing, infant mortality, and menarche.[10]

Family and community were the foci of the various projects within the ✓ IFCH, and the staff showed a keen interest in social structure, family relationships, poverty, migration, witchcraft, traditional healers, nutrition, and work. At a time when medical anthropology was not yet an organized subdiscipline, the IFCH was training staff to analyze and take account of local belief systems and patterned behavior. The anthropological sophistication of the IFCH physicians can be seen in a transcript of a case conference (Chesler et al. 1962), in which they discussed cultural differences in illness care and management among White, Zulu, and Indian families. The participants in the conference questioned and evaluated the cultural acceptability of their explanations to patients, and they explored the instances in which they endorsed, accepted, or rejected those beliefs of their patients which differed from their own. S. Kark reports that they were assisted in their discussions by Hilda Kuper, a South African anthropologist who had had experience among the Swazi of Swaziland and the Zulus of Durban (S. Kark: personal communication; see also Kuper 1984).

The Karks continued their training in epidemiology and social science: they received Nuffield fellowships enabling them to study at Oxford from

1947—1948. Their time at Oxford was divided between John Ryle's new Institute of Social Medicine[11] and the Institute of Social Anthropology headed by E. E. Evans-Pritchard. They studied epidemiology at Ryle's Institute, and worked with Evans-Pritchard, Meyer Fortes, and Max Gluckman, the primary forgers of British Social Anthropology at that time. The Karks also worked with a group of students who went on to become eminent anthropologists: John Barnes, Clyde Mitchell, Elizabeth Colson, Paul and Laura Bohannan; and Morris Carstairs, a psychiatrist. The Karks analyzed much of their Polela data in Gluckman's methodology seminar and in discussions with Fortes and Evans-Pritchard. In that setting they were able to refine their ideas about a socially oriented epidemiology (S. and E. Kark: personal communication), but changing politics made it difficult to apply these new ideas in South Africa.

The attempt to develop a South African National Health Service was already under siege by the late 1940s. Opposition from the South African Medical Association moved George Gale, the Chief Health Officer of the Ministry of Health and one of the main sponsors of the health center service and the work of the Karks and their colleagues, to state publicly that the health centers "would not be allowed to encroach upon the legitimate rights of private practice" (Gale 1946:330). Three years later, facing increasing criticism that social medicine involved an attempt to *socialize* medicine, Gale had to separate explicitly the operations of the health centers from the concept of social medicine:

In view of the ambiguities, misunderstandings and controversies which have arisen from the use of the term social medicine, it has been decided, by the present Minister of Health himself, to discontinue its use in connection with Government Health Centres. Henceforth, therefore, the term used will be simply 'Health Centre practice'. (Gale 1949: 633)

Conservative politics led the National Health Service movement to fail in South Africa. The South African government of the middle 1940s had questioned the prevailing policy of racial separation, but this government was defeated in the general elections of 1948. The new government then developed its infamous policy of apartheid, and two conservative supporters of apartheid were chosen Prime Minister in the 1950s. Work became increasingly difficult for activists interested in social equality and in social medicine: in 1956 apartheid was used to segregate "White" from "Non-White" blood for transfusions (letters, South African Medical Journal [SAMJ] 30: 1024). Apartheid was applied to the medical profession in 1957, when the Nursing Act prohibited "White" nurses and midwives from being supervised by "Non-Whites" (Stein et al. 1957).

During the 1950s many of the dissenters began to emigrate. The Karks left South Africa in 1958 when Sidney Kark was invited to be Professor and Chair of the Department of Epidemiology at the University of North Carolina at Chapel Hill. The department was to be strengthened under the leadership of Sidney Kark, John Cassel (who had already emigrated from South Africa), John Fulton (a dental epidemiologist), and Ralph Patrick Jr. (an anthropologist). S. Kark had already made a tentative commitment to become a World Health Organization Visiting Professor at the Hebrew University Hadassah Medical School, should the University widen its program in Social Medicine and Public Health (S. Kark: personal communication). When this plan came to fruition in 1959, Kark left for his assignment in Jerusalem, and Cassel was appointed as Chair in the Department of Epidemiology at Chapel Hill.

The Human Resources and Intellectual Legacy of the IFCH

When the government closed the IFCH it signalled the end of the South African experiment in social medicine, but it also ensured that the IFCH staff, ideas, and methods would spread worldwide. Many members of the IFCH team emigrated in the 1950s and early 1960s; a list of their names would read almost like a *Who's Who* of contemporary research and action in social medicine and social epidemiology.

The Karks emigrated to Israel in 1959, and were joined there by other IFCH staff who had been invited to serve in the expanded program at Hebrew University. They began work in what soon evolved into the Department of Social Medicine (later the School of Public Health and Community Medicine) at the Hebrew University-Hadassah Medical School in Jerusalem. The Karks and their colleagues continued to emphasize the need to include the social sciences in medical research. The former IFCH members worked on designing innovative health education programs, investigating the health effects of status inconsistency and social class, using surveys in community medicine, describing lay medical decision-making and client behavior in clinics, evaluating the effectiveness of midwives, and designing community medicine projects to diagnose, treat, and prevent heart disease, hypertension, and diabetes. (See Figure 1 for a list of names and citations.) The Karks' ideas on how to incorporate epidemiology and social science into the delivery of health services to communities are presented in S. Kark's 1974 text *Epidemiology and Community Medicine,* and more recently in his 1981 text *The Practice of Community-Oriented Primary Health Care.* Kark's model of community-oriented primary care has been promoted as a workable goal for medicine in the United States (Mullan 1982).

Other South Africans associated with the IFCH went elsewhere. Some went to Uganda and Kenya where they founded preventive medicine programs similar to those of the IFCH. Others came to the United States to apply their IFCH experiences to work in community health centers and major universities.

The work of the IFCH had also attracted foreign nationals, two of whom were important to the growth of social medicine and social epidemiology in

USA:
U.N.C. Chapel Hill:
  (John Cassel) (see text)
  (Phillips) (1977, 1979)
  (Steuart) (1975)
  (Slome) (1976, 1977)

Duke:
  (Salber) (1975, 1981)

Harvard:
  Harry Phillips (1967)
  Eva Salber
  H. D. Cohn (1975)

UCLA:
  (Hilda Kuper) (1962, 1984)
  Guy Steuart

Israel:
  (Syndey Kark) (see text)
  Emily Kark (see text)
  Guy Steuart (1965)
  J. H. Abramson (1966, 1979, 1982)
  B. Gampel (1967)
  J. Chesler (1962)
  C. Slome

IFCH
&
POLELA

East Africa:
  G. Gale (1949)
  J. W. Bennett (1965, 1973, Matovu et al. 1971)

Note: Parentheses indicate the most recent affiliations of those who worked at more than one institution after the IFCH. Dates in parentheses are references.

Fig. 1.   The Intellectual Legacy of the IFCH. (A partial list of staff affiliations and representative references.)

the United States. Anthropologist Norman Scotch spent 18 months at the IFCH doing post-doctoral research on Zulu hypertension (e.g. Scotch 1960, 1963b), and now directs the School of Public Health at Boston University. Jack Geiger did a clerkship at the IFCH when he was a medical student at Case Western, and later published on the social factors in arthritis and in hypertension (Scotch and Geiger 1962, 1963). In the United States he became influential in the social medicine and community health center movements (e.g. Geiger 1971 — Geiger clearly acknowledged his indebtedness to S. Kark and his colleagues; 1984: 17).

The ideas and methods initiated at Polela and the IFCH thus spread throughout the world, and helped spawn similar projects in other areas. The themes of this research movement in part resembled those of 19th century social medicine: health was seen as a social concern; social and economic conditions were shown to have an important effect on health and disease; and both individual and social (group) interventions were seen as necessary to promote health and prevent disease (Rosen 1947: 678—683). However, the work of Polela and the IFCH added to these principles the realization that epidemiologic and social science methods could be used to understand the extent of community health problems, to direct the focus of curative and preventive measures, and to evaluate the effectiveness of these measures. Perhaps most important from an anthropological point of view, the IFCH experience taught its staff the importance of gaining cultural understanding

(Kark and Kark 1962), as I will explain in the following discussion of John Cassel's work. This emphasis can be seen clearly in many of the projects and publications that resulted after the project halted and its staff scattered throughout the world.

The next section will explore one of the research programs that grew out of Polela and the IFCH: the work of John Cassel and his colleagues at the University of North Carolina, Chapel Hill. Several of the research efforts mentioned above also deserve extended treatment, but Cassel's work is the most important contribution to social epidemiology.

III. STUDYING SOCIAL CHANGE AND ADAPTATION: THE WORK OF JOHN CASSEL (1921–1976)

John Cassel was born in South Africa to an upper-middle class household (his mother was a physician, and his father a dentist). He studied medicine at the University of the Witwatersrand, and on entering the South African Health Center Service was sent with his wife Margaret, a nurse, to the IFCH for training. In 1948 Cassel was selected by S. Kark to join the Polela Health Center. J. Cassel was a physician at Polela for four years, and M. Cassel served as a nurse.

The importance of the Polela experience to Cassel's later work cannot be overestimated. His close contact with the health problems of the Polela community, and the fact that his own attempts at curative and preventive care were sometimes hampered by competition from traditional medical beliefs and practices, helped him to develop an interest in the social and cultural components of health. This interest is most clearly stated in anthropological terms in his chapter (in Kark and Steuart 1962) entitled 'Cultural Factors in the Interpretation of Illness: A Case Study' (Cassell 1962). Cassel presented this case study "as an illustration of the insight provided by knowledge of the cultural patterning and social situation into behavior which would otherwise appear as a series of inexplicable unrelated acts" (1962: 238). He described how two related kin groups in Polela managed cases of pulmonary tuberculosis, cervical cancer, and persistent headaches, and showed how knowledge of a series of related witchcraft accusations helped explain the management strategies chosen by these groups, and by a missionary who also became involved in the case.

A more general description and analysis of the importance of cultural understanding in the Polela project was given in Cassel's lead chapter in Paul's classic 1955 text *Health, Culture and Community*. There Cassel analyzed the different levels of Zulu resistance to the Polela staff's curative and preventive efforts. Attempts by the staff to change attitudes toward food; to increase production and consumption of vegetables, eggs, and milk; to treat pulmonary tuberculosis; or to combat soil erosion — each met higher levels of resistance. The male labor out-migration created by South African labor regulations brought syphilis and tuberculosis into the community, and made long-term treatment of working-age males problematic. Local unemployment and population pressure, combined with traditional food preferences and land use patterns better adapted to another time and place, helped make soil erosion a serious problem and malnutrition a common diagnosis (Cassel 1955: 35; Kark and Cassel 1952: 136; Kark 1944: 41). Understanding which cultural patterns were easiest to modify allowed the workers at Polela to target their efforts toward reasonable goals; knowing who held power in the community allowed them to focus their actions on the most significant potential change-agents in the community. Important health improvements were seen throughout the course of the project, especially in infant mortality, incidence of infectious diseases, and prevalence of malnutrition.

Cassel left South Africa in 1952 on a Rockefeller Foundation fellowship to study public health at the University of North Carolina at Chapel Hill. He joined the School of Public Health there in 1954, and became Chair of the Department of Epidemiology in 1959. The University of North Carolina soon developed a strong joint faculty in the social sciences and epidemiology. The anthropologist Ralph Patrick was hired in the epidemiology department in 1958, and the psychologist C. David Jenkins in 1959. The sociologist and anthropologist Berton Kaplan joined the School of Public Health in 1962, and the epidemiology department in 1967. The medical sociologist Robert N. Wilson joined the Chapel Hill epidemiology department in 1963, and held a joint appointment in sociology. From 1966 to 1972 Wilson chaired the Department of Mental Health in the School of Public Health.

Research from Chapel Hill

At Chapel Hill Cassel further developed the ideas from his Polela experience. In Polela, social and behavioral factors had had a clear impact on health. In North Carolina, Cassel confronted a largely agricultural state in the process of developing a post-war industrial base. The impact of society and culture on health was not as dramatic or life-threatening in North Carolina as it was in Polela. Nonetheless, the series of studies undertaken by Cassel in North Carolina would eventually show the equally significant health effects of such diffuse social processes as social and cultural change and adaptation.[12]

Although psychological studies are not a focus of this paper, it is important to note that similar work on the specifically *mental* health effects of social and cultural disorganization were taking place concurrently under the leadership of Alexander and Dorothea Leighton at Cornell and Harvard. (D. Leighton subsequently taught at UNC Chapel Hill.) The Leightons' work on mental illness and that on physical illness at Chapel Hill took place at a time when anthropologists were growing interested in the concepts of acculturation (Beals 1953) and culture change (Lange 1965). However, while theories about the nature and effects of social and cultural change became increasingly important in social epidemiology (Cassel 1964), the applied epidemiological studies that explored the health consequences of such change had little impact on further theorizing in anthropology.

Many of the ideas that would guide Cassel's research for the next decade were expressed in a 1960 paper he co-authored with Ralph Patrick and C. David Jenkins, where they began to develop a conceptual framework for analyzing the social and cultural processes relevant to health. This paper was one of the first social epidemiological papers to separate explicity the social system from the cultural system. Acknowledging the work of the anthropologist Clifford Geertz, the authors stated that culture refers to "the fabric of meaning in terms of which people interpret their experience and guide their action", while the term social structure (which they equate with society) refers to "the way that group life is ordered, the persistent and regular social relationships of people" (1960: 945). These distinctions were not made in detail, but Cassel et al. employed them in order to differentiate between the appropriateness of cultural norms, and three different forms of social organization within which norms applied: occupation, family, and social class. Specific hypotheses were to be tested within each of these three arenas. Thus this paper showed the growing theoretical sophistication of researchers in social epidemiology — with the increasing general acceptance of the etiological importance of the social and cultural environment, it became more important to develop theoretical models which could account for the obvious (and alarming) complexity of this environment.

In the 1960 paper Cassel et al. proposed an epidemiological study of the changes in health status that might accompany changes from a rural agricultural to an industrial way of life. This study, designed to take place in a manufacturing plant in a small Appalachian town, was to compare three groups of people: agricultural workers, first generation factory employees, and second and third generation factory employees. Cassel et al. hypothesized, first, that the first generation workers, those experiencing the greatest cultural change, would have poorer health status than the other groups; and second, that less family solidarity and greater incongruity between cultural background and current social situation would be most closely associated with poor health and adjustment.

The results of this 1960 proposal were published in 1961 (Cassel and Tyroler 1961) and confirmed many of the hypotheses from the 1960 paper. Using measures of general morbidity and of absenteeism due to illness, Cassel and Tyroler showed that the health status of factory workers who were the first to move into the industrial area was lower than the health status of factory workers whose relatives had already been employed in the factory.

Further tests of the 1960 hypotheses came in 1964 and 1971. In 1964 Tyroler and Cassel described the effects of urbanization on coronary heart disease mortality, by comparing urbanizing rural residents with urban residents. In 1971, Neser, Tyroler, and Cassel estimated at the county level the extent of social disorganization in the black population in North Carolina, and compared these estimates with rates of stroke mortality. They found a consistent increase in mortality associated with increased levels of social disorganization in each of four age groups. These gradients did not change significantly when they were stratified according to economic level, access to medical care, or geographic features such as water or soil type.

Cassel's research interests ranged widely (see the annotated bibliography of his selected works done by members of the Chapel Hill Epidemiology Department, Ibrahim et al. 1980). He had a strong interest in health services research (e.g. Hulka et al. 1972), and participated in the famous Evans County Heart Study,[13] which examined social and clinical risk factors for heart disease. His conceptualization of the effects of the social environment on host resistance (1976) is his classic work; the paper had been cited more than 400 times within 7 years of publication (Syme 1983). Less well known were two projects with strong anthropological components: a project on the Polynesian island of Ponape, studying the health effects of culture change (see Patrick and Tyroler 1974); and a project for the Peace Corps in Malawi, training and supervising Peace Corps Volunteers in tuberculosis control (McKay: personal communication).

Other anthropologically-oriented projects occurred at North Carolina. Berton Kaplan, who joined the Epidemiology Department in 1967, had done a dissertation in Sociology at Chapel Hill in 1962 (published 1971) which used participant observation techniques. Kaplan focused on the health consequences of culture change in an urbanizing mountain community in Western North Carolina. Kaplan has held a joint appointment in the Anthropology Department at Chapel Hill since 1966; from 1966—1967 he directed the Medical Anthropology Program.[14]

Robert Wilson, a member of the Sociology Department, also collaborated with the epidemiologists at Chapel Hill. The second part of his book on Medical Sociology (Wilson 1970) contains four chapters on social epidemiology. In addition, he co-edited two books on social psychiatry (Leighton et al. 1957; Kaplan et al. 1976). Herman A. Tyroler, hired by Cassel in the early 1960s, also played (and continues to play) a strong part in the Chapel Hill investigations. He initiated the 1962 study on social change and health consequences, and also later collaborated with Ralph Patrick in presenting data from the Ponape study (Patrick and Tyroler 1974).

Arthur Rubel was a graduate student at Chapel Hill who was strongly influenced by the epidemiology taught there. Rubel's Ph.D. was in anthropology, but he minored in epidemiology, and reports that his training in epidemiology there was his most significant exposure to the scientific method (Rubel: personal communication). Rubel's paper 'The Epidemiology of a Folk-Illness' (1964) represents an early attempt to apply the analytic categories of epidemiology to anthropological research on a folk illness called *susto*. His work on *susto* has continued, and he has refined his use of epidemiologic methods (see Collado et al. 1983; Rubel et al. 1984).

In the early 1970s members of the Chapel Hill epidemiology department began to publish on the protective health effects of social support. Epidemiological work since the 1930s had returned to the study of the host, but Cassel's work helped to demonstrate the importance of host susceptibility and resistance. Social support has since become a popular focus for studies in social epidemiology, but its anthropological origins have largely been forgotten. Some authors have been careful to distinguish between social networks and social support (e.g. Berkman and Syme 1979), and to acknowledge the influence of anthropological theories and research. The primary theoretical groundwork for recent studies in social networks was laid in the 1950s and 1960s by such authors as Barnes (1954), Young and Willmott (1957), Bott (1957), and Mitchell (1969). At Chapel Hill, Nuckolls et al. (1972) did early work on the health effects of social support, using pregnancy prognosis as the outcome variable. Kaplan et al. (1977) wrote one of the first major review papers on the topic. The members of the Chapel Hill epidemiology department have published an exhaustive review of the social support literature (Broadhead et al. 1983).

The work of Cassel and his colleagues at Chapel Hill has had a profound impact on social epidemiology. If the South African work is broadly typified as concerned with how to provide health care to communities, the Chapel Hill work might be typified as being concerned with developing epidemiological strategies to measure the health effects of social and cultural change. The new social medicine practiced in South Africa had its roots firmly (and knowingly) planted in a 19th century sociological epidemiology; the Chapel Hill research on the effects of social and cultural change had an unacknowledged affinity with this same 19th century work. For example, the previous chapter notes Virchow's 19th century thesis that epidemic diseases were markers of cultural change. While considering the contemporary epidemics of the industrial world — cancer, heart disease, stroke, other chronic diseases, accidents — a repetition of Virchow's words gives them an added significance: "The history of artificial epidemics is therefore the history of disturbances which the culture of mankind has experienced. Its changes show us with powerful strokes the turning points at which culture moves off in new directions" (quoted in Rosen 1947: 681).

IV. ANTHROPOLOGY AND EPIDEMIOLOGY: OTHER MODERN THEMES

Collaborative work in the 20th century between anthropology and epidemiology was not confined to the IFCH and Chapel Hill; these were chosen for more detailed treatment because they trained many of the important figures in modern social epidemiology, and because they had a strong anthropological component in their theories and methods. But at least two later U.S. experiments in providing health care duplicated many aspects of the IFCH: the Navajo-Cornell Field Health Research Project (known as the Navajo-Many Farms Project) in Arizona from 1955 to 1962 (see Adair and Deuschle 1970); and the Tufts-Delta Health Center in Mound Bayou, Mississippi from 1965 to the present (see e.g. Geiger 1971, 1984). Like the IFCH, each of these was designed to deliver health care to rural populations, and each developed innovative methods that combined the social sciences with medicine and epidemiology.

Many projects duplicated or challenged the etiologic conclusions of the researchers at the University of North Carolina: a broader review of U.S. social epidemiology from 1950 to 1970 would include the work on stressful life events by Holmes, Rahe, and Masuda at the University of Washington, and by the Dohrenwends at Columbia; work on social stress by Hinkle and Wolff at Cornell and by Levine and Scotch at Boston University; work on social networks, social mobility, and acculturation by Berkman, Marmot, and Syme at the University of California Berkeley; and work on social class by Hollingshead and social support by Kasl at Yale. These are just a few of the many U.S. research centers doing work in social epidemology today, but their researchers have backgrounds in sociology rather than in anthropology.

Collaborative projects between anthropologists and epidemiologists began to proliferate in the late 1950s. This was a time of redefinition in epidemiology, manifested in an article by Milton Terris (1962) in the American Journal of Public Health, and an accompanying editorial by Anthony Payne.[15] Terris argued that the field of epidemiology was "returning in large measure to the physicochemical and sociological orientation of the first half of the 19th century, but on a much sounder scientific basis than was possible at that time" (1962: 1375).

A number of epidemiology textbooks in the late 1950s defined the field as applying to any and all diseases, infectious or chronic, and also stated the importance of the social environment as a factor in disease etiology (MacMahon, Pugh, and Ipsen 1960; Morris 1957; J. Paul 1958; Reid 1960; Taylor and Knoweldon 1957). In a separate but complementary literature, several authors discussed the potential contribution of the social sciences to public health and medicine (e.g. Anderson 1969; Foster 1961; Hasan and Prasad 1960; Jaco 1958; Rubin 1960; Suchman 1963; Susser 1964; Susser and Watson 1962; Vijil 1959; and Wardwell and Bahnson 1964). Early literature reviews in the developing field of medical anthropology also started to discuss epidemiology at about this time (see especially Caudill 1953: 789; Polgar 1962: 162—64; and Scotch 1963a: 41—47).

In 1958 A. Fleck, then a County Commissioner of Health in New York State, and F. Ianni, an anthropologist, wrote a paper entitled 'Epidemiology and Anthropology: Some Suggested Affinities in Theory and Method'. This paper was the first to state explicitly that the disciplines of anthropology and epidemiology had important parallels. Published in a journal of applied anthropology, the paper provoked little comment by epidemiologists (Fleck: personal communication; Ianni: personal communication). It emphasized the social aspects of the research by Panum, Snow, and other 19th century epidemiologists, and also discussed some of the difficulties of modern-day collaboration between anthropologists and epidemiologists. One primary difficulty cited by Fleck and Ianni was that anthropologists working in applied sociomedical research were commonly included only as consultants: they had little control over the nature of the questions being asked and learned little about epidemiology. Another problem they cited was that epidemiologists historically had been too concerned with disease agents: Fleck and Ianni had high hopes for what they called an emerging "neo-ecological approach" in epidemiology, which placed greater emphasis on multiple causality and on the importance of the environment. They made the provocative remark that "The epidemiologist must be and is a social anthropologist with his particular interest being nosology" (1958: 39, nosology is the science of disease classification). An example of the kind of research envisioned by these authors was just beginning in Chapel Hill under the guidance of John Cassel.

Another important collaboration between an epidemiologist and an anthropologist began in the late 1950s at the University of Manchester, where Mervyn Susser (epidemiologist) and Walter Watson (social anthropologist) co-authored a pioneering 1962 text entitled *Sociology in Medicine*.[16] This text, revised in 1972 and 1985, provides one of the first and most comprehensive surveys of concepts and literature in the social sciences and epidemiology. Manchester also saw the development of an emerging school of medical anthropology in the United Kingdom, through the work of medically oriented social scientists such as Derek Allcorn and Ronald Frankenburg, and socially oriented physicians such as Joyce Leeson.[17] The Social Medicine Unit of the Medical Research Council also sponsored work by epidemiologists and social scientists, for example Jeremy Morris worked there with social scientists such as Allcorn and E. M. Goldberg; and physicians such as R. F. L. Logan and J. B. Loudon.[18] Thus social epidemiology also was evolving in England, particularly under the guidance of Morris (1959; 1979; Morris et al. 1966), but the field there involved sociologists far more commonly than it did anthropologists (J. Morris: personal communication, Firth 1978).

Why did this dramatic increase in interdisciplinary exchange happen in the 1950s and early 1960s? At least six reasons can be given: the growing numbers of international studies in epidemology; increasing migration and pace of change of human populations; growing epidemiological and anthropological interest in studies of migrant groups; a resurgence of interest in human behavior as an important etiological variable; uncertainty as to why effective preventive or curative treatments were not being used by more people; and the creation of private and public sources of research funds that both created and responded to these various projects.

(1) *International Studies*. Anthropology became more relevant to epidemiology in the late 1950s and 1960s, when many epidemiological studies were being done overseas to get comparative information on disease distributions and etiology. Conditions such as hypertension, obesity, atherosclerosis, diabetes, and cancer appeared to have different epidemiological profiles in different world regions (Doll 1980; Gear 1959; Haenszel and Correa 1975; Keys and Anderson 1955; Mann et al. 1964; Reid 1975). Studies were designed to assess the respective contributions of social and genetic inheritance to these diseases in different parts of the world. Adequate theories and measures of effects of the social environment had to be developed for these culture specific studies. The work by Norman Scotch (1960, 1963b) on Zulu hypertension has already seen mentioned — it was done at the IFCH in South Africa — but it deserves mention again at this point as a pioneer of these measures and theories.

(2) *Social Change*. The growth in studies of social change and acculturation that occurred in North American anthropology from the 1930s through the 1960s made the field more accessible and useful to epidemiologists. Beginning with the Social Science Research Council's formation of a Committee on Acculturation in 1935 (see Redfield, Linton and Herskovits 1936), anthropologists in the United States embarked on more than three decades of debate and redefinition about the concept of acculturation. Social anthropological research on acculturation gradually fell out of favor after the mid-1960s (though it continued in psychological anthropology); social anthropologists like Robert Murphy at Columbia declared that acculturation studies had mistakenly singled out acculturation as a special class, when it was really a necessary aspect of social structure (Murphy 1964).

Many epidemiological uses of social science concepts were not subsequently critiqued by social scientists, and were not viewed by social scientists as empirical tests of their hypotheses. It would be provocative to consider, for example, what new questions and theories might have been developed had the North Carolina research results been discussed by the critics of the acculturation literature.

(3) *Migrant Groups*. Researchers interested in the health effects of social and cultural change conducted studies of migrant groups in an attempt to capitalize on "natural experiments" (much like Snow or Durkheim) in which the influence of genetic and social factors on disease could be separated (e.g. Beaglehole et al. 1977; Cassel 1974; and the collected papers in Lewitter 1980). In the 1960s various anthropologists became consultants and designers of these migrant studies: the Ponape project with Ralph Patrick has already been mentioned; it also involved J. Fischer, who had co-authored

the 1961 paper on *kuru*. Anthropologists such as Margaret Clark helped develop an acculturation scale in a study of the effects of acculturation on coronary heart disease among Japanese migrants (Marmot and Syme 1976). The anthropologist Paul Baker and his colleagues began a large project documenting health changes among Samoan migrants to Hawaii and California (McGarvey and Baker 1979; see also Janes, this volume).

(4) *Behavior and Etiology.* The expansion of epidemiology into international comparisons was not the only reason — or forum — for the growing involvement of anthropology. To understand how diseases are transmitted one needs to know how hosts come into contact with agents, but the "diseases of development" provide few obvious agents. Smoking, drinking, eating, and other behaviors appeared to have significant etiological importance, but appeared to be part of a complex web of interacting causal factors. As behaviorally complex diseases of development became more prevalent, it became more important for anthropologists and epidemiologists to study human behavior as an etiological variable. It was necessary to go beyond the conventional disciplinary boundaries of epidemiology in order to conceptualize and measure these factors adequately. A significant example of such behavioral research on heart disease etiology and control is the volume edited by Syme and Reeder (1967).

(5) *Modifying Behavior.* Yet another factor drawing anthropologists and other social scientists into epidemiological research was the seemingly refractory nature of human behavior. It was difficult enough to establish that behavioral factors played causal roles in the etiology of chronic noninfectious diseases, but to intervene on such behaviors was even more problematic. Social scientists had clear expertise in evaluating and designing effective interventions, as well as in exploring the effects of the social environment on health. For example, anthropologists such as Francis Ianni and Ralph Patrick, Jr. participated in separate evaluations of polio vaccine acceptance in New York and in Florida (Ianni et al. 1960; Johnson et al. 1962). Many social scientists contributed to a volume on community resistance to fluoridation edited by Benjamin Paul and others (Paul 1961; Paul et al. 1961).

(6) *Funding Sources.* The increasing availability of private and federal funding was a critical stimulus fostering the growing involvement of the social sciences in epidemiology in the 1950s and 1960s. The work at Polela and at the Institute of Family and Community Health in the late 1940s and 1950s had been funded partly by the Rockefeller Foundation through the efforts of John Grant, and much of the early work at Hebrew University was funded by the World Health Organization (Kart and Steuart 1962: v–vi). Benjamin Paul's Social Science Program at the Harvard School of Public Health was initiated and funded largely by the Russell Sage Foundation (B. Paul: personal communication). The National Institutes of Health started a Human

Ecology Study Section in 1960, which provided much of the funding for
domestic research projects in social epidemiology (S. L. Syme: personal
communication).

These are just a few reasons why collaboration between the social sciences
and epidemiology increased during the 1950s and 1960s. Other technological, theoretical, and administrative categories that were mentioned as
being important in the development of 19th century epidemiology also apply
to events in the 20th: that is, the development of new statistical procedures
(for example, path analysis and multiple regression techniques) made analyses of multivariate relationships more feasible, and in conjunction with
general access to high-speed computers allowed researchers to examine
various models of multicausal relationships. (Mervyn Susser recently has
written a review of the historical evolution of epidemiologic methods
[1985b].) New administrative procedures for tracing study participants, and
developing and funding large scale cohort studies (for example: Framingham,
Massachusetts; Tecumseh, Michigan; Evans County, Georgia; Hagerstown,
Maryland) also increased the volume of research done and the complexity of
the models developed. Finally, much as the move from generalized to
localized pathology allowed 19th century researchers to conceptualize illness
in different terms, so also did the growing 20th century interest in ecology
help to motivate new studies in the social environment.

Epidemiology, Medical Ecology, and the Social Environment

In the 1950s some epidemiologists became interested in medical ecology, an
analytical perspective that focuses on "the study of the populations of man
with special reference to environment and to populations of all other
organisms as they affect his health and his numbers" (Audy 1958: 102). This
interest was evident as early as 1936 (Dudley 1936), but it began to grow
rapidly both during and after World War II. Here the field of *geographical
epidemiology* (discussed in the previous chapter) again became important: in
their new incarnation as medical geographers, the practitioners of geographical epidemiology played important roles during World War II, when important battles were fought against tropical diseases in South East Asia (e.g., the
work of Ralph Audy [1968] on scrub typhus).

The definitional line between medical geography and medical ecology is
vague; Jacques May, a well-known medical geographer, has proposed that
medical geography be replaced with the words "human ecology of health and
disease" (May 1978 [1952]: 212). Medical geography emphasizes the spatial
aspects of disease distribution, while medical ecology stresses the organizational aspects of disease distribution. In contrast to a medical geographer's
questions about place and time, a medical ecologist might investigate the
manifestations of a disease at different ecological levels — at organismic,

individual, community, or population levels — and might consider the interactions among these levels (see Brody and Sobel 1979).

One of the most significant results of the exchanges among medical ecology, medical geography, and epidemiology in the 1950s was that researchers were given further theoretical justifications for including the social environment in the study of the distribution and determinants of diseases. John Gordon wrote in 1949 that "the part exerted by the socio-economic environment is probably the most neglected of any epidemiological influence." In 1958 Gordon wrote that "The notable addition to the content of epidemiology under the influence of ecology is in relation to the social environment" (1958:351). In a 1960 text entitled *Human Ecology and Health*, Edward Rogers, a Professor of Public Health at the University of California at Berkeley, wrote in a similar vein:

Public health has always been concerned with man and his environment and, in this sense, oriented toward human ecology — though in a somewhat limited fashion at first. Today, however, the significance and the meaning of the term *environment* have acquired new proportions. ... Environment in this sense includes, of course, not only the material and spatial aspects of man's world but the nonmaterial web of human social relations called culture which profoundly influences man's state.[19] (1960: vii, emphasis in the original)

In 1965, the Geographic Epidemiology Unit at the Johns Hopkins School of Hygiene and Public Health embarked on an ambitious international comparative research project, designed to study the ecology of disease in five developing countries. The project team drew its members from the disciplines of epidemiology, social anthropology, entomology, sanitary engineering, public health nursing, and laboratory science. Studies from three countries were eventually published: Peru (Buck et al. 1968), Chad (Buck et al. 1970), and Afghanistan (Buck et al. 1972). The role of the social anthropologist in these studies was to collect contextual socioeconomic and cultural data, and to facilitate the acceptance of the project within each study area. An interview schedule was designed which could be used cross-culturally, and was translated into the respective national languages. Key informants were interviewed in order to obtain information about the different villages and cultures.[20]

This project illustrates the use of anthropology to aid in entry into the field, and to incorporate information on the socio-cultural environment into an ecologically-minded research effort. Despite mention of the type and schedule of agricultural work, recency of settlement, frequency of out-migration and in-migration, and rapidity of social change, few systematic attempts are made in these three works to correlate the socio-cultural environment with the descriptive epidemiology of tropical disease. The social and cultural information serves as context, but the purpose of the research effort was descriptive rather than analytic.[21]

Research at Harvard University also helped to promulgate an involvement of the social sciences in epidemiology. John Gordon was writing there on epidemiology as medical ecology, and was forcefully presenting a case for including the social sciences in epidemiological research (Gordon 1952; 1953; 1958; 1966; Gordon et al. 1952). The anthropologist Benjamin Paul headed the Social Science Program at the Harvard School of Public Health from 1951—1962 (see Paul 1963), and trained students in an anthropological approach to public health. Ralph Patrick, Norman Scotch, Jack Geiger, Frederick Dunn, Steven Polgar, and Edward Wellin were just a few of the people influenced by Paul at Harvard. Paul's text *Health, Culture and Community* (1955) was used as a training manual both at Harvard and elsewhere in the world, and it taught thousands of students that socio-cultural factors were important components of public health programs.

This section has concentrated on centers in the United States where specifically anthropological collaborations took place with epidemiology. A complete review of U.S. social epidemiology from 1950 to 1970 would examine the growth and development of human population laboratories (Kessler and Levin 1970), and work on topics such as stressful live events, social support, social stress, social discontinuities, and social factors in the etiologies of hypertension, cancer, psychiatric illness, and coronary heart disease.

V. SUMMARY AND CONCLUSIONS

Nineteenth century research into the social aspects of disease causation covered three broad areas: the development of the concepts of the *host* and the *social environment* in sociological epidemiology, and the accompanying emphasis on the *social origins of disease* and the need for *social treatments* as developed in social medicine; the refinement of categories of *place* and *time* in geographical/historical epidemiology; and the use of *field surveys* and *qualitative observations* in biological/parasitological epidemiology.

These 19th century areas were also addressed in 20th century research: put broadly, the work we discussed from Polela and the IFCH used the terms of social medicine; that from Chapel Hill concentrated on sociological epidemiology; and that from Johns Hopkins concentrated on geographical epidemiology. Distinct conceptions of culture and society were employed in each of these cases, as were distinct conceptions of the proper role of the social sciences in epidemiological research.

At the IFCH in the South Africa of the 1940s and 1950s, as at Navajo-Many Farms in the United States of the 1950s and 1960s, and at Mound Bayou in the 1960s and 1970s, research was centered on the provision of care: etiologic investigations focused on those factors that might be readily influenced by the staff of the health unit. What these three projects had in common was that each was designed to provide services to disenfranchised populations; populations whose health profiles and incomes were below average, and whose health beliefs and practices differed from those of the groups in power. It is ironic that these experiments in social medicine, and in the employment of social science in medicine — both marginal activities in the United States and South Africa — were given chances to prove themselves only on marginalized populations. It is not merely ironic, but tragic, that these programs were successful but were nonetheless targeted for extinction or for crippling budget cuts.

The work at Chapel Hill provides an example of research centered on etiology, and more theoretically on the means by which the concepts and methods of the social sciences might be used in epidemiological research. The Chapel Hill group attempted to develop theoretical models that were anthropologically and sociologically sophisticated, capable of being tested with epidemiological methods, and also capable of being applied in public health practice. This approach can be contrasted with research efforts in which anthropologists were hired to specialize in the behavioral parts of epidemiologic surveys, such as work at the Geographical Epidemiology Unit at John Hopkins, where social research provided social context to epidemiological descriptions, and facilitated the research process itself.

Despite the appearance of a dynamic and lively history of collaborative efforts between anthropology and epidemiology, every successful collaboration between these fields actually represents many missed opportunities. In fact, contrary to the spirit of the collaborative efforts presented here, ideas like the following are still commonly seen in the mainstream literature of these disciplines:

(1) Science consists only of quantitative observations.

— (From an epidemiology text) "However full of insight an investigator's considerings may be, they are unlikely, if not supported by observations objectively recorded in quantitative terms, to form a basis for the considerings of successive generations of investigators" (MacMahon and Pugh 1970:6).

(2) Social science does not produce such observations.

— (From a historical review of epidemiology) "Exploitation of the relationship between social and biological factors is inhibited as much as anything by the failure of the social sciences to provide data comparable to those of the biological sciences, data susceptible to statistical analysis" (Gordon 1952:126).

(3) Anthropology is as much art as science, and *should not* produce quantifiable observations.

— (From an eminent reviewer of British social anthropology) "The implication of my present essay is quite the reverse; the data which derive from fieldwork are subjective and not objective. I am saying that every anthropological observer, no matter how well he/she has been trained, will see something that no other such observer can recognize, namely a kind of harmonic projection of the observer's own personality. And when these observations are 'written up' in monograph or any other form, the observer's personality will again distort any purported 'objectivity'.

   So what should be done? Nothing. Anthropological texts are interesting in themselves and not because they tell us something about the external world" (Leach 1984: 22).

   If one accepts these polarized statements as fair descriptions of main-stream disciplinary attitudes then there is little room for interdisciplinary cooperation. But to be fair, the history of anthropology and epidemiology is neither one of antagonism nor one of close cooperation. As I have said, it is rather a history of benign neglect. By emphasizing collaborations and theoretical connections I have not painted a false portrait, but rather an overly-flattering one. The most common style of interdisciplinary research in the near future will continue to consist of individual investigators reaching beyond their respective disciplines to borrow concepts and methods. More programmed collaboration between anthropologists and epidemiologists awaits greater knowledge of past collaborative successes, greater sensitivity to the potential contributions of other disciplines, and greater understanding and tolerance of the respective merits of qualitative and quantitative research methods.

   On what topics might future collaborators focus? Many of the projects and themes discussed in this chapter illustrate areas that would be improved by continued collaborative work. For example, anthropologists can contribute to the design and maintenance of epidemiologic surveillance procedures. They can assist in producing valid and reliable data by helping to phrase interview questions using native terms and concepts, and by raising questions about potential interviewer effects and informant recall biases. They can collaborate in designing epidemiologic studies by employing their knowledge of cross-cultural variability to help conceptualize variables. Given the increasing contemporary interest in host-related factors in disease etiology, anthropologists can contribute to more complex and robust theories of the health-related effects of social networks, social class, social disorganization, and other variables employed in modern epidemiologic studies. Finally, they can suggest resolutions to the potentially conflicting goals of cross-cultural generalizability and culture-specific applicability of research findings.

   Epidemiologists can contribute to anthropology by serving as consultants and critics of study designs and analytic techniques, by clarifying the relation-ships between independent social and behavioral variables and postulated outcomes, and by providing anthropologists with statistically defensible sampling strategies and study designs which can empirically test various theories of the health effects of social and cultural variables.

   We have seen that anthropologists and epidemiologists have studied behavioral factors in disease causation as well as specific adaptations to prevalent diseases, shared research hypotheses and theories, and collabo-rated to complete cross-cultural field projects. Continuing interdisciplinary cooperation will transform benign neglect into a more active and general collaboration.

ACKNOWLEDGEMENTS

This paper could not have been written without help from many sources. I am particularly indebted to the following persons who so kindly (and copiously) responded to my requests for information: Aaron Antonovsky, Frederick Dunn, John Fischer, Andrew Fleck Jr., William Foege, Francis Ianni, Berton Kaplan, Emily and Sidney Kark, Solomon Katz, Kazuyoshi Kawata, Shirley Lindenbaum, David McKay, Jeremy Morris, Benjamin Paul, Eric Peritz, Harry Phillips, Arthur Rubel, Eva Salber, Norman Scotch, Harvey Smith, Zena Stein, Guy Steuart, Howard Stoudt, Robert Straus, Mervyn Susser, S. Leonard Syme, Anthony Wallace, Walter Wardwell, and Robert Wilson. My thanks also to the following for comments on earlier drafts of this paper: Frederick Dunn, Sydney Kark, Lynn Morgan, Zena Stein, Mervyn Susser, S. Leonard Syme, Robert Wilson, Frank Zimmerman, the editors, and an anonymous reviewer.

I gratefully acknowledge the financial support received from the following sources: NIMH research fellowship number F31 MH09039, the Wenner-Gren Foundation for Anthropological Research, the Rennie Endowment at the University of California, Berkeley, and the Schepp Foundation.

Portions of this paper were presented at the 1985 Annual Meeting of the American Anthropological Association in Washington, D.C.

NOTES

1. I shall use the general term "social epidemiology" in this account, and avoid using a number of other specific modifiers. Sociocultural, behavioral, psychosocial, and cultural epidemiology have all been proposed as general terms in the literature I review, but so far have added little clarification. The important distinction here is between an epidemiology with a distinct interest in social and cultural factors, and an epidemiology without such an interest.

2. Anthropology's focus on culture is sometimes distinguished from sociology's focus on social interaction or social structure. The latter refers to the institutionally defined, persistent ordering of human relationships. The boundary between these two disciplines is sometimes arbitrary, especially since today they share many concepts and methods. In the past anthropologists worked on a relatively small scale, studying tribes, villages, or at largest, political units like counties or townships. Sociologists worked on a larger scale, studying aggregate national-level phenomena, or studying particular roles or institutions. In keeping with the scale of their respective studies, anthropologists have tended to collect data through participating in the daily life of their chosen field site for extended periods of time (called "participant observation"), and to use qualitative descriptive techniques (labelled "*ethnographic*") that emphasize detail and range of behavior. Sociologists have used survey techniques that require quantitative analysis and emphasize modal behavior. Anthropological comparisons are commonly cross-cultural in scope; the

field of *ethnology* consists of such comparisons of different cultural practices and social structures. On the other hand, sociological comparisons are commonly intra-cultural.

By now much of this has changed: the difference between anthropology and sociology today lies in literature and employment as much as in method. Separate journals and academic departments help maintain operational differences between anthropology and sociology, although the substantive theoretical differences are not always large. Some sociologists (e.g., Charles Bosk, Erving Goffman, Anselm Strauss) have done work that is frequently indistinguishable from anthropology. Some British anthropologists state that they study social structure, while sociologists study social relations, or state that anthropology is a kind of 'comparative sociology' (Radcliffe-Brown 1952). Others state that social anthropology is itself a branch of sociology (Mair 1972). These divisions, their antecedents, and their consequences are detailed in Harris 1968; Murphy 1976; and Ortner 1984.

3. Social factors will be defined in this paper as aspects of the enduring, institutionally-defined ordering of human relationships. These factors include descriptive categories such as class, education, age, and occupation, as well as more abstract conceptual categories such as acculturation, social networks, social disorganization, and status inconsistency. Behavioral factors will be defined as physical actions that have some effect upon the environment. I will use the term behavioral factors here to describe physical actions such as preparing food, smoking, drinking, exercising, or contacting water or soil. The content of behavior is itself largely culturally and socially determined.

4. Ernest Hooton, in his study of the Pecos Pueblo (1930), began an era of epidemiological categorizations of disease in the field of paleopathology (see Ubelaker 1982). Al Damon, a physical anthropologist in the epidemiology department at Harvard, produced many thoughtful analyses of the categories of race, sex, and ethnic group as used in physical anthropology and in epidemiology (see, e.g., Damon 1964; 1969). He also collaborated with H. W. Stoudt on a series of anthropometric measures (see Stoudt et al. 1960). Stoudt's experience later resulted in an article on the reliability of specific epidemiologic measures of obesity (Seltzer et al. 1970).

5. Work in mental illness has involved anthropological techniques at least since Emil Kraeplin's 1904 work comparing German and Javanese differences in the nature and frequency of mental disorder. The largest and most complex project undertaken in psychiatric epidemiology was the work of the Leightons and their colleagues, first at Cornell, and later at Harvard (A. Leighton 1959; A. Leighton et al. 1963; D. Leighton et al. 1963; Hughes et al. 1963). It took place in Stirling County, Nova Scotia, and was later compared to a similar project in Abeokuta, Nigeria. The Stirling County study drew on the disciplines of psychiatry, sociology, medicine, anthropology, and epidemiology to assess the effects of sociocultural conditions and individual experiences on psychiatric symptoms. A. Leighton has recently discussed the early development of his research focus (Leighton 1984). Grob has recently (1985) published a historical review of psychiatric epidemiology, but he pays no particular attention to an anthropological contribution.

6. *Kuru* is a slow virus infection common in the 1950s—1960s among the Fore people of highland New Guinea. This disease absorbed the labors of anthropologists, neurologists, pathologists, and epidemiologists for some time before its cause was finally isolated. (It was spread through the handling and consumption of infected human brain tissue.) A. and J. Fischer coined the term "cultural epidemiology" in their 1961 paper on the disease, and emphasized that cultural factors, especially those which influenced contact between human hosts and disease agents, were relevant to epidemiology.

D. Carlton Gajdusek, who won a Nobel prize for his research on *kuru*, has written vividly about the search for a causal agent (see Farquhar and Gadjusek 1981; Gajdusek 1977), but has neglected the contribution that others have made to the enterprise (see Lindenbaum 1982). Although the etiological investigation of kuru is an important chapter in the collaboration between anthropologists and epidemiologists, many details of the effort remain to be told.

7. See the following general descriptions of the project: Kark and Kark 1981a and 1981b; Kark and Kark 1962; Slome 1962; and S. Kark 1951. See also the progress reports from the project: e.g., Gale 1946, 1949; Gear 1943; S. Kark 1942, 1944; S. Kark and Cassel 1952.

8. See the 1934 paper by George Gale on traditional health beliefs, and also Kark and Kark 1981a.

9. See chapters by Jacobson, Slome, Gampel, Ward, and Abramson in Kark and Steuart 1962.

10. See papers such as 'Infant Rearing in Different Culture Groups', by the anthropologist Hilda Kuper (1962: 93—113); 'A Comparative Study of Infant Mortality in Five Communities', by S. Kark and Chesler (1962: 114—134); and 'The Menarche in African and Indian Girls', by E. Kark (1962: 178—185).

11. Ryle was appointed in 1943 to be the first Professor of Social Medicine at Oxford. See his book *Changing Disciplines*, Oxford University Press, 1948.

12. I am indebted to David McKay for suggesting the importance of the transition occurring in post-War North Carolina.

13. See the collected papers published in 1971 in the *Archives of Internal Medicine* 128: 887—975, and in 1980 in the *Journal of Chronic Diseases* 33(5).

14. See Goethals and Kaplan 1968 for an outline of the theory guiding the inclusion of anthropology and epidemiology in the UNC Chapel Hill program.

15. This sort of discussion seems to occur in epidemiology about every twenty years — the 1960s discussion followed the debates of twenty years earlier about what the field meant and what its proper scope of investigation included (see the editorial [*American Journal of Public Health* 1942] and subsequent letters [Vol. 32, Nos. 4, 6, 7—9, 11] on this topis). It also preceded a similar discussion in the 1980s (see Greenberg 1983; Marmot 1976; Rothman 1981; Stallones 1980; and Terris 1983).

16. For a description of the evolution of this work see Susser (1985a). Mervyn Susser and Zena Stein, South Africans not specifically affiliated with the IFCH, nonetheless shared many of the goals and orientations of the IFCH as described here. Their work in South Africa, England, and the U.S. has stressed the importance of social factors in epidemiologic studies (see e.g. Susser and Stein 1962; Stein and Susser 1967; Susser 1968; Stein 1985).

17. See for example Allcorn (1955), Frankenburg (1980), Frankenburg and Lesson (1973), Leeson (1960).

18. See Goldberg (1958), Logan (1964), Loudon (1976).

19. Thanks to S. Leonard Syme for directing me to this work.

20. The methodological appendix to the first volume (Buck et al. 1968: 121—128) contains a series of instructive anecdotes concerning the project's local reception.

21. For recent examples of the analytic rather than descriptive utilization of this behavioral approach in medical geography, see Armstrong (1973, 1976) on what he calls "self-specific environments", and also Roundy (1978). For similar applications in anthropological research, see Alland (1969, 1970), and Dunn (1979).

REFERENCES

Abramson, J. H.
  1962 The 'Marshlands' Health Service. *In* A Practice of Social Medicine. S. L. Kark and G. Steuart (eds.), pp. 335—360. Edinburgh: E. & S. Livingstone.
  1966 Emotional Disorder, Status Inconsistency and Migration. Milbank Memorial Fund Quarterly 44 (1): 23—48.

1979 Survey Methods in Community Medicine: An Introduction to Epidemiologic and Evaluative Studies. Edinburgh: Churchill Livingstone.

Abramson, J. H., R. Goffin, J. Habib et al.
1982 Indicators of Social Class: A Comparative Appraisal of Measures for Use in Epidemiologic Studies. Social Science and Medicine 16: 1739—1746.

Ackerknecht, E. H.
1948 Anticontagionism between 1821 and 1867. Bulletin of the History of Medicine 22: 562—593.

Adair, J. and K. W. Deuschle
1970 The People's Health: Medicine and Anthropology in a Navajo Community. New York: Appleton-Century-Crofts.

Alland Jr., A.
1969 Ecology and Adaptation to Parasitic Diseases. In Environment and Cultural Behavior: Ecological Studies in Cultural Anthropology. A. P. Vayda (ed.), pp. 80—89. Garden City, NY: Natural History Press.
1970 Adaptation in Cultural Evolution: An Approach to Medical Anthropology. New York: Columbia University Press.

Allcorn, D. H.
1955 The Social Development of Young Men in an English Industrial Suburb. Ph.D. Dissertation, University of Manchester.

American Journal of Public Health
1942 Editorial: What and Who Is an Epidemiologist? 32: 414.

Anderson, D, O.
1969 The Social Sciences and Public Health Programs — An Epidemiologist's View. Canadian Journal of Public Health 60: 1—6.

Armstrong, R. W.
1973 Tracing Exposure to Specific Environments in Medical Geography. Geographical Analysis 5: 122—132.
1976 The Geography of Specific Environments of Patients and Non-Patients in Cancer Studies, with a Malaysian Example. Economic Geography 52: 161—170.

Audy, J. R.
1958 Medical Ecology in Relation to Geography. British Journal of Clinical Practice 12(2): 102—110.
1968 Red Mites and Typhus. (University of London Heath Clark Lectures, 1965) London: Athlone Press.

Barnes, J. A.
1954 Class and Committees in a Norwegian Parish Island. Human Relations 7: 39—58.

Beaglehole, R., C. E. Salmond, A. Hooper et al.
1977 Blood Pressure and Social Interaction in Tokelauan Migrants in New Zealand. Journal of Chronic Diseases 30: 803—812.

Beals, R.
1953 Acculturation. In Anthropology Today. A. L. Kroeber (ed.), pp. 621—641. Chicago: University of Chicago Press.

Bennett, F. J., G. A. Saxton, J. S. W. Lutwama et al.
1965 The Role of the Rural Health Centre in the Teaching Programme of a Medical School in East Africa. Journal of Medical Education 40: 690—699.

Bennett, F. J., N. A. Barnicot, J. Woodburn et al.
1973 Studies on the Viral, Bacterial, Rickettsial and Treponemal Disease in the Hadza of Tanzania, with a Note on Injuries. Human Biology 45: 245—272.

Berkman, L. and S. L. Syme
1979 Social Networks, Host Resistance, and Mortality: A Nine-Year Follow-Up of Alameda County Residents. Americal Journal of Epidemiology 109: 186—204.

Bott, E.
1957 Family and Social Network. (Revised ed. 1971.) London: Tavistock.

Broadhead, W. E., B. H. Kaplan, S. A. James et al.
  1983 The Epidemiologic Evidence for a Relationship Between Social Support and Health.
         American Journal of Epidemiology 117: 521—537.
Brody, H. and D. S. Sobel
  1979 A Systems View of Health and Disease. *In* Ways of Health. D. S. Sobel (ed.), pp.
         87—104. New York: Harcourt Brace Jovanovich.
Buck, A. A., R. I. Anderson, K. Kawata et al.
  1972 Health and Disease in Rural Afghanistan. Baltimore: York Press.
Buck, A. A., R. I. Anderson, T. T. Sasaki et al.
  1970 Health and Disease in Chad: Epidemiology, Culture, and Environment in Five
         Villages. Baltimore: Johns Hopkins University Press.
Buck, A. A., T. T. Sasaki, and R. I. Anderson
  1968 Health and Disease in Four Peruvian Villages: Contrasts in Epidemiology. Balti-
         more: Johns Hopkins University Press.
Cassel, J. C.
  1955 A Comprehensive Health Program among South African Zulus. *In* Health, Culture,
         and Community. Case Studies of Public Reactions to Health Programs. B. D. Paul
         (ed.), pp. 15—41. New York: Russell Sage Foundation.
  1962 Cultural Factors in the Interpretation of Illness. A Case Study. *In* A Practice of
         Social Medicine. S. L. Kark and G. W. Steuart (eds.), pp. 238—244. Edinburgh: E.
         & S. Livingstone.
  1964 Social Science Theory as a Source of Hypotheses in Epidemiological Research.
         American Journal of Public Health 54: 1482—1488.
  1974 Hypertension and Cardiovascular Disease in Migrants: A Potential Source of Clues?
         International Journal of Epidemiology 3(3): 204—206.
  1976 The Contribution of the Social Environment to Host Resistance. American Journal
         of Epidemiology 104: 107—123.
Cassel, J. C., R. C. Patrick Jr., and C. D. Jenkins
  1960 Epidemiologic Analysis of the Health Implications of Culture Change. A Concep-
         tual Model. Annals of the New York Academy of Sciences 84(17): 938—949.
Cassel, J. C. and H. A. Tyroler
  1961 Epidemiological Studies of Culture Change I: Health Status and Recency of Indus-
         trialization. Archives of Environmental Health 3: 25—33.
Caudill, W.
  1953 Applied Anthropology in Medicine. *In* Anthropology Today. A. L. Kroeber (ed.),
         pp. 771—806. Chicago: University of Chicago Press.
Chapin, C. V.
  1928 The Science of Epidemic Diseases. Scientific Monthly 26: 481—493.
Chesler, J., M. Cormak, A. Singh, et al.
  1962 Three Cases of Gastro-Enteritis in Infants. A Family Doctor Case Conference. *In* A
         Practice of Social Medicine. S. L. Kark and G. W. Steuart (eds.), pp. 143—154.
         Edinburgh: E. & S. Livingstone.
Cohn, H. D. and W. M. Schmidt
  1975 The Practice of Family Health Care: A Descriptive Study. American Journal of
         Public Health 65: 375—383.
Collado Ardon, R., A. J. Rubel, C. W. O'Nell, et al.
  1983 Letter; A Folk Illness (Susto) as an Indicator of Real Illness. The Lancet, 10 Decem-
         ber, 1362.
Damon, A.
  1964 Some Host Factors in Disease: Sex, Race, Ethnic Group and Body Form. American
         Journal of Physical Anthropology 22: 375—382.
  1969 Race, Ethnic Groups and Disease. Social Biology 16: 69—80.
Doll, R.
  1980 The Epidemiology of Cancer. Cancer 45: 2475—2485.

Douall, J. A.
  1952 The Bacteriological Era, 1876—1920. *In* The History of Amercian Epidemiology. F. H. Top (ed.), pp. 74—113. St. Louis: C. V. Mosby.
Dudley, S.
  1936 The Ecological Outlook on Epidemiology. Proceedings of the Royal Society of Medicine 30(1): 57—70.
Dunn, F. L.
  1979 Behavioral Aspects of the Control of Parasitic Diseases. Bulletin of the World Health Organization 57(4): 499—512.
Elkind, H. B.
  1938 Is There an Epidemiology of Mental Disease? American Journal of Public Health 28: 245—250.
Farquhar, J. and D. C. Gajdusek (eds.)
  1981 Early Letters and Fieldnotes from the Collection of D. Carlton Gajdusek. New York: Raven Press.
Firth, R.
  1978 Social Anthropology and Medicine — A Personal Perspective. Social Science and Medicine 12B: 237—245.
Fischer, A. and J. L. Fischer
  1961 Culture and Epidemiology: A Theoretical Investigation of Kuru. Journal of Health and Human Behavior 2: 16—25.
Fleck, A. C. and F. A. J. Ianni
  1958 Epidemiology and Anthropology: Some Suggested Affinities in Theory and Method. Human Organization 16(4): 38—40.
Foster, G.
  1961 Public Health and Behavioral Science: The Problems of Teamwork. American Journal of Public Health 51: 1286—1293.
Frankenburg, R.
  1980 Medical Anthropology and Development: A Theoretical Perspective. Social Science and Medicine 14B: 197—207.
Frankenburg, R. and J. Leeson
  1973 The Sociology of Health Dilemmas in the Post-Colonial World. *In* Sociology and Development. E. deKadt and G. Williams (eds.). London: Tavistock, pp. 255—278.
Frost, W. H.
  1941 Papers of Wade Hampton Frost, M. D.. A Contribution to Epidemiology Method. K. F. Maxcy (ed.). New York: Commonwealth Fund.
Gajdusek, D. C.
  1977 Unconventional Viruses and the Origin and Disappearance of Kuru. Science 197: 946—960.
Galdston, I.
  1951 Social Medicine and the Epidemic Constitution. Bulletin of the History of Medicine 25: 8—21.
Gale, G. W.
  1934 Native Medical Ideas and Practices in Relation to Native Medical Services. South African Medical Journal 8: 748—753.
  1946 Health Centre Practice, Promotive Health Services and the Development of the Health Centres Scheme. South African Medical Journal 20: 326—330.
  1949 Government Health Centres in the Union of South Africa. South African Medical Journal 23: 630—636.
Gampel, B.
  1962 The 'Hilltops' Community. *In* A Practice of Social Medicine. S. L. Kark and G. W. Steuart (eds.), pp. 292—308. Edinburgh: E. & S. Livingstone.

1967 The Behavior of Mothers to the Examination of Their Babies. Developmental Medicine and Child Neurology 9: 59—63.

Gampel, B., C. Slome, N. Scotch et al.
1962 Urbanization and Hypertension among Zulu Adults. Journal of Chronic Diseases 15: 67—70.

Gear, H. S.
1943 The South African Native Health and Medical Service. South African Medical Journal 17(11): 167—172.
1959 World Epidemiology and Health Statistics. South African Medical Journal 33: 228—231.

Geiger, H. J.
1971 A Health Center in Mississippi — A Case Study in Social Medicine. In Medicine in a Changing Society. L. Corey, S. E. Saltman, and M. F. Epstein (eds.), pp. 157—167. St. Louis: C. V. Mosby.
1984 Community Health Centers: Health Care as an Instrument of Social Change. In Reforming Medicine: Lessons of the Past Quarter Century. V. W. Sidel and R. Sidel (eds.), pp. 11—32. New York: Pantheon Books.

Goethals, P. and B. H. Kaplan
1968 Medical Anthropology at the University of North Carolina: A Preliminary Note. Proceedings of the Southern Anthropological Society 1: 55—63.

Goldberg, E. M.
1958 Family Influences and Psychosomatic Illness. An Inquiry into the Social and Psychological Background of Duodenal Ulcer. London: Tavistock.

Gordon, J. E.
1949 The epidemiology of accidents. American Journal of Public Health 39: 504—515.
1952 The Twentieth Century — Yesterday, Today, and Tomorrow (1920—   ). In The History of American Epidemiology. F. H. Top (ed.), pp. 114—167. St. Louis: C. V. Mosby.
1953 Evolution of an Epidemiology of Health, Parts I, II, and III. In The Epidemiology of Health. I. Galdston (ed.), pp. 24—73. New York: New York Academy of Medicine.
1958 Medical Ecology and the Public Health. American Journal of the Medical Sciences 235(3): 336—359.
1966 Ecologic Interplay of Man, Environment and Health. American Journal of the Medical Sciences 252: 341—356.

Gordon, J. E., O'Rourke, F. L. W. Richardson et al.
1952 The Biological and Social Sciences in an Epidemiology of Mental Disorder. American Journal of the Medical Sciences 223: 316—343.

Greenberg, B. G.
1983 The Future of Epidemiology. Journal of Chronic Diseases 36: 353—359.

Greenwood, M.
1935 Epidemics and Crowd Diseases, An Introduction to the Study of Epidemiology. New York: Macmillan.

Grob, G. N.
1985 The Origins of Psychiatric Epidemiology. American Journal of Public Health 75: 229—236.

Haenszel, W. and P. Correa
1975 Developments in the Epidemiology of Stomach Cancer Over the Past Decade. Cancer Research 35: 3452—3459.

Hamer, W. H.
1929 Epidemiology Old and New. New York: Macmillan.

Harris, M.
1968 The Rise of Anthropological Theory. New York: Thomas Crowell.

Hasan, K. A. and B. G. Prasad
  1960 The Role of Anthropology in Social and Preventive Medicine. Journal of the Indian
        Medical Association 35: 22—26.
Hooton, E. A.
  1930 The Indians of Pecos Pueblo, a Study of their Skeletal Remains. New Haven: Yale
        University Press.
Hughes, C. C., M.-A. Tremblay, R. N. Rapoport et al.
  1963 People of Cove and Woodlot: Communities from the Viewpoint of Social Psy-
        chiatry. New York: Basic Books.
Hulka, B. S., L. L. Kupper, and J. C. Cassel
  1972 Determinants of Physician Utilization: Approach to a Service-Oriented Classifi-
        cation of Symptoms. Medical Care 10: 300—309.
Ianni, F. A. J., R. M. Albrecht, W. E. Boek et al.
  1960 Age, Social, and Demographic Factors in Acceptance of Polio Vaccination. Public
        Health Reports 75(6): 545—556.
Ibrahim, M. A., B. H. Kaplan, R. C. Patrick Jr. et al.
  1980 The Legacy of John C. Cassel. American Journal of Epidemiology 112: 1—7.
Jaco, E. G. (ed.)
  1958 Patients, Physicians, and Illness. New York: The Free Press.
Jacobson, Z.
  1962 Case Note-Book of the 'Riversend' Community. In A Practice of Social Medicine. S.
        L. Kark and G. W. Steuart (eds.) pp. 256—268. Edinburgh: E. & S. Livingstone.
Jelliffe, D. B. and F. J. Bennett
  1960 Indigenous Medical Systems and Child Health. Journal of Paediatrics 57: 248—261.
Johnson, A. L., C. D. Jenkins, R. C. Patrick Jr. et al.
  1962 Epidemiology of Polio Vaccine Acceptance. Florida State Board of Health Mono-
        graph 3.
Kaplan, B. H.
  1971 Blue Ridge: An Appalachian Community in Transition. Morganton: Center for
        Appalachian Studies, University of West Virginia.
Kaplan, B. H., R. N. Wilson, and A. H. Leighton (eds.)
  1976 Further Explorations in Social Psychiatry. New York: Basic Books.
Kaplan, B. H., J. C. Cassel, and S. Gore
  1977 Social Support and Health. Medical Care 15(5): 47—58.
Kark, E.
  1962 The Menarche in African and Indian Girls. In A Practice of Social Medicine. S. L.
        Kark and G. W. Steuart (eds.), pp. 178—185. Edinburgh: E. & S. Livingstone.
Kark, S. L.
  1942 A Health Service among the Rural Bantu. South African Medical Journal 16(10):
        197—198.
  1944 A Health Unit as Family Doctor and Health Adviser. South African Medical
        Journal 18(3): 39—46.
  1951 Health Centre Service. In Social Medicine. E. H. Cluver (ed.), pp. 661—700. South
        Africa: Central News Agency.
  1974 Epidemiology and Community Medicine. New York: Appleton-Century-Crofts.
  1981 The Practice of Community-Oriented Primary Health Care. New York: Appleton-
        Century-Crofts.
Kark, S. L. and J. C. Cassel
  1952 The Pholela Health Centre: A Progress Report. South African Medical Journal
        26(6): 101—104, 132—136.
Kark, S. L. and J. Chesler
  1962 A Comparative Study of Infant Mortality in Five Communities. In A Practice of
        Social Medicine. S. L. Kark and G. W. Steuart (eds.), pp. 114—134. Edinburgh: E.
        & S. Livingstone.

Kark, S. L. and E. Kark
  1962 A Practice of Social Medicine. *In* A Practice of Social Medicine. S. L. Kark and G.
    W. Steuart (eds.), pp. 3—40. Edinburgh: E. & S. Livingstone.
  1981a Community Health Care in a Rural African Population. *In* A Practice of Com-
    munity-Oriented Primary Care. S. L. Kark, pp. 194—213. New York: Appleton-
    Century-Crofts.
  1981b Community-Oriented Primary Health Care of Infants in Rural Polela. *In* A Practice
    of Community-Oriented Primary Care. S. L. Kark, pp. 214—246. New York:
    Appleton-Century-Crofts.
Kark, S. L. and G. W. Steuart (eds.)
  1962 A Practice of Social Medicine. A South African Team's Experiences in Different
    African Communities. Edinburgh: E. & S. Livingstone. `
Kessler, I. I. and M. L. Levin (eds.)
  1970 The Community as an Epidemiologic Laboratory: A Casebook of Community
    Studies. Baltimore: Johns Hopkins Press.
Keys, A. and J. T. Anderson
  1955 The Relationship of the Diet to the Development of Atherosclerosis in Man.
    Symposium on Atherosclerosis. National Academy of Sciences, Publication 338. pp.
    181—197.
Kuper, H.
  1962 Infant Rearing in Different Culture Groups. *In* A Practice of Social Medicine. S. L.
    Kark and G. W. Steuart (eds.), pp. 93—113. Edinburgh: E. & S. Livingstone.
  1984 Function, History, Biography: Reflections on Fifty Years in the British Anthro-
    pological Tradition. *In* Functionalism Historicized: Essays on British Social Anthro-
    pology. G. W. Stocking (ed.), pp. 192—213. Madison: University of Wisconsin
    Press.
Lange, C. H.
  1965 Culture Change. *In* Biennial Review of Anthropology. B. J. Siegel (ed.). Stanford:
    Stanford University Press.
Leach, E. R.
  1984 Glimpses of the Unmentionable in the History of British Social Anthropology.
    Annual Review of Anthropology 13: 1—23.
Leeson, J. E.
  1960 A Study of Mentally Handicapped Children and their Families. Medical Officer
    104: 311—314.
Leighton, A. H.
  1959 My Name is Legion. Foundations for a Theory of Man in Relation to Culture. New
    York: Basic Books.
  1984 Then and Now: Some Notes on the Interaction of Person and Social Environment.
    Human Organization 43: 189—197.
Leighton, A. H., J. Clausen, and R. N. Wilson (eds.)
  1957 Explorations in Social Psychiatry. New York: Basic Books.
Leighton, A. H., A. T. Lambo, C. C. Hughes et al.
  1963 Psychiatric Disorder among the Yoruba. Ithaca, NY: Cornell University Press.
Leighton, D. C., J. S. Harding, D. B. Macklin et al.
  1963 The Character of Danger: Psychiatric Symptoms in Selected Communities. New
    York: Basic Books.
Lewitter, F. I. (ed.)
  1980 Genetic Epidemiology in an Anthropological Context: A Symposium. Medical
    Anthropology 4(3): 291—422
Lindenbaum, S.
  1982 Review of Kuru: Early Letters and Fieldnotes from the Collection of D. Carlton
    Gajdusek, by J. Farquhar and D. C. Gajdusek. Journal of the Polynesian Society
    91(1): 150—152.

Logan, R. F. L.
    1964 Studies in the Spectrum of Medical Care. *In* Problems and Progress in Medical
          Care. G. McLachlan (ed.), pp. 3—55. London: Nuffield Provincial Hospitals Trust.
Loudon, J. B. (ed.)
    1976 Social Anthropology and Medicine. London: Academic Press.
MacMahon, B., T. F. Pugh, and J. Ipsen
    1960 Epidemiologic Methods. Boston: Little, Brown and Company.
MacMahon, B. and T. F. Pugh
    1970 Epidemiology: Principles and Methods. Boston: Little, Brown and Company.
Mair, L.
    1972 An Introduction to Social Anthropology (2nd ed.). New York: Oxford University
          Press.
Mann, G. V., R. D. Shaffer, R. S. Anderson et al.
    1964 Cardiovascular Disease in the Masai. Journal of Atherosclerosis Research 4: 289—
          312.
Marmot, M. G.
    1976 Facts, Opinions, and Affaires du Coeur. American Journal of Epidemiology 103:
          519—526.
Marmot, M. G. and S. L. Syme
    1976 Acculturation and Coronary Heart Disease in Japanese-Americans. American Jour-
          nal of Epidemiology 104: 225—247.
Matovu, H., F. J. Bennett, and J. Namboze
    1971 Kasangati Health Centre: A Community Approach. East Africa Medical Journal 48:
          33—39.
May, J. M.
    1978 History, Definition, and Problems of Medical Geography: A General Review.
          (Report to the Commission on Medical Geography of the International Geographi-
          cal Union, 1952.) Social Science and Medicine 12D: 211—219.
McGarvey, S. T. and P. T. Baker
    1979 The Effects of Modernization and Migration on Samoan Blood Pressures. Human
          Biology 51: 461—479.
Medalie, J. H.
    1978 Family Medicine: Principles and Applications. Baltimore: Williams and Wilkins.
Medalie, J. H. and U. Goldbourt
    1976 Angina Pectoris among 10,000 Men. II. Psychosocial and Other Risk Factors as
          Evidenced by a Multivariate Analysis of a Five Year Incidence Study. American
          Journal of Medicine 60: 910—921.
Mitchell, J. C.
    1969 The Concept and Use of Social Networks. *In* Social Networks and Urban Situations.
          J. C. Mitchell (ed.), pp. 1—50. Manchester: Manchester University Press.
Morris, J. N.
    1957 Uses of Epidemiology (1st ed.). Edinburgh: E. & S. Livingstone.
    1959 Health and Social Class. The Lancet 7 February: 303—305.
    1979 Social Inequalities Undiminished. The Lancet 13 January: 87—90.
Morris, J. N., A. Kagan, D. C. Pattison et al.
    1966 Incidence and Prediction of Ischaemic Heart-Disease in London Busmen. The
          Lancet 10 September: 553—559.
Mullan, F.
    1982 Community-Oriented Primary Care. An Agenda for the '80s. New England Journal
          of Medicine 307: 1076—1078.
Murphy, R.
    1964 Social Change and Acculturation. Transactions of the New York Academy of
          Sciences 26: 845—854.
    1976 The Dialectics of Social Life. New York: Columbia University Press.

Neser, W. B., H. A. Tyroler, and J. C. Cassel
    1971 Social Disorganization and Stroke Mortality in the Black Population of North Carolina. American Journal of Epidemiology 93: 166—175.
Nuckolls, K. B., J. C. Cassel, and B. H. Kaplan
    1972 Psychosocial Assets, Life Crisis, and the Prognosis of Pregnancy. American Journal of Epidemiology 95: 431—441.
Ortner, S. B.
    1984 Theory in Anthropology since the Sixties. Comparative Studies in Society and History 26: 126—166.
Patrick Jr., R. C., and H. A. Tyroler
    1974 Some Health Consequences of Modernization in Ponape. Paper presented at the 73rd Annual Meeting of the American Anthropological Association, Mexico City, November.
Paul, B. D. (ed.)
    1955 Health, Culture and Community. New York: Russell Sage.
Paul, B. D.
    1961 Fluoridation and the Social Scientist: A Review. The Journal of Social Issues 17(4): 1—12.
    1963 Teaching Cultural Anthropology in Schools of Public Health. In The Teaching of Anthropology. D. W. Mandelbaum, G. W. Lasker, and E. A. Albert (eds.), pp. 503—512. American Anthropological Association Memoir No. 94.
Paul, B. D., W. A. Gamson, and S. S. Kegeles (eds.)
    1961 Trigger for Community Conflict: The Case of Fluoridation. The Journal of Social Issues 17(4).
Paul, J. R.
    1958 Clinical Epidemiology. Chicago: University of Chicago Press.
Payne, A. M.-M.
    1962 The Scope and Methods of Epidemiology. American Journal of Public Health 52: 1502—1504.
Phillips, H. T.
    1967 Planning for Community Health. Lancet 1: 893.
    1977 Preventive Medicine, USA — What's in It for Us? Journal of Health Politics, Policy and Law 2: 411—426.
Phillips, H. T. and A. G. Beza
    1979 The Use of Health Surveys in Health Systems Agency Planning (Editorial). American Journal of Public Health 69: 221—222.
Phillips, H. T. and E. J. Salber
    1955 Some Social Aspects of Paediatrics. South African Medical Journal 29: 499—503.
Polgar, S.
    1962 Health and Human Behavior: Areas of Interest Common to the Social and Medical Sciences. Current Anthropology 3(2): 159—205.
Radcliffe-Brown, A. R.
    1952 Structure and Function in Primitive Society. New York: Free Press.
Redfield, R., R. Linton, and M. Herskovits
    1936 Memorandum for the Study of Acculturation. American Anthropologist 38: 149—152.
Reid, D. D.
    1960 Epidemiological Methods in the Study of Mental Disorders. Public Health Papers, No. 2. Geneva: World Health Organization.
    1975 International Studies in Epidemiology. American Journal of Epidemiology 102: 469—476.
Rogers, E. S.
    1960 Human Ecology and Health: An Introduction for Administrators. New York: Macmillan.

Rosen, G.
1947   What is Social Medicine? A Genetic Analysis of the Concept. Bulletin of the
        History of Medicine 21: 674—733.
Rothman, K.
1981   The Rise and Fall of Epidemiology, 1950—2000 A.D. New England Journal of
        Medicine 304: 600—602.
Roundy, R.
1978   A Model for Combining Human Behavior and Disease Ecology to Assess Disease
        Hazard in a Community: Rural Ethiopia as a Model. Social Science and Medicine
        12D: 121—130.
Rubel, A. J.
1964   The Epidemiology of a Folk Illness: Susto in Hispanic America. Ethnology 3: 268—
        283.
Rubel, A. J., C. W. O'Nell, and R. Collado Ardon
1984   Susto: A Folk Illness. Berkeledy, CA: University of California Press.
Rubin, V. (ed.)
1960   Culture, Society, and Health. Annals of the New York Academy of Sciences 84(17):
        783—1060.
Ryle, J.
1948   Changing Disciplines. Oxford: Oxford University Press.
Salber, E. J.
1962   Birth-Weights of South African Babies. In A Practice of Social Medicine. S. L. Kark
        and G. W. Steuart (eds.), pp. 155—159. Edinburgh: E. & S. Livingstone.
1975   Caring and Curing: Community Participation in Health Services. New York: Prodist.
1981   Where Does Primary Care Begin? The Health Facilitator as a Central Figure in
        Primary Care. Israel Journal of Medical Sciences 17: 100—111.
Scotch, N. A.
1960   A Preliminary Report on the Relation of Sociocultural Factors to Hypertension
        Among the Zulu. Annals of the New York Academy of Sciences 84: 1000—1009.
1963a Medical Anthropology. In Biennial Review of Anthropology. B. J. Siegel (ed.), pp.
        30—68. Stanford: Stanford University Press.
1963b Sociocultural Factors in the Epidemiology of Zulu Hypertension. American Journal
        of Public Health 53: 1205—1213.
Scotch, N. A. and H. J. Geiger
1962   The Epidemiology of Rheumatoid Arthritis. A Review with Special Attention to
        Social Factors. Journal of Chronic Diseases 15: 1037—1067.
1963   The Epidemiology of Essential Hypertension. A Review with Special Attention to
        Psychologic and Sociocultural Factors. II: Psychologic and Sociocultural Factors in
        Etiology. Journal of Chronic Diseases 16: 1183—1213.
Seltzer, C. C., H. W. Stoudt, B. Bell et al.
1970   Reliability of Relative Body Weight as a Criterion of Obesity. American Journal of
        Epidemiology 91: 339—350.
Slome, C.
1962   Community Health in Rural Pholela. In A Practice of Social Medicine. S. L. Kark
        and G. W. Steuart (eds.), pp. 269—291. Edinburgh: E. & S. Livingstone.
Slome, C., W. M. Lednar, D. E. Roberts et al.
1977   Should James Go to School? Mother's Responses to Symptoms. Journal of School
        Health 47: 106—110.
Slome, C., H. Wetherbee, M. Daly et al.
1976   Effectiveness of Certified Nurse-Midwives. A Prospective Evaluation Study. Ameri-
        can Journal of Obstetrics and Gynecology 124: 177—182.

Stallones, R.
  1980 To Advance Epidemiology. Annual Review of Public Health 1: 69—82.
Stein, Z. A.
  1985 A Woman's Age: Childrearing and Childrearing. American Journal of Epidemiology 121: 327—342.
Stein, Z. A. and M. W. Susser
  1967 The Social Dimensions of a Symptom: A Sociomedical Study of Enuresis. Social Science & Medicine 1: 183—201.
Stein, Z. A., M. W. Susser, A. Kushlick et al.
  1957 Nursing Act 1957 (Letter). South African Medical Journal 31: 736.
Steuart, G. L.
  1965 Health, Behavior and Planned Change: An Approach to the Professional Preparation of the Health Education Specialist. Health Education Monographs 20: 3—26.
  1975 Beyond the Individual for the Practice of Social Medicine: Household Networks as Etiologic-Diagnostic Units. In Topias and Utopias in Health. S. Ingman and A. Thomas (eds.), pp. 85—97. The Hague: Mouton.
Steward, J. H.
  1955 Theory of Culture Change. The Methodology of Multilinear Evolution. Urbana, IL: University of Illinois Press.
Stoudt, H. W., A. Damon, and R. A. McFarland
  1960 Heights and Weights of White Americans. Human Biology 32: 331—341.
Suchman, E. A.
  1963 Sociology and the Field of Public Health. New York: Russell Sage.
Susser, M. W.
  1964 The Uses of Social Science in Medicine. The Lancet 29 August: 7357—7361.
  1968 Community Psychiatry: Epidemiologic and Social Themes. New York: Random House.
  1973 Causal Thinking in the Health Sciences: Concepts and Strategies of Epidemiology. London: Oxford University Press.
  1985a Preface. In Sociology in Medicine. M. W. Susser, W. Watson and K. Hopper (eds.). London: Oxford University Press.
  1985b Epidemiology in the United States after World War II: The Evolution of Technique. Epidemiologic Reviews 7: 147—177.
Susser, M. W. and Z. A. Stein
  1962 Civilization and Peptic Ulcer. The Lancet i: 115—119.
Susser, M. W. and W. Watson
  1971 Sociology in Medicine (1st ed. 1962). London: Oxford University Press.
Syme, S. L.
  1983 The Social Environment and Disease: Towards a Proper Epidemiology. Paper presented at the 16th Annual Meeting of the Society for Epidemiologic Research. Winnipeg, Canada. June 17.
Syme, S. L. and L. C. Reeder (eds.)
  1967 Social Stress and Cardiovascular Disease. Milbank Memorial Fund Quarterly 45, Part 2.
Taylor, I. and J. Knowelden
  1957 Principles of Epidemiology. Boston: Little, Brown and Company.
Terris, M.
  1962 The Scope and Methods of Epidemiology. American Journal of Public Health 52: 1371—1376.
  1983 The Complex Tasks of the Second Epidemiologic Revolution: The Joseph W. Mountin Lecture. Journal of Public Health Policy 4: 8—24.

1985 The Changing Relationships of Epidemiology and Society: The Robert Cruickshank Lecture. Journal of Public Health Policy 6: 15—36.

Tyroler, H. A. and J. C. Cassel
1964 Health Consequences of Culture Change. II. The Effect of Urbanization on Coronary Health Mortality in Rural Residents. Journal of Chronic Diseases 17: 167—177.

Ubelaker, D. H.
1982 The Development of American Paleopathology. *In* A History of American Physical Anthropology 1930—1980. F. Spencer (ed.), pp. 337—356. New York: Academic Press.

Vijil, C.
1959 Public Health and Social Science. Copenhagen: Ejnar Munksgaard.

Ward, N. T.
1962 The Health of 'Forestville'. *In* A Practice of Social Medicine. S. L. Kark and G. W. Steuart (eds.), pp. 309—334. Edinburgh: E. & S. Livingstone.

Wardwell, W. I. and C. B. Bahnson
1964 Problems Encountered in Behavioral Science Research Utilizing Retrospective Epidemiological Data. American Journal of Public Health 54: 972—981.

Wilson, R. N.
1970 The Sociology of Health: An Introduction. New York: Random House.

Young, M. and P. Willmott
1957 Family and Kinship in East London. London: Routledge and Kegan Paul.

SECTION II

INFECTIOUS DISEASES

MARILYN K. NATIONS

EPIDEMIOLOGICAL RESEARCH ON INFECTIOUS DISEASE: QUANTITATIVE RIGOR OR RIGORMORTIS? INSIGHTS FROM ETHNOMEDICINE*

INTRODUCTION: AN ENLIVENED DATA SET

Epidemiology often forsakes the richness of a people's way of living for quantitative rigor. And, although statistical calculations may be built on valid mathematical models, they run a serious risk of being inaccurate by excluding a vital human element: the way people *really* approach illness and cope with death.

The business community suffers a similar plight. In the bestseller *In Search of Excellence,* Peters and Waterman (1982) caution the corporate world against the 'Paralysis through Analysis Syndrome'. That is, the affliction of building analytic models that are too complex to be useful, too unwieldy to be flexible, and too precise to capture "sloppy" personal interactions and other "messy human stuff" (p. 31). The warning is a suitable one for the traditional epidemiologist as well, whose models are often inadequate reflections of the complexities of human health behavior. In doing anthropological fieldwork in the town of Pacatuba in northeastern Brazil I was witness time and again to this weakness of traditional epidemiology. In Pacatuba, stories similar to the one presented below are not uncommon. There, on the pages of Pacatuba's death registry, an account of Dona Fatima's infant daughter's death is missing. But, for this poor Brazilian mother, no event is more noteworthy.

Losing a Life

Quickly before death set in, the infant girl's tiny hands were tied around a matchbox in an attitude of prayer and her eyes pried open to see God. Then her body was placed on a crude wooden table in her home to remain, in the light of votive candles, until the next day when she would rest in a homemade coffin. Dona Fatima, the infant's mother, collapsed in her hammock, her only comfort the thought that her daughter no longer suffered: she was now an

* Field research was made possible by the Federal University of Ceará, the Maternidade Escola Assis Chateaubriand, the University of Virginia, Division of Geographic Medicine, and the W. K. Kellogg Foundation. Additional support was provided by the National Center for Health Services Research, OASH (Grant number 1 RO3 HSO4437-01) and the Pan American Health Organization. Projects are currently being supported by Primary Health Care Operations Research and The Edna McConnell Clark Foundation.

Craig R. Janes et al. (eds.), Anthropology and Epidemiology, 97—123.
© 1986 *by D. Reidel Publishing Company.*

"angelhino" — a little angel innocent of sin — and, as such, she would fly directly to heaven avoiding purgatory where adults must languish to expiate their sins before reaching their destination. Still, Dona Fatima could not sleep. It was only three years since her son had died of the same *doenca de crianca* — "illness of the child". Now Fatima stared at the body of her only daughter, questioning God's plan in taking the two children from her.

She had done everything she knew to protect her baby from the common childhood illnesses in Pacatuba: *quebranto* (evil eye), *susto* (fright disease), *sombra* (spirit intrusion) and *quintura* (intestinal heat). She had planted a *pihao* bush outside the house, strung a gold-leaf charm on a red ribbon and tied it to the child's wrists, been careful not to even expose her intentionally to loud noises or cross-roads, and never allowed her outside on the hot ground without sandals. After such symptoms as vomiting or diarrhea, Fatima collected medicinal leaves and roots and prepared the proper teas. When the baby had not improved, she went to Dona Mocina, an elderly *rezadeira* or "praying woman", who began the appropriate healing ceremony. The old woman's incantations, herbal preparations and healing powers had always cured her four oldest children, but the baby was weak and playued by an unusually powerful *quebranto* cast upon her by a menstruating woman, or so Dona Mocina had diagnosed. Every village mother knows this kind of curse can kill within a day, so Fatima spent her savings on an expensive antibiotic, but this too failed. The infant's fontanelle had already fallen, diarrhea and vomiting increased, her lips became dry and cracked, and, worst of all, her glazed eyes sank deeply into their sockets, giving her "angel eyes", the omen of death. When Fatima realized traditional remedies were unavailing, she borrowed money from her *comadre* to purchase a bus ticket to Fortaleza. Though she had travelled to the capital several times as a maid, she was still bewildered by its high-rise buildings, rushing crowds and noisy traffic. Carrying the dying baby in her arms, Fatima descended from the bus and walked past rows of offices and specialty medical clinics. She could not read the signs on the buildings, but knew from the past that these places did not treat "illness of the child". It was only after a ten-block walk that she came to her destination. After waiting nearly three hours, her infant, now nearly lifeless, was lifted from her arms by strangers in white. "There is not much hope for this one", they scolded, "you cannot wait until they are half dead and then expect us to perform a miracle!" Fatima lowered her head and nodded in silence; only God knew she had done everything to save her baby. The hospital attendants shaved smooth spots on her infant's head and repeatedly thrust a needle into her scalp. At last they tapped the small, blue vein and administered a balanced electrolyte solution in hopes of reversing the effects of severe dehydration.

Later, Fatima and her child returned home. The infant's fate was now in God's hands. Fatima would go to church at sunrise and make a vow to San Francisco to crawl on her knees to his shrine in Canede, to cut off her hair, to carve a wooden statue — anything if only her daughter would be allowed to live. But instead, Fatima felt only a heaviness in her arms; her baby was dead, now a "little angel". In all her twenty-seven years Fatima had never known such a weight as her dead child. She covered the child's bruised head with the old sheet she used as a blanket.

Morning came quickly. A crowd, mostly women and children, gathered around the wooden table. Prayers were recited, and Fatima said farewell to her baby. Four boys carried the open casket filled with flowers covering all but the child's face and hands, and led the procession of school children through the streets to the community cemetery. Fatima's husband lowered the sky-blue coffin into the ground then furiously shovelled dirt over his right shoulder. Exhausted, he walked away — never once looking back.

Posing Questions to the Epidemiologist

A central contention of this chapter is that for epidemiology to achieve its purpose within Third and Fourth World nations, a recognition of folk-defined illnesses is a necessary step. For example, it is critical to answer the following questions: How do such folk-defined illnesses as "evil eye" and "illness of the child" relate to biomedical syndromes — diarrhea and dehydration — which are identified by epidemiologists as the leading causes of childhood mortality in Pacatuba (Guerrant et al. 1983), in Northeast Brazil (Puffer and Serrano 1973), and worldwide (Walsh and Warren 1979)? How can one guarantee that the death of an unnamed "angel" become part of the epidemiologist's data set? How can the epidemiologist identify risk factors without a grass-roots view of the victim's daily life? The answers do not lie solely in stacks of computer print-outs or complicated mathematical formulas. These statistical tools — often detached — must be enlivened by the real life observations of the anthropologist.

A HISTORY OF OFFERINGS FROM THE SOCIAL SCIENCES

Uniting the Fields

That a promising partnership between anthropology and epidemiology can be forged is not a novel idea. Theoretical and methodological affinities between these fields were pointed out to anthropologists as early as 1958 by Fleck and Ianni (1958). As they saw it, a common meeting ground for the two disciplines rested on the concept of multiple causation of disease. In sharp contrast to the widely accepted "Doctrine of Specific Etiology", this new approach maintained that getting sick depends upon a complex inter-action of many variables — one of which is the disease agent (Dubos 1965). Other factors in this "causal network", as Dunn (1975) has labelled it, include the host's general metabolic state and immune response, the political and economic environment, and cultural beliefs and practices. These multiple factors or "insults" impinge directly on an individual or group causing its level of health to rise and fall accordingly (Audy 1971; Dunn 1976b). To stay healthy, people must balance these multiple factors. Exposure to a pathogen does not necessarily result in infection, infection is not always sufficient to cause illness, and the impact that illness has on the overall health of an individual is not a constant (Audy 1971). When one or more insults outweighs the coping ability of the individual or group, the scale is tipped in favor of disease. A true appraisal of human illness, Fleck and Ianni argue, must "consider all elements of the environment and, must focus upon man, the host, rather than upon the parasite which invades him or the disease state which afflicts him (1958: 39)". The theoretical underpinnings of this multi-factorial approach have been more fully developed by, among others, Audy (1971), Dubos (1959, 1965), May (1960), and Armelogos et al. (1978).

Alland (1966), however, argues that the dictum which includes *all* human behavior in disease analysis, is overwhelming, vague and non-directional. In sharpening this model, two anthropologists have constructed schema which allow the investigator to dissect any broad behavioral category into discrete, manageable units for analysis. Dunn (1976b) bases his classification of a behavior on three criteria: (1) it either enhances or undermines ones health; (2) it is a deliberate or non-deliberate health action; (3) it is influenced by the community or outside of it (pp. 22—23). He has successfully applied this conceptual template to an analysis of behavioral factors contributing to *Wuchereria* and *Brugia* infections in Malaysia (1976a). Nurge (1975) orga-nizes key risk factors in the virulence and transmission of a wide array of infectious diseases including measles, diptheria, trachoma, hookworm and gonorrhea according to the potential impact of familial, social and environ-mental factors. Despite efforts of medical ecologists to promote a multi-factorial model of disease causationl, infectious diseases continue to be analyzed, for the most part, by following a "biologistic" approach (Fabrega 1972). This paradigm does not integrate human behavioral factors with the biological correlates of such behavior and its social and cultural determi-nants.

The absence of sociocultural data in traditional studies of infectious diseases in not surprising given the longstanding separation of social and biological sciences. Each discipline had developed its own rich body of knowledge according to a specific methodological paradigm and, thus, the two have rarely intersected. Yet, anthropology — dedicated to the study of social and cultural systems — has an enormous contribution to make to the expansion of the otherwise reductionist, biologistic portrayal of infectious diseases. By observing and participating fully in the life of people being studied by the epidemiologist, the anthropologist is trained to record the details of day-to-day events and family relations, to elicit local attitudes, beliefs and values and to take notice of larger socioeconomic forces which impinge on the community. Together, these grassroots insights into the culture enable the anthropologist to evaluate social inputs in terms of their relative importance as determinants of disease transmission.

Investigating Sociocultural Factors in the Regulation of Infectious Diseases

A few outstanding studies have demonstrated how specific cultural beliefs and practices expose people to (or protect them from) the foci of disease transmission, and directly contribute to (or inhibit) infection. These provide the strongest evidence to support the inclusion of sociocultural variables in etiologic models of infectious diseases. Dietary customs, child care patterns, religious practices, migration patterns, agricultural techniques, kinship relations and traditional medical treatments, to name but a few, have been implicated by social scientists as critical factors in the natural history of a number of infectious diseases.

Dietary Customs: The Far Eastern dietary custom of eating "drunken crabs", is responsible, according to Fan (1964) for the spread of the Oriental lung fluke, *Paragonimus westermani.* Native recipes for this popular hors d'oeuvre call for freshwater crabs and crayfish to be soaked in brine, vinegar, or wine, then consumed. But when improperly cooked, encysted metacercariae are ingested along with the crustaceans. Similarly, traditional dishes of fermented pork prepared by migrants to New York have been responsible for recent outbreak of trichinosis (Imperato et al. 1974). Schantz et al. (1977) report a higher risk of infection from the *Trichinella* nematode in German-, Italian-, Polish- and Portuguese-Americans than in the United States population at large. Homemade spiced pork sausages, prepared according to traditional ethnic recipes are a culinary specialty of these groups, but also a source of parasitic infection.

Two exotic examples of food habits which increase risk of infectious diseases are geophagia, or dirt eating, and cannibalism. Children with appetites for dirt or clay are at higher risk for toxocariasis; of 100 children ages 1 to 6 included in this study, those who ate feces, soil or grass were 20 times more likely to have elevated *Toxocara* antibody levels than children who did not eat non-food items (Glickman et al. 1981). The cannibalistic custom of South Fore Women of New Guinea, who ritually eat the (often) partially-cooked brains of their deceased kinswomen, has grave epidemiological consequences. Gajdusek (1973) showed how this cannibalistic custom transmitted a slow virus which resulted in kuru, a degenerative neurological disease.

Closer to home, in our own University of Virginia Outpatient Clinic, dietary habits proved to be the critical transmission factor in one mysterious case. A 32-year old black woman presented to our clinic with fever, chest pains and a cough which recurred eight or nine times in the course of a year.

Chest X-rays showed traces of pulmonary infiltrates; blood tests were normal except for an elevated eosinophil count. The case finally made sense when the clinical anthropologist conducted an interview with the patient. The fact that she insisted on a pregnancy test instead of a remedy for her respiratory complaints was the tip-off. Asked why, the woman related that she suspected that she was pregnant because the quantity of dirt she usually ate had increased dramatically to 3—4 cups a day! Moreover, it was dark, red clay she preferred, and the best was located near her outdoor latrine. Careful re-examination of the X-rays confirmed the telltale signs of geophagia: small rocks in the stomach. Given this evidence, the unusual diagnosis of *Toxocara canis* was made. This soil borne parasite migrates through the lungs during its life cycle and causes the symptoms presented by this patient.

Child Care Patterns: The child care practices of the Turkana of Kenya have been linked by Nelson (1972) to high incidence of the larval stage of *Echinococcus granulosus* — hydatid disease. Among these nomadic pastoralists, "dog nurses" are used to care for the young. The animals are trained to lick the child clean after defecation or vomiting, and to provide warmth and protection while the baby sleeps nuzzled in its fur. This traditional practice brings the child and the infected dog into close contact. During "nursing duties", infective eggs stuck around the dog's muzzle (due to licking its own anus) are transferred to and ingested by the child.

Religious Practices: The Muslim ritualistic practice of washing before prayer increases the exposure risk of endemic populations to bilhariasis (Farooq 1966). The exposure of skin during cleansing to water which harbors infective cercariae increases the chance of cercarial penetration and infection. Kochar et al. (1973) demonstrated the relationship of Hindu religious beliefs to hookworm infections in rural West Bengal. A popular text in Hindu households orders that the first act, after rising and chanting the first morning prayer, is defecation; omission of these acts is sinful. Yet, it is precisely at this time, when the sun has not yet dried the damp soil, that active hookworm larvae are present on the soil surface. Contact and penetration of the larvae through the soles of the feet of the most disciplined Hindu is thus facilitated. In contrast, however, it was also noted that the actual practice of ablution probably prevent hookworm infection. Because defecation is considered a ritually defiling act, it must be immediately followed by purification. The body is washed promptly, which not only reduces the time feet are exposed to larvae but also washes many away.

Migration Patterns: Migration patterns have been associated with the spread of a number of communicable diseases. In Ethiopia, for example, a boost in trade, encouraged by expanding communication, has drawn many carriers of infectious diseases to a single location far from their homelands. Such activities often intensify and enlarge the parasitic cycles of illnesses including cholera, schistosomiasis, yellow fever and trypanosomiasis (Roundy 1973).

Agricultural Techniques: Agricultural practices have had a major impact on the historical course of infectious diseases ever since the first farmers gathered with their livestock in permanent settlements. Close contact with animal hosts and with fellow farmers fuels an infection/reinfection cycle which characterizes such diseases as smallpox, measles and influenza. The etiologic agents of these diseases are similar to those agents commonly afflicting domestic animals (Cockburn 1967).

In an ecological analysis of malaria, Livingstone (1958) linked the felling of forests, establishment of permanent settlements, cultivation of high-yield crops and associated multiplication of mosquito breeding places to a sharp rise in the occurrence of malaria among the people of west Africa. Later, Wiesenfeld (1967) traced a change in the agricultural practices of sub-Saharan Africans to a change in the frequency of the sickle-cell gene. He suggested that slash and burn cultivation increases the number of breeding places available to the major vector of malarial parasitism, *Anopheles gambiae.* Because of the protective benefits conferred by the sickle-cell gene in the fight against malaria, Weisenfeld's observation suggested a close relationship of social change to major genetic and health change.

Kinship Relations: The differing intensities of social relationships or inter-actions between people has been explored as a critical factor in the trans-mission of infectious diseases (eg. Dunn 1969). In many societies, kinship beliefs determine who associates with whom, and to what extent. Among the Fore of New Guinea, for example, the kinship system is such that many kin in a residential group share no biological ties. Unaware of this fact, early investigators thought that kuru was a genetic disorder carried by a male-recessive gene (since they observed many more incidents of kuru in women than in men). However, it appears that because the female kin affected are unrelated genetically, their common practice of cannibalism was indeed the cause of infection (Lindenbaum 1979).

Medical Practices: Traditional medical practices and treatments thought to protect man from illness have also been implicated in the transmission of parasitic diseases. In southern Africa, Nelson (1972) describes a popular medical practice which contributes to the very serious disease in man, cysticercosis. A brewed medicament from proglottids of the pork tapeworm, *Taenia solium,* is prepared for the patient suffering from, ironically, tape-worm infection. Direct ingestion of the infectious *T. solium* eggs in the gravid proglottids is held responsible for the rare development of the cysticercosis stage in man. This final illustration is, perhaps, most intriguing to the medical anthropologist since it is the community's indigenous health-care system which introduced and has since reinforced the practice among its members. For this reason it is important to consider how ethnomedicine — or popular medical beliefs and practices — has contributed to the epidemiology of infectious diseases.

ETHNOMEDICINE AND EPIDEMIOLOGY AS PARTNERS

Examining Ethnomedicine

Medical anthropologists have long shared a curiosity for the health beliefs and behaviors which exist outside the mainstream of medicine. Ethnomedicine is the formalized area of study which grew out of this curiosity. Hughes defines the term as "those beliefs and practices relating to disease which are the products of indigenous cultural development and not explicitly derived from the conceptual framework of modern medicine (1968: 87)". Thus, an ethnomedical study explores what has come to be called "the popular health culture" of the members of a society (Polgar 1962). Although not always recognized, a body of beliefs about disease, its relation to other aspects of life, its causes, and its cures, exists in all human groups. These health beliefs and their behavioral derivatives have evolved over much time as adaptive responses to the particular diseases that threaten each culture.

In an attempt to review, systematically, the major contributions of ethnomedicine to the epidemiology of infectious diseases, it seems best to divide the field into three (sometimes overlapping) areas: disease recognition, etiology and management. Each of these components of a given medical system is two-sided in that it has the potential to either enhance or hinder the health level of a community.

Lay Recognition of Infectious Diseases: Working within the limited framework of its own historical health experiences, every culture is responsible for creating a process with which to recognize and classify illnesses. Clearly, the entire folk decision-making process must be viewed in a cultural context. Cultures regularly are called upon to differentiate between serious dysfunctions and those that are minor, transient, or "natural". Common ailments of childhood and conditions that are endemic or regularly prevalent in an area are often explained as "natural". They may be treated with home remedies or, in many cases, go untreated. Of particular interest to the epidemiologist is that word of such illnesses may never reach beyond the walls of the victim's rural home — and rarely past the boundaries of the village.

Gillies (1976) reports that among the Ogori tribes, curers are not expected to intervene in cases of malaria, hepatitis or yellow fever. The common cold, seasonal diarrhea, measles, malaria and smallpox are regarded by the Zulu people as illnesses that "just happen" and thus require no outside intervention or consultation by local healers (Ngubane 1976). Young

Egyptian boys in the Nile Delta north of Cairo commonly excrete blood-stained urine due to infestation with a pathogenic blood fluke, *Shistosoma mansoni*. Yet, the endemic population does not recognize these boys as "diseased"; the child excreting unstained urine is the anomaly.

The human body has many ways of telling an individual that he/she is suffering from infection and that a special kind of attention is required to rid the body of disease. In many traditional societies, lay conceptions about human anatomy and the way in which the body fights off illness have been uncovered by the anthropologist. The first step in curing the ills of a community is, clearly, to first recognize the lay conceptions upon which a people base their recognition of a disease, then negotiate an acceptable approach.

When measles victims contract diarrhea in rural Bangladesh, mothers choose not to administer the often life-saving oral rehydration therapy available to their child in the belief that the body is actually flushing out unwanted impurities (Shahid 1983: 153). They commonly make an effort to hasten the eruption of measles based on a similar theory that the rash, held inside the intestines, must surface in order to properly cleanse the body. External applications of *nim* and *lai* leaves are used while patients are forced to ingest both nim and *karala* leaves (Shahid 1983).

Among the villagers of northeastern Brazil there exists a lay conception that the lung is connected directly to the intestinal tract. As a result, mucous and blood in the stool are not recognized as indicators of serious enteric infection, but rather of the inevitable release of mucal build-up in the lungs. Rather than seeking medical attention for the diarrhea, mothers choose to treat their infant's cold (Nations 1982).

Accurate recognition of an infectious disease changes according to the cultural setting in which it appears. Oral thrush (*Candida albicans*) is considered an essentially benign and transient condition in the United States. Mexicans, however, fear the infection— nicknamed "Algodon: The white sign of danger" — because it is, indeed, associated with high mortality in some areas (Mull and Mull 1983).

The folk definition and recognition of a condition as "serious" can reveal a number of clues to the epidemiologist about the nature of the disease under investigation. Under this topic of discussion falls a report of the cholera epidemic in Mali. Word of this "new" illness reached Mali in 1970 across the Guinean border — where it had hit for the first time in history. Descriptions of its acute onset, rapid clinical course, dramatic signs and symptoms, and high case fatality ratio dubbed the disease "Apollo". After all, what name conveyed the feeling of speed better than that of the recently launched U.S. space mission? The type and magnitude of the epidemic was unlike anything the Malians had encountered before. Traditional healers blamed the disaster on the whims of an overpowering God against whom their non-western remedies would have little success. But, vaccinations had proved effective against earlier attacks of measles and smallpox, so they supported the nationwide immunization program (Imperato 1974).

Lay Etiology of Disease: Belief systems of a culture influence the second step in the decision-making process as well: what is the causative agent cited for the illness and how should it be treated? Western industrial countries with belief systems based in "scientific-technological" values offer treatment such as anti-helminthic drugs, insecticides, and surgery directed at biological agents of disease. Other cultures, with different ideological input, attribute parasitic disease to imbalances in the equilibrium of a healthy body, soul loss, movement of real or imaginary parts of the body from their normal position, magical origins, or the "will of God", to name a few. Treatment, in keeping with these basic beliefs, is directed at specific "culture-bound" agents and can be understood only in light of the accepted etiology.

In many parts of the world measles is considered the handiwork of larger than life, malevolent gods rather than that of microscopic viruses. To the Bambari of Mali, for example, the ultimate cause of measles, prompted by excessive exposure to wind, is spiritual. Female witches (*nenenyi*) are held chiefly responsible for the thousands of young lives taken each year (Imperato 1968). Smallpox, in the eyes of the traditional Hindu medical system, is a punishment inflicted by Sitali Devi — the goddess of smallpox (Morinis 1978). Hindu rituals are designed to win the favor of the displeased goddess. Victims offer her cool water (since she dislikes heat), clean the house (since she forbids dirt), and make personal amends for any religious or social failings. Vaccination by the modern medical community has entered the collective health picture without displacing firmly established Hindu rituals. One protects villagers from the virus while the other "renders cosmic forces at work both comprehensible and manageable (Morinis 1978: 59)". The people of South India call smallpox, measles, chickenpox, and other similar diseases *ammai* and blame them on the goddess Mariammai. The annual festival for the goddess is considered the only safe protective measure against illness. Victims refuse biomedicine either to ward off disease or relieve symptoms. In accord with the wishes of the elders, who diagnose such diseases, victims hang *neem* leaves, clean house and eat only those foods defined as "cool" by the Indian community (Mather 1972).

Even in western societies, medical/religious beliefs alter the course of infectious diseases. One example, among many in the United States, occurred recently on an Illinois university campus where Christian Scientists responded to a measles outbreak by assuring students that "death and disease have no real existence because they are not created by God" (The Washington Post 1985). These teachings had a significant impact on the spread of the measles epidemic because students were not immunized. Many sought healing through prayer and refused medical treatment even after the onset of infection.

Few ethnomedical studies specifically deal with childhood diarrhea in terms of the folk decision-making process. One study is my own in north-eastern Brazil which I will discuss further on in some detail. Another was done in South India by Lozoff et al. in 1975. Beliefs about the cause of childhood diarrhea among medical personnel and Indian families differ significantly. Open-ended interviews with fifty-six families in Vellore, India revealed that the most common folk explanation for diarrhea was "heat in the body", producing stools with froth, pus or blood. Severe dehydration was conceived as an entirely independent condition caused by ritual impurity or pollution. As a result, popular treatments for diarrhea and dehydration require either a rebalancing of the hot-cold equilibrium, or ritual purification of the child's body, respectively. The authors argue that modern rehydration therapy must be adusted to meet the essential requirements of both folk and biomedical belief systems (Lozoff et al. 1975)

Lay Treatment of Disease: Just as etiologies differ drastically between cultures, so too do the treatments chosen to free the affected individual from illness. The attitudinal system of the endemic population detemines to whom the patient will go for treatment, the type of treatment accepted, preventive measures followed, and the success of intervention on the part of extra-community medical systems.

The high frequency of the hepatitis B antigen (HB Ag) in South African Bantu seems in part due to the scarification of the skin by witch-doctors. Findings which compared scarred and unscarred Bantu suggest that the use of unsterilized instruments during tribal ceremonies may be a factor responsible for spreading the HB Ag in certain populations (Kew et al. 1973).

The use of lead-containing preparations in traditional practices presents a significant health hazard to a substantial section of the world's population. In Nigeria, the native doctor ("Babalawo") and the local herbalist ("Eleweomo") are frequently the only practitioners available to manage the outbreak of infectious diseases. Little is known about the pharmacological content of the remedies they choose, but studies have revealed alarming concentrations of lead in the widely used treatment, "tiro" (Healy et al. 1984).

Traditional medicine, its preparations and practices, plays a major role in many sub-cultures of the United States. Analyses of Asian folk remedies in the U.S. have revealed fatal levels of lead in such materials as "ghasard", a brown power given to some children on a daily basis as a tonic (MMWR 1984: 645). Lead containing folk remedies have been identified as the culprit in poisoning cases among Hmong and Mexican-Hispanic children as well (MMWR 1984: 644). Two toxic ethnomedical subtances, *greta* and *azarcon*, have recently been discovered in the Southwest U.S. They are, respectively, lead oxide and lead tetroxide, and have been used for at least four generations in the treatment of a Mexican-American culture-bound syndrome, *empacho*. Both compounds are far more toxic than swallowing elemental lead, and have been linked with over fifteen cases of clinically identified lead poisonings in the Southwest (Trotter 1985).

In the urban-north U.S. a voodoo medicinal potion has been implicated in the death of at least one young, black worshipper (Saphir 1967). Another study has linked the consultation of herbalists by both urban and rural blacks with subsequent poisoning (Buchanan and Cane 1976).

When the harmful properties of some ethnomedical treatments are considered, epidemiologists and social scientists alike are tempted to regard the entire package of traditional remedies as inferior to western, biomedical ones. However, efforts to locate, isolate, and analyze a number of natural remedies whose effectiveness has been proven over centuries have ended in some convincing and truly fascinating information for the western scientist. Such efforts resulted in the discovery of quinine, which has been used for centuries to treat malaria in tropical regions of the world. The natural chemical — which comes directly from the bark of the cinchona tree in Asia and Africa — has been successfully synthesized in many western laboratories (Kubo 1982). Amazon healers prescribe another tree bark derivative — veronica — to treat the parasitic disease schistosomiasis. Prescription drugs made from synthetic chemicals are available to treat schistosomiasis, but these are so strong that they may damage or destroy essential body tissue (Kubo 1982). A natural substance with no side effects, veronica may prove useful not only as a curative measure, but as the basis of an insecticide (antifeedant) directed at the disease's deadly vector, a water snail. Focusing on the eradication of the snail vector, several naturally occurring molluscicides have been isolated in the lab (Kubo 1983b; Kubo 1984b; Kubo 1984c). In the jungles of South America, the small, bitter fruit of the olive tree is the weapon of the people in their fight against malaria. Two components of the molluscicidal agent found in fruit have been extensively studied in hopes of expanding their use from the South American villages to threatened populations worldwide (Kubo 1984c).

In the East African bush, Bwana Mganga (tribal medicine men) offer herbal teas brewed from the orange berry of the *Maesa lanceolata* bush to cholera victims. Those in danger of being infected sip the tea daily as a precautionary measure. In the lab, analysis led chemists to "maesanin", a compound whose anti-bacterial activity evokes a non-specific host defense reaction (Kubo 1983a).

In rural India, curry is made from a spicy tasting bark from the warburgia bush which also provides local healers with a treatment for stubborn fungal infections. Labs in the U.S. have isolated a chemical from the warburgia bush which dramatically enhances the effectiveness of low-dose antibiotics. In certain areas of the world where such infections are considered serious (such as the previously discussed candidiasis), the discovery could prove life-saving (Kubo 1984b).

In Kenya, African natives dump large quantities of cashew fruit into the ponds where mosquitoes and aquatic snails breed. This leftover from Africa's cashew nut export business holds, for the local community, a powerful insecticide and barrier against disease. The chemical, identified as anacardic acid is deadly to the mosquitoes that carry malaria and the snails that transmit schistosomiasis (Kubo 1984a).

Among the Hausa of northern Nigeria, herbal pharmacopoeia has proven an effective weapon against malarial infection. Laboratory studies have tested the hypothesis that the chemical components of the traditional remedies actually increase levels of intracellular oxidation and, in this way, interfere with parasite development. Data suggest that this action is indeed of therapeutic value in the prevention and/or treatment of malaria (Etkin 1979).

Applying Ethnomedicine Nationwide

The inadequacy and ineffectiveness of existing tropical disease control measures worldwide prompted the establishment of the Special Program for Research and Training in Tropical Diseases, co-sponsored by the UNDP/ World Bank/WHO in 1980 (Rosenfield et al. 1981). The program's aims are two-fold. Investigators have called for the improvement of existing tools used to combat certain priority diseases intimately associated with poverty conditions (malaria, schistosomiasis, filariasis, trypanosomiasis, leprosy and leishmaniasis). And, in hopes of developing effective "new" tools, they have supported programs that identify social aspects of disease causation, transmission and control. The program is innovative in its emphasis on using the methods and orientations of the behavioral sciences in parasitic disease research and control programs (Dunn 1979). The program's goals have been well received. Dunn stresses that comprehensive studies ought to incorporate quantitative data with observational data in order to be effective. They would give meaning to traditional practices and provide a rationale for planning programs designed to either modify disease-related behaviors or the environment.

The trans-disciplinary perspective which is the foundation for the UNDP/ WB/WHO program is one which has also given rise to a nation-wide attack on schistosomiasis in China. Recognizing the importance of traditional remedies, as well as the strength with which spiritual beliefs are rooted in the Chinese culture, China's anti-schistosomiasis campaign was guided by the celebrated policy of "walking on two legs" (Cheng 1971). That is, the treatments and practices of both Chinese and Western medical systems were used in the campaign's control measures starting in the 1950s. Those dedicated to coping with huge numbers of infected people realized that the success of their program rested on an ability to understand the firmly established Chinese system of health care. An enormous network of health workers was set in action to study disease etiology and treatments. People in endemic areas, understandably, attributed their suffering to "natural" and supernatural events: unfavorable "wind and water" or "evil spirits" (Cheng 1971). Education programs were instituted in the most rural areas, and studies of the indigenous, natural treatments were conducted in the labs. For example, Chinese healers have orally given ground, dried pumpkin seed (*Cucurbita moschata*) to their schistosomiasis patients for years (Cheng 1971). The striking therapeutic effects of this cure and other natural preparations have been analyzed and described in biochemical terms. This kind of approach is a vital one for a country truly dedicated to eliminating the long-standing separation of two drastically different — but equally important — medical systems.

CREATIVE CONTRIBUTIONS OF ETHNOMEDICINE TO THE EPIDEMIOLOGY OF INFECTIOUS DISEASE

A number of specific areas can be identified in which an ethnomedical perspective can guard against epidemiology becoming bound by its own rigor; areas where sensitivity to cultural factors can foster a reasonable approach to analysis, and in which conclusions can more closely mirror reality. In descriptive epidemiology — or the subfield that accounts for what diseases are present, when and where — there are three areas where an ethnomedical perspective is relevant: first, in the detection of mortality and establishment of death rates; second, in the detection of morbidity and generation of attack rates; and third, in the identification of high risk populations for selective treatment and referral. In analytic epidemiology — or the subfield which probes the hows and whys of disease patterns — it is the identification of behavioral risk (or health promotive) factors in which an ethnomedical perspective can add tremendous insight.

To illustrate how knowledge of an individual's health perceptions, beliefs and actions can contribute creatively to each of these tasks, and to research in infectious diseases in general, I present data gathered from field research on acute and chronic enteric infections in northeastern Brazil. This work was conducted in Fortaleza, Brazil in collaboration with the University of Virginia Division of Geographic Medicine and the Universidade Federal do Ceara School of Medicine.

Detecting Mortality and Establishing Accurate Causes of Death

Mortality rates are the pulse by which a country's health is measured; they alert planners not only to the adequacy of a nation's medical resources, but also serve as a general index of socio-economic development. Hence, it is upon death rates that decision-makers formulate national and even global health strategies, allocate resources, and base health research. With such an important function, it seems odd that mortality statistics, especially in developing nations, remain inadaquate. As of 1970, reliable national mortality statistics were available for only about 35% of the world's population (World Health Organization 1970). Many epidemiologists are well aware of these shortcomings in current analytic approaches and are among the first to claim that new methods to accurately grasp childhood deaths are needed. This problem is explicitly recognized by the following, all-too-familiar disclaimer: "due to unrecorded early infant deaths, especially in rural areas, these rates may underrepresent actual childhood mortality in this region". Such serious underreporting of infant mortality is the case in northeastern Brazil. In one rural community we carefully researched mortality on a house to house basis. Only 14 out of 49 childhood deaths occurring during 1984 were on record at the official death registry (J. McAuliffe p. c.). But, is this problem of underrepresentation simply a logistical one, such as not having enough money or manpower to conduct thorough mortality reviews, as we are generally lead to believe? Or does the problem equally rest on the inappropriateness of current epidemiologic survey methods used to identify and record the occurrence of death? Both of these are important factors which work to limit the accuracy of health statistics, but the latter is central and often overlooked.

In the earliest phase of a survey, epidemiologists are called upon to calculate an ideal sample size based on statistical models derived from observed and expected mortality rates. Clearly, an expected value which misses its mark will throw off all subsequent calculations. And, it threatens to turn out a sample size far from the ideal: so large that it costs the investigator unnecessary time and money, or so small that it fails to provide convincing conclusions. New methods of estimating deaths in underdeveloped areas, including the observational techniques characteristic of anthropology, might be adopted to more reliably approximate expected mortality rates.

Most mortality rates are based on data from official death registries (eg. Puffer and Serrano 1973). Yet, "hidden" deaths often occur, are dealt with within the popular realm and, hence, go undetected by the official system. The reasons for this are many: inaccessibility of registry offices, lack of education and knowledge about the system, suspicion that records will be used by the government for taxation or military purposes, and fear on behalf of squatters or illegal aliens to reveal their identity, among others (Basch 1978). For example, one community-based mortality surveillance conducted in rural Indonesia by the World Health Organization's Diarrheal Diseases Control Division was believed, by locals, to have missed a substantial number of infant deaths (M. Merson, p. c.). This is a serious methodological flaw if these rates are to serve as baseline data to document the impact of WHO's Oral Rehydration Programs.

One solution to this dilemma is for the researcher to probe the local funerary culture in order to learn the ethnomedical beliefs and practices surrounding early and childhood death and burial. Does, for instance, the culture in question practice intentional infanticide or simply neglect selected children, leaving them to the ravages of one of many infantile illnesses, as has been reported among the Chaga of East Africa (Raum 1940)? If infanticide is practiced, is it the direct result of moral transgressions by the parent(s) (eg. an illegitimate pregnancy, pre-marital or extra-marital relations) such that the formal announcement of death carries with it social repercussions? Where are infants and children buried? Does the burial site for children differ from adults as is the case among the Ngoni of Africa who bury one twin under the veranda of the hut so as to, presumably, keep it close to the surviving twin (Read 1968)? Are newborns named immediately after birth or do they remain in a liminal or ambiguous state for some time, as is also reported among the Ngoni (Real 1968)? Moreover, is their incorporation as individuals into the society so limited that their early death is of less consequence to the family and, hence, less likely to be reported when epidemiologists ask parents to "name their children who have died?" At the grassroots level, what types of people are responsible for providing medical care to infants during the perinatal period and who is involved directly in mourning or burial rituals?

Providing answers to these and other questions relating to childhood death is one aspect of ethnomedical research. In northeastern Brazil, for example, I learned in several instances involving illegitimate births that these newborns were not named, but simply referred to as *angelinhos* (little angels) who, because they had not yet sinned, were expected by parents to fly straight to heaven. "Little angels", I was told, "were not of this world, but were already in God's keeping". Given this belief, it is barely surprising that mothers neglected the secular task of registering their infants' deaths with the official state registrar or church. Economic sanctions also prevented proper death registration; mothers had to walk to town, pay a registration fee, and risk losing the child's food supplements (her own too, if she was nursing) provided by the state. The deaths of these little angels remained "hidden", except, of course, to the traditional healer (*rezadeira*) who was treating them, neighbors who lit votive candles as tributes, the local craftsman who built the rustic wooden coffin, the school children who carried the open boxes in processions through the village streets, and the men and cemetery keeper who dug the graves and buried the *angelinhos*. These are *not* the people who customarily report vital statistics to health bureaucracies.

Just as an ethnomedical perspective can be critical in identifying who died, it can also illuminate causes of death. In January of 1980, our UVA project physician/epidemiologist reviewed the deaths of 43 project children with their parents in order to determine a most probable cause of death. By taking a formal medical history, the physician established that diarrhea/dehyration was by far the leading cause of death, followed by respiratory problems, measles, perinatal complications and others. Three months later, in April, I visited the same families studied by the UVA physician/epidemiologist. This time, however, the aim was to elicit what Kleinman (1978) has called the parent's own explanatory model of their child's health problem and cause of death. As Table I shows, rarely did the biomedical and ethnomedical perspectives on the causes of death agree. Instead, villagers believed deaths attributed by biomedicine to diarrhea and dehydration were caused by things ranging from, for example, supernatural illnesses like fright disease (*susto*) and evil eye (*quebranto*) to teething (*denticao*) and contaminated milk. Deaths judged by physicians to have resulted from respiratory problems were popularly believed to be caused by "taking birth in the nose" or "conditions

TABLE I

Biomedical and ethnomedical causes of 43 childhood deaths in Pacatuba, Brazil 1980

Biomedical	Ethnomedical	
Most probable cause of death as determined by physician/epidemiologist (*n* = 46)	Cause of death elicited from family by medical anthropologist (*n* = 62)	
DIARRHEA/DEHYDRATION (32)	'Fright disease'	(18)
	'Evil eye'	(8)
	'Illness of the child'	(8)
	'Teething'	(4)
	'Swollen belly'	(2)
	'Wind in umbilical cord; cord didn't fall off'	(1)
	'Weakness from cold vapor rising from floor'	(1)
	'Born sick'	(1)
	'Contaminated milk'	(1)
	'Worms'	(1)
RESPIRATORY PROBLEMS (3)		
— respiratory obstruction (1)	'Taking birth in nose'	(1)
— inflammed throat, cough, fever (1)	'White balls in throat'	(1)
— penumonia (1)	'Condition of hospital'	(1)
MEASLES (3)	'Strong wind entered child's body'	(2)
	'Cold'	(1)
	'Agitated blood'	(1)
	'Fright disease with fever'	(1)
PERINATAL (3)		
— birth trauma (1)	'Fright disease attacking baby in womb'	(1)
— premature birth (2)	'Mother's sadness during pregnancy'	(2)
OTHER (5)		
— intestinal obstruction (1)	'Swollen belly'	(1)
	'Prison of feces/urine'	(1)
— disseminated canidiasis (1)	'White balls in mouth'	(1)
— anemia (1)	'Lack of blood'	(1)
— accident (2)	'Accident' (fire, drowning)	(2)

in the hospital". Death due to premature birth was thought by local women to be caused by "the mother's saddness during pregnancy". Only in the case of "accidents" did doctors and villagers agree exactly.

Clearly, knowing the family's explanation of death, the symptoms associated with each folk illness, and, when feasible, correlations of folk with biomedical diagnostic criteria can aid and direct epidemiologists in their retrospective reconstruction of circumstances surrounding a child's death. It is also important to realize that many cultures consider dissection of the dead abhorrent and contrary to religious beliefs. Establishing an exact cause of death in these cases is often impossible (Basch 1978).

Detecting Morbidity and Establishing Accurate Attack Rates

Assessing the level of sickness in a community and calculating the number of illness episodes suffered per person per year is often done by epidemiologists, who typically conduct weekly or even daily prospective household surveillance. This was the case in the UVA-UFC study. Village mothers kept a clipboard which displayed a picture of each child in the family. Beside the photo was a box for each day of the week in which she was to mark an "X" on the days her child suffered diarrhea and a "0" when no diarrhea was present. Once a week a Brazilian medical student would visit the house, review the data and collect the form. At this time stool samples were collected. These samples were later subjected to microbiologic analysis and classified according to the biomedical scheme as: (1) a noninflammatory or secretory diarrhea characterized by *V. cholerae* and enterotoxigenic *E. coli*; (2) an inflammatory diarrhea or dysentery characterized by *Shigella* and *Campylobacter jejuni*; or (3) a penetrating diarrhea caused by such pathogens as *Samonella typhi*. These data were then analyzed quantitatively to yield both age- and pathogen-specific attack rates for diarrhea.

Although these analytic steps represent standard procedure for epidemiologic studies of infectious diseases, the essential methodologic question is this: Do these statistically impressive epidemiologic conclusions flow from a valid and reliable data set? That is, do survey data capture the actual occurrence of sickness in the household, especially when village mothers' perceptions of illness are based in a different etiologic system? Dona Maria, for instance, reported to the investigating medical student that Carlos, her son, did not have diarrhea on the morning I stayed with the family. Soon after the student left, Carlos defecated a liquid stool streaked with blood and mucous. Questioned tactfully about the discrepancy in her reporting, Dona Maria replied that "Carlos doesn't have diarrhea, he has *quintura*" (intestinal heat). Clearly, this village mother's folk taxonomy of gastrointestinal illness differed significantly from our project physician's notions. She believed that diarrhea was a symptom of at least five folk illnesses — evil eye (*quebranto*), fright disease (*susto*), spirit intrusion (*encosto*), illness of the child (*doenca da crianca*) and intestinal heat (*quintura*) — each with their own social meaning, physical symptoms and even stool characteristics. However, the medical student never asked about these problems. Maybe, she reasoned, "they just didn't want to know about these things".

As Dona Maria's response illustrates, any epidemiologic survey which hopes to reasonably mirror household illness patterns must begin with a thorough understanding of the popular folk medical taxonomy. Next, suspected correlations, or even partial points of overlap between the popular and biomedical etiologic systems should be explored. For example, we are currently testing the hypothesis that the folk illness "intestinal heat" (or the accumlation of excesssive heat in the intestine) — with its characteristic symptoms of blood, mucoid stools, fever and abdominal cramping — correlates closely with inflammatory diarrhea or dysentery. Such information will allow the epidemiologist to design surveillance questionnaires that include inquiries into locally-recognized illness and so increase the likelihood that specific symptoms, such as diarrhea, are detected and are reflected in attack rates.

The Identification of High Risk Indicators for Selective Treatment and Referral

A major goal of descriptive epidemiology is to characterize, on the basis of morbidity and mortality data, that portion of the population which is at highest risk for a particular disease. Until now, epidemiologists have neglected the consideration of folk illnesses in helping to identify those persons at high risk for developing clinical disease. Because common and deadly conditions such as malnutrition and diarrhea pose such a danger to infants' survival, it is not surprising that indigenous medical systems have evolved special labels for the most serious, life threatening conditions. The "*runche*" child — literally "the crying one", for example, is easily recognized by adults living in rural Nepal; he/she is miserable, whinny, hard to live with and refuses to eat — behaviors which worsen following episodes of diarrhea, fever, or measles. The traditional recognition of this folk illness (*runche*) resulted in the earlier and faster diagnosis of undernutrition by physicians, without requiring costly individual nutritional assessments (Bomgaars 1976). In Brazil we discovered similar cultural clues to identify children at high risk for severe dehydration. Children with the folk illness "fallen fontenelle" (when the soft spot on the top of the head has sunken deep into the skull) and those with "eyes of angels" who "looked towards God with glazed-over eyes", were the same children doctors judged to have severe dehydration and to be in need of immediate rehydration and transfer to urban hospitals for supervised care.

The astute epidemiologist can seize upon such longstanding and widely recognised "omens of death" to help generate high risk profiles for common infectious diseases. From these, selective medical interventions can be developed and referral pathways can be built linking traditional healers with back-up biomedical care without ever introducing unfamiliar diagnostic skills such as the widely advocated skin tugor test and medical jargon such as "dehydration".

The Identification of Behavioral Risk Factors and the Generation of Testable Hypotheses

Analytic epidemiology wrestles with the hows and whys of existing patterns in human disease; its mission includes identifying potential risk (or protective) factors, and then examining their correlation with disease outcomes. The standard analytic approach often encountered in infectious disease research includes examining the relationship of well-recognized socioeconomic factors such as income, education, nutritional status, maternal literacy, housing type or size and water source with infection and morbidity. Sometimes with multiple regression analysis, the number of factors examined at once may become quite complex. However, given the entire range of the human condition, are *these* simple social and economic factors the most sensible to examine; are *they* the ones most closely tied to the disease transmission process? Is it even possible to consider the totality of factors which bear on the course of disease while designing research protocols, often thousands of miles away from the field? Without in-depth knowledge of the social, cultural and ecological context of the research setting, the answer is no. Only with detailed anthropological observations of people going about life as usual is it possible to achieve a good understanding of the complex causal chains in disease etiology.

In Brazil, that meant following and observing children as they played, scavenged food, took baths in the river, received herbal cures from the local Voodoo healer and defecated on the kitchen floor when the rains began. These ethnographic descriptions, grounded in popular health beliefs and practices, provide the creative spark that ignites a chain of thought leading to hypothesis formulation and can eventually lead to documenting powerful links between socio-cultural factors and disease.

For example, during many informal conversations with indigenous healers about children's health in rural Brazil, I was repeatedly warned by them of a change that was occuring in the traditional practice of prolonged breast-feeding, and the negative effect the shift to bottlefeeding was having on infants' health. Healers bluntly told me that "a crianca que nao amama, morre!" (the child that does not breastfeed, dies!). Following up on this clue, I examined, retrospectively, the pregnancy and breastfeeding histories of 53 project mothers, representing 307 child feeding experiences (Nations 1982). What I "rediscovered" was that for the first time in this community, a dramatic decline was occurring in both the initiation and duration of breastfeeding. The decline began around 1955 and by 1980, 54% of wealthier project women and 10% of the very poorest mothers did not even initiate lactation. Of the 90% of the poorest women who did breastfeed, breastmilk substitutes including *minguas,* or cereals made from commercially-prepared rice, corn, wheat flakes or manioc root mixed with powdered milk formulas, as well as teas and other weaning foods, were now being introduced almost immediately after birth, an average of only two weeks postpartum.

This observation prompted us to hypothesize that the change in the traditional practice of prolonged breasfeeding would have a significant impact on the incidence of diarrheal diseases. To test this hypothesis we correlated the daily prospective diarrhea records of 15 project newborns with feeding methods for a total of nearly 5,000 days of observation. We discovered that when infants were breastfeed exclusively, they spent fewer than 2% of their days with diarrhea. When infants were fed weaning foods — formulas, cereals, teas — together with breastmilk, they experienced a significant increase in illness, spending nearly 10% of their days with diarrhea. In the first 6 weeks after breastfeeding was stopped altogether, a further significant increase in diarrhea occurred. These children spent over 20% of their days with diarrhea. This represents more than a ten fold increase in the risk of diarrhea with weaning. We then proposed that the increased risk bottlefeeding poses for infants was due to at least two factors: increased exposure to environmental contaminants, particularly highly polluted village water supplies used to dilute formulas, and to the loss of protective factors contained in mother's milk. Our laboratories documented both the rapid proliferation of fecal coliforms in milk formulas mixed with river water and the presence of measurable antibody titers in mothers' milk and colostrum against enterotoxigenic *E. coli* and rotaviruses — the two most frequent enteric pathogens identified in this community.

Insights from the popular medical realm were central to our research; these ethnomedical clues led us to examine a factor — changing infant feeding practices — that had not been planned in the initial project design. The results proved timely. The Brazilian National Breastfeeding Promotion Program had just begun, and our data were utilized to help convince local Brazilian physicians to promote breastfeeding as an important preventive strategy for diarrhea. But, village healers only laughed as our team pored over mounds of data sheets for long hours, then rejoiced in the findings. After all, hadn't they told us so?

Our anthropological observations of household ethnomedical practices relating to child care have suggested many more questions including the following: What impact, if any, does the widespread ritual practice of expressing and discarding antibody-rich colostrum at the base of the clay household water pot have on childrens' health and on diarrheal illnesses in particular? Does the common widespread practice of dirt-eating (geophagia) by village children play a significant role in the transmission of soil borne parasites such as *Ascaris lumbricoides, Strongyloides stercoralies,* or *Toxocara canis*? The list of ethnomedically-derived hypotheses is virtually limitless. The focus, however, is on the direct link of ethnomedical beliefs and practices to real life observations among people who actually suffer the illnesses epidemiologists describe and analyze.

CONCLUSION: IMPLICATIONS OF COLLABORATIVE EFFORTS BETWEEN ANTHROPOLOGY AND EPIDEMIOLOGY FOR INFECTIOUS DISEASES RESEARCH

By joining forces, the medical anthropologist and the epidemiologist can bring the strengths of both of their disciplines to bear on critical health problems worldwide, such as the widespread infectious diseases. With the inclusion of an ethnomedical perspective into the field of epidemiology, however, I foresee major methodological as well as theoretical implications. Likely we will witness the sharpening of mortality surveillance methods so that they are tied more closely to local cultural settings and are less dependent on official death records. Community resources will be tapped more often to form mortality networks comprised of people involved directly with childhood death such as the traditional healer, midwife, coffin maker, grave digger, cemetery keeper, the local merchant or vender who sells candles, grave wreaths and other religious items, and neighborhood children who help bury their unfortunate playmates.

Another implication of this merger may well be the restructuring of morbidity surveillance methods which incorporate ethnomedical illnesses and lead to the construction of what Pfifferling has called a "folk-perceived morbidity profile (1975)". The utility of such an emic assessment for medicine, however, will rest on demonstrating its correlation (even in the broadest sense) with biomedical taxonomies.

When tapped as a shorthand and cost-effective method to identify serious illnesses for referral, epidemiologic research on cultural indicators of high risk, such as those discussed above, will almost certainly fuel the development of innovative rural health care delivery models. This implication, will be realized in the very near future given the recent thrust towards primary health care and the ever-growing involvement of lay healers in providing basic medical interventions, such as oral rehydration therapy.

Theoretically, lending weight to peoples' health beliefs and practices in epidemiology will press us to rethink widely accepted Western biomedical schemata of disease classification and etiology, such as the standard International Classification of Diseases (ICD-9-CM). It will force us to wrestle conceptually, once again, with multiple causes of illnesses, as social factors achieve explanatory prominence in the study of infectious diseases. It will demand that epidemiologists deal with the often "soft" and "untidy" qualitative data that will challenge even the most sophisticated linear mathematical model. In short, it represents a significant paradigm shift. Epidemiology will require a headlong plunge into resolving, once and for all, what Dunn has previously called the "epidemiological paradox" — that is, the epidemiologist's "decreasing ability to deal quantitatively with causal assemblages as their size and complexity increase, and as their scope extends into the psychosocial domains (Dunn 1975)".

How often I have heard the frustrations inherent in this "epidemiologic paradox" expressed by colleagues while investigating infectious diarrhea in Brazil. *If* only we could guarantee that all drinking water in this neighborhood comes from the Sao Joao river, *then* we could pinpoint the transmission of enteric pathogens to water. *If* only we could assume that the village childrens' total food intake comes from meals eaten at home, *then* we could show a clear relationship between dietary intake, diarrhea and malnutrition. However, women make choices every day about the sources of water they will use based on its availability, distance from the house, color, taste, clarity, movement or exposure to the sun, and poor children often scavenge for food from friends, neighbors and anywhere else they can find it. Simplification for the purpose of statistical analysis is often difficult, if not impossible when dealing with complex human behavior.

Perhaps having to deal with ethnomedical data will force us to capture the whole health picture and to stress the interrelatedness of each part in contributing to disease. Indeed, if such a paradigm shift is not forthcoming, I fear epidemiologic *rigor* in infectious diseases research will be more akin to *rigor*mortis.

REFERENCES

Alland, A., Jr.
   1966 Medical Anthropology and the Study of Biological and Cultural Adaptation. American Anthropologist 68(1): 40—51.
Armelogos, G. J., A. Goodman, and K. H. Jacobs
   1978 The Ecological Perspective in Disease. *In* M. Logan and E. Hunt (eds.), Health and the Human Condition, pp. 71—83. North Scituate, Mass.: Duxbury Press.
Audy, R. J.
   1971 Measurement and Diagnosis of Health. *In* P. Shepard and D. McKinley (eds.), Environ/Mental: Essays on the Planet as a Home, pp. 140—162. New York: Houghton Mifflin.
Basch, P. F.
   1978 International Health. New York: Oxford University Press.
Bomgaars, M. R.
   1976 Undernutrition: Cultural Diagnosis and Treatment of Runche. JAMA 236(22): 2513.
Buchanan, N. and R. D. Cane
   1976 Poisoning Associated with Witchdoctor Attendance. JAMA 50: 1138—1140.

Cassel, J.
    1964 Social Science Theory as a Source of Hypotheses in Epidemiological Research.
          American Journal of Public Health 55: 1482—1488.
Cheng, T. A.
    1971 Schistosomiasis in Mainland China: A Review of Research and Control Programs
          Since 1949. The American Journal of Tropical Medicine and Hygiene 20(1): 26—
          53.
Cockburn, T. A.
    1967 Infectious Diseases: Their Evolution and Eradication. Springfield, Ill.: Charles C.
          Thomas.
    1978 Commission on Professional and Hospital Activities. The International Classifica-
          tion of Diseases. 9th revision. (ICD-9-CM). Ann Arbor, Mich.: Edwards Bros., Inc.
Dubos, R.
    1959 Mirage of Health. Garden City: Doubleday-Anchor.
    1965 Man Adapting. 1970 printing. New Haven: Yale University Press.
Dunn, F. L.
    1969 Social Relationships, Kinship and Communicable Transmission. Proceedings of the
          VIIIthe International Congress of Anthropological and Ethnological Sciences, 1968,
          Tokyo and Kyoto. Science Council of Japan. Vol. 1, Anthropology, section A-7,
          Medical Anthrlopology, p. 243.
    1975 Causal Assemblages in Epidemiology as Sources of Hypotheses in Anthropological
          Research. Paper presented at the American Anthropological Association, Medical
          Anthropology Symposium, December 4.
    1976a Human Behavioral Factors in the Epidemiology and Control of *Wuchereria* and
          Brugia Infections. Bulletin of the Public Health Society 10: 34—44.
    1976b Human Behavioral Studies in Parasitic Disease Research and Control. Assignment
          Report. Dept. of International Health and the George Williams Hooper Foundation,
          School of Medicine, University of California, San Francisco, pp. 1—44.
    1979 Behavioral Aspects of the Control of Parasitic Diseases. Bulletin of the World
          Health Organization 57(4): 499—665.
Etkin, M. L.
    1979 Indigenous Medicine Among the Hausa of Northern Nigeria: Laboratory Evaluation
          for Potential Therapeutic Efficacy of Antimalarial Plant Medicinals. Medical An-
          thropology. 3(4): 401—429.
Fabrega, H., Jr.
    1972 Medical Anthropology. *In* B. Siegal, (ed.), Biennial Review of Anthropology, pp.
          167—229. Stanford: University Press.
Fan, P. C. and O. K. Khaw
    1964 Relationship of Food Habits to Human Infection with *Paragonimus westermani*.
          Chinese Medical Journal 11: 55—64.
Farooq, M. and M. B. Mallah
    1966 The Behavioral Pattern of Social and Religious Water-Contact Activities in the
          Egypt-49 Bilharziasis Project Area. Bulletin of the World Health Organization 35:
          377—387.
Fleck, A. C. Jr. and F. A. Ianni
    1958 Epidemiology and Anthropology: Some Suggested Affinities in Theory and Method.
          Human Organization 16(4): 35—40.
Gajdusek, D. C.
    1973 Kuru in the New Guinea Highlands. *In* J. D. Spillane (ed.), Tropical Neurology, pp.
          377—383. New York: Oxford University Press.
Gillies, E.
    1976 Causal Criteria in African Classifications of Disease. *In* J. B. Loudon (ed.), Social
          Anthropology and Medicine, pp. 358—395. New York: Academic Press.

Glickman, L. T. et al.
    1981 Pica Patterns, Toxocariasis and Elevated Blood Lead in Children. American Journal
           of Tropical Medicine and Hygiene 30: 77—80.
Guerrant, R. L. et al.
    1983 Prospective Study of Diarrheal Illness in Northeastern Brazil: Patterns of Disease,
           Nutritional Impact, Etiologies and Risk Factors. Journal of Infectious Disease
           148(6): 986—997.
Healy, M. A., M. Aslam, and O. A. Bamgboye
    1984 Traditional Medicine and Lead-containing Preparations in Nigeria. Public Health
           98: 26—32.
Hughes, C. C.
    1968 Ethnomedicine. In The International Encyclopedia of Social Sciences, 10: 87—93.
           New York: Free Press/MacMillan.
Imperato, P. J.
    1968 Traditional Beliefs About Measles and its Treatment Among the Bambara of Mali.
           Tropical and Geographical Medicine 21: 62—67.
    1974 Cholera in Mali and Popular Reactions to Its First Appearance. Journal of Tropical
           Medicine and Hygiene 77(12): 290—296.
Imperato, P. J. et al.
    1974 Trichinosis Among Those Living In New York City. JAMA 227: 526—529.
Kew, M. C. et al.
    1973 The Witch Doctor and Tribal Scarification of the Skin and the Hepatitis B Antigen.
           South African Medical Journal 47: 2419—2420.
Kleinman, A., L. Eisenberg, and B. Good
    1978 Culture, Illness, and Care: Clinical Lessons from Anthropologic and Cross-Cultural
           Research. Annals of Internal Medicine 88: 251—258.
Kochar, V. K. et al.
    1973 Human Factors in the Regulation of Parasitic Infections: Cultural Ecology of Hook-
           worm Populations in Rural West Bengal. In F. Haley et al. (eds.), Medical Anthro-
           pology, pp. 287—311. Paris: Mouton Publishers.
Kubo, I.
    1982 Pharmacies in the Jungle. In World Book (eds.), The Science Year, pp. 126—137.
           Childcraft International Inc.
    1983a Antibacterial Quinone's Structure Determined. Tetrahedron, p. 3825.
    1983b Structure of Mukaadial: A Molluscicide from the Warburgia Plants. Chemistry
           Letters, pp. 979—980.
    1984a Fighting Two Deadly Diseases. The New York Times. December 4, 1984.
    1984b Molluscicides and Insecticidal Activities of Isobutylamides Isolated from Fagara
           macrophylla. Experientia Basel, Switzerland 40: 340—341.
    1984c Molluscicides from Olive europaea and their Efficient Isolation by Countercurrent
           Chromatographics. Journal of Agricultural and Food Chemistry 32: 687.
    1984d Plant Extract Fights Fungus. Science News 125: 375.
    1984 Lead Poisoning: Associated Death from Asian Folk Remedies. Morbidity and
           Mortality Weekly Report 33(45): 638, 643—645.
Lindenbaum, S.
    1979 Kuru Sorcery. Los Angeles, Mayfield Publishing Co.
Livingstone, F.
    1958 Anthropological Implications of Sickle Cell Gene Distribution in West Aftrica.
           American Anthropologist 60: 533—562.
Lozoff, B.
    1975 Infection and Disease in South Indian Families: Beliefs about Childhood Diarrhea.
           Human Organization 34: 353—358.

Mather, R. J. and T. J. John
 1972 Popular Beliefs About Smallpox and Other Common Infectious Diseases in South
      India. Tropical and Geographical Medicine 25: 190—196.
May, J. M.
 1960 The Ecology of Human Diseasē. Annals of the New York Academy of Sciences
      84(17): 789—794.
Morinis, E. A.
 1978 Two Pathways in Understanding Disease: Traditional and Scientific. WHO Chroni-
      cle 32: 57—59.
Mull, D. S. and J. D. Mull
 1983 Algodoncillo: White Sign of Danger. Medical Anthropology Quarterly 14(4): 9—13.
Nations, M. K.
 1982 Illness of the Child: The Cultural Context of Childhood Diarrhea in Northeast
      Brazil. Ph. D. Dissertation, Department of Anthropology, University of California,
      Berkeley.
Nelson, G. S.
 1972 Human Behavior in the Transmission of Parasitic Disease. In E. U. Cunning and C.
      A. Wright (eds.), Behavioral Aspects of Parasitic Transmission, pp. 109—121. New
      York: Academic Press, Inc.
Ngubane, H.
 1976 Some Aspects of Treatment Among the Zulu. In J. B. Loudon (ed.), Social Anthro-
      pology and Medicine, pp. 318—357. New York: Academic Press.
Nurge, E.
 1975 Anthropological Perspective for Medical Students. Human Organization 34(4):
      348—351.
Peters, T. J. and R. H. Waterman, Jr.
 1982 In Search of Excellence: Lessons from America's Best-Run Companies. New York:
      Harper and Row.
Pfifferling, J. H.
 1975 Some Issues in the Consideration of Non-Western and Western Folk Practices as
      Epidemiological Data. Social Science and Medicine 9: 655—658.
Polgar, S.
 1962 Health and Human Behavior: Areas of Interest Common to the Social and Medical
      Sciences. Current Anthropology 3: 159—205.
Puffer, R. R. and C. V. Serrano
 1973 Patterns of Mortality in Childhood. Washington, D. C.: Pan American Health Orga-
      nization. Publication PAHO No. 262.
Raum, O. F.
 1967 Chaga Childhood: A Description of Indigenous Education in an East African Tribe.
      London: Oxford University Press (original 1940).
Read, M.
 1968 Children of Third Fathers: Growing Up Among the Ngoni of Malawi. New York:
      Holt, Rhinehart and Winston.
Rosenfield, P. L., Widstrand, C., and A. D. Ruderman
 1981 Social and Economic Research in the UNDP/World Bank/WHO Special Pro-
      gramme for Research and Training in Tropical Diseases. Social Science and
      Medicine 15A: 529—538.
Roundy, R. W.
 1973 The Cultural Geography of Communicable Disease Transmission in Ethiopia. H. G.
      Marcus (ed.). Monograph No. 3, pp. 427—441. Occasional Papers Series, African
      Studies Centre, Michigan State University, East Lansing.

Rubel, A. J.
   1964   The Epidemiology of a Folk Illness: *Susto* in Hispanic America. Ethnology. 3: 268—283.
Saphir, J. R. et al.
   1967   Voodoo Poisoning in Buffalo, N. Y. JAMA 202(5): 437—438.
Schantz, P. M., D. D. Juranek, and M. G. Schultz
   1977   Trichinosis in the United States, 1975. Increase in Cases Attributable to Numerous Common-Source Outbreaks. Journal of Infectious Diseases 136: 712—715.
Shahid, N. S. et al.
   1983   Beliefs and Treatment Related to Diarrheal Episodes Reported in Association with Measles. Tropical and Geographical Medicine 35: 151—156.
Trotter, R. T., II
   1985   Greta and Azarcon: A Survey of Episodic Lead Poisoning from a Folk Remedy. Human Organization 44(1): 64—72.
Walsh, J. A. and K. S. Warren
   1979   Selective Primary Health Care: An Interim Strategy for Disease Control in Developing Countries. The New England Journal of Medicine 301: 967—970.
   1985   Students Confined to Illinois Campus Unless Immunized. The Washington Post. Section G-11, March 2, 1985.
Wiesenfeld, S. L.
   1967   Sickle-Cell Trait in Human Biological and Cultural Evolution. Science 157: 1134—1140.
   1970   World Health Organization. Programmes of Analysis of Mortality Trends and Levels. Technical Report Series, No. 440, p. 36.

PETER KUNSTADTER

ETHNICITY, ECOLOGY AND MORTALITY IN
NORTHWESTERN THAILAND

INTRODUCTION

This paper describes mortality transitions, morbidity patterns and risk factors
in several types of communities, identified on the basis of ethnographic
research, within an ethnically differentiated population in an ecologically
varied portion of northwestern Thailand. Community type is the basic unit of
comparison. Disaggregation of the population according to type of community shows that fertility and mortality patterns are systematically associated with ethnicity and ecology (location and basic economy) of these
communities. Populatiors in the study area allow control of ecological and
ethnic variability by comparing, for example, the same ethnic group in
different ecological settings (Northern Thai in Town, Suburb, and Lowland
Rural communities, and different ethnic groups in the same ecological setting
(e.g., Highland Skaw Karen, Po Karen, and Lua' with similar swidden
economies).

The basic methodological tactic of controlled comparisons between
groups has been used in a variety of epidemiological (e.g., Syme et al. 1975),
social anthropological (e.g., Eggan 1954; Kunstadter 1984a) and human
biological studies (e.g., Baker 1977: 22ff; 1982: 213 ff). The present study is
unusual in combining the natural experiment approach of migration studies
(same ethnic group in different environments) with intergroup comparisons
in similar environments. The study is descriptive and demonstrates differences between types of communities. Hypotheses concerning the causes of
the differences are suggested (e.g., with respect to access to medical care
facilities and prevalence of behavioral risk factors), but these hypotheses, or
alternative ones which might involve genetic differences between ethnic
groups, have not been tested.

Mortality rates in human populations are a consequence of interactions
with their social and natural environments and their demographic structure.
Populations are exposed to hazards including disease organisms and vectors
in their environments. People also increase or decrease hazards by their own
behavior including their methods of satisfying human needs through patterns
of housing, food production, distribution and preparation, birthing, weaning,
sanitation, health care, recreation and other customs. Both environmental
and cultural differences are reflected in their life chances.

One of the most dramatic concomitants of socioeconomic development
has been the decline in death rates and consequent increase in life expectancy associated with the control of infectious diseases and the reduction of

125

Craig R. Janes et al. (eds.), Anthropology and Epidemiology, 125—156.
© 1986 *by D. Reidel Publishing Company.*

fluctuations in the food supply. These changes appear statistically as reductions in crude and age-specific death rates (especially at younger ages), a fall in the relative and absolute importance of infectious diseases as causes of death, and an increase in the relative importance of external and degenerative causes of death.

The decline in death rate fuels the population explosion and may be associated with transitional changes in fertility and migration, as people respond to changes in population size and concentration. As detailed historical studies are carried out in the West, and as more experience is gained in non-Western populations undergoing socioeconomic development, the linkages between mortality, fertility and socioeconomic development appear to be much more varied than when the classic theory of the demographic transition, based on national aggregate figures from Western Europe and North America, was first outlined 40 years ago. Likewise data are beginning to appear which allow us to test generalizations about the mortality transition which have been based on Western experience under very different cultural and environmental conditions. In particular, the role of cultural differences is now being considered as an important determinant of the demographic response to socioeconomic change (e.g., Coale, Anderson and Harn 1979).

This chapter analyses data from types of communities representing a range of ethnic and ecological differences in northwestern Thailand. Thus we can examine the nature and pace of mortality changes in situations where socioeconomic development has been widespread and in some places rapid, but uneven, and in which there are important cultural differences. Current levels of vital rates in the study area cover a range from high to low fertility and mortality. Mortality changes since the early 1950s are examined in terms of rates and causes of death, using information from a census, and reproductive histories. Mortality transitions in the different types of communities have followed different paths, both in terms of the pace of change, and causes which predominate at different mortality levels. The different patterns of mortality transition are associated with ethnic differences in behavior, and with rate of socioeconomic change in these communities. Some of the demographic differences, demonstrated in earlier studies (Kunstadter 1971), have persisted for many years.

SOURCES OF DEMOGRAPHIC AND HEALTH DATA

Most of the demographic data discussed in this chapter are from communities surveyed in 1981 in Mae Sariang and adjacent Mae La Noi districts of Mae Hongson Province, northwestern Thailand. Several additional highland Po Karen villages and one lowland rural Northern Thai village were surveyed in Mae Sariang District in 1982. A morbidity survey in 1984 covered one lowland suburban, one lowland Northern Thai, and one highland Lua' village, all of which had been surveyed previously, plus one highland Hmong village in Chiang Mai Province, from which demographic data were also collected. Demographic data from all survey dates for communities of the same type (e.g., Po Karen) were aggregated for the demographic analyses presented in Tables I—V.

SOCIOECONOMIC DEVELOPMENT AND HEALTH PROGRAMS IN THE STUDY AREA

Northwestern Thailand is an ethnically and ecologically diverse area. It can be divided ecologically into lowlands and highlands. Lowlands are usually narrow valleys, at an elevation of 200 to 400 meters. The population is predominantly Northern Thai, but especially in Mae Hongson Province, there are also large numbers of lowland Skaw Karen villages. Irrigated rice was traditionally the major staple crop. Highlands are rolling and sometimes steep hills, dissected by small valleys. The village of highland populations, representing several distinct ethnic minority groups ("hilltribes"), are generally found at elevations from about 600 to 2000 meters. The traditional staple crop was upland (swidden) rice, sometimes supplemented at lower elevations by irrigated rice, and at higher elevations by cash crops, especially opium. Characteristics of the various types of communities are described in more detail below.

Mae Sariang District is in a part of northwestern Thailand which was crossed by trade routes between Burma and the valley of the Mae Ping, but was relatively isolated until an all weather road was completed to the district town in 1965. Subsequently a network of access roads has connected lowland villages with the town or the main highway. Starting in the late 1970s a system of dry season roads reached a number of highland villages. Improved transportation and communication has greatly increased access to markets, and was associated with rapid commercial development in the town, and with proliferation of government services. The narrow valley of the Mae Yuam, in which the district town is located, was once a rice deficit area, but an irrigation system built beginning in about 1969 now allows year-round cropping in much of the area it serves, and many farmers in the valley north and south of the town now plant a dry season cash crop as well as their traditional rainy season subsistence rice crop.

Major public health services in the area included smallpox vaccination and eradication, following a severe epidemic at the end of the Second World War. Malaria control reduced mortality from that cause alone from an annual rate of about 5/1000 to about 0.5/1000 in the early 1950s within a few years, according to records in the Regional Malaria Office in Chiang Mai. A small missionary hospital was established near the district town in the early 1960s to supplement the government second class health station in town, and a modern first class government hospital was opened in the late 1970s in one of the suburbs. Border Police supplied small amounts of modern curative medicine in the highlands. On rare occasions the Border Police also arranged for medical evacuation by helicopter from some of these villages. Beginning in about 1980 health stations were established in some of the highland villages. Piped water was supplied to the town and many of the suburbs in the mid-1970s. Piped water supplies were also provided, more slowly, in many of the rural lowland communities and a few of the highland villages.

Primary and secondary schools were founded in town and surrounding suburbs several generations ago, and small primary schools were also set up in some of the larger rural lowland villages shortly after World War Two. Primary schools were established in some of the highland villages beginning in about 1960, and staffed by Border Patrol Police, who also served as agricultural development agents. Highland village schools were integrated into the national educational system at the end of 1960, and 1970s, at about the same time as the compulsory education was increased from four to six primary grades.

Development projects in the highlands accelerated in the late 1970s. They aimed primarily at agricultural improvements, including expansion of irrigation. As noted, they have also built roads, upgraded schools, supplied paramedical personnel, and improved the domestic water supply in some villages. The developments were generally less elaborate and reached the highlands after they had been completed in the lowlands.

DESCRIPTION OF COMMUNITY TYPES

Demographic and health data in this chapter are analysed in terms of community types which have distinctive ethnic compositions and histories, and which display differences in patterns of demographic change.

In the lowland valley the *district town* has a mixed ethnic population, including mostly Northern Thai, but also some Central Thai, Shan, Chinese, Indians and others. The town is an administrative, educational, religious and market center. Most town dwellers are merchants or civil servants.

Suburban communities surrounding the town were once separate villages, occupied mainly by rice farmers. The town's activities have expanded rapidly in the past 20 years, and many of the suburbs have coalesced as a result of rapid population growth due both to natural increase and migration. Migrants to the suburbs include substantial numbers of Skaw Karen and Lua' and, in recent years, some Po Karen from nearby hill villages, and a rapidly growing number of lowland Thais from other parts of Thailand. Farmers now form a small proportion of the suburban population; most adult residents are wage workers or civil servants.

The rural lowland valley is settled with Northern Thai and Skaw Karen villages of irrigated rice farmers. Many of the *lowland rural Northern Thai* villages in this area, including the one surveyed in this study, are occupied by people whose ancestors were ethnically Lua', but who have "become Northern Thai" within the past three or four generations.

Lowland rural Skaw Karen villages are occupied by wet rice farmers who have been settled in this area for well over 100 years. They are predominantly animists, in contrast with other lowland populations who are predominantly Buddhist. Their language is completely distinct from the Thai language.

Highland Skaw Karen villages were founded in this area early in the 19th century by a few Skaw Karen settlers coming from the west. Early migrants often intermarried with Lua', and then established their own rapidly growing villages in swidden lands which at first they rented from Lua' villages. They now have a mixed swidden and wet rice subsistence economy, supplemented by a little wage work, especially in the lumbering industry. Most of these people are animists, but some are Christians.

Highland Po Karen villages, located to the south of the main highway from Hot to Mae Sariang, have been settled in this area for well over 100 years. Some are located on the sites of old Lua' villages. Their subsistence economy is similar to that of the highland Skaw Karen villages, but they have become involved in the wage labor market only recently. Po Karens are generally poorer than Skaw Karens. Most Po Karens are animists. Their language is related to, but not mutually intelligible with Skaw Karen.

Highland Lua' are the autocthonous population in the area, speaking a Mon-Khmer language and living in villages which have been settled in approximately the same location for many hundreds of years. Most of the highland Lua' are animists, but some are Christians. Lua' villages have subsistence economies which are traditionally based on swiddening, but in recent years have increasing amounts of wet rice farming and wage work.

Highland Hmong generally live at higher elevations and greater distances from town than the other highland groups in the study area. They speak a language unrelated to the other groups in the study. They have a mixed economy traditionally based on rice, maize and a cash crop of opium grown on swidden fields. Unlike the other types of communities, which are permanent settlements, Hmong communities have tended to be temporary aggregates of households which may split and move in search of new land. Also unlike the other groups, who traditionally build their houses supported off the ground on posts, Hmong build their houses on the ground. Hmong houses are large by comparison with the other groups, and generally contain extended families with a mean size well over 10, twice as large as the households of the other groups.

METHODS OF STUDYING DIFFERENCES AND CHANGES IN MORTALITY

Questionnaire surveys were conducted in communities representing different ethnic and ecological settings in 1981, 1982, and 1984. Every household was covered in each of the surveyed communities. A total of 17,240 people were covered in over 40 communities. The reported cause of death was recorded for 104 individuals who were reported to have died in the 12 months prior to the date of survey. Reproductive histories were gathered from all ever-married women in the surveyed communities. They included reports of 15,019 births, and 2,606 deaths of children born to these women. A morbidity survey in 1984 covered four communities and recorded information on risk factors and on reported illnesses and symptoms of all household members in the seven days prior to survey.

Demographic results of these surveys are summarized in Table I, which shows total population surveyed (Table IA), age composition of the population (Table IB), and vital rates, based on vital events in the 12 months prior to the date of survey divided by the population as of date of survey (Table IC). Age-standardized death rates were calculated using the population of the town for the standard age distribution.

Very few deaths in the study area are medically certified, so we relied on the respondents' descriptions or reports of cause of death, which usually included major symptoms and circumstances (e.g., accident, long illness). We were generally able to code the reported cause of death, following categories in the 9th Revision of the International Classification of Diseases (WHO 1977). These classes were in turn combined into Major Groups of Causes of Death, following the classification of the Population Bulletin of the United Nations, No. 6, 1962, pp. 73—76, slightly expanded from the modification by ECAFE (United Nations [ECAFE] 1973: 43—46). Deaths reported in the 12 months prior to the surveys, as well as those reported in reproductive histories, were tabulated by these major types of cause. The tabulations were further broken down by time period to show differences and changes in causes of death.

Morbidity data were collected from two sources. Diagnoses of out-patients and inpatients were taken from the records of the Mae Sariang Christian Hospital (Sawyer 1982), and a survey was conducted in March — April 1984 in one suburban community, one lowland rural Northern Thai village, one highland Lua' village, and one highland Hmong village. The purpose of this survey was to explore the range of conditions from lowland to highland. It was not possible to include representatives of all community types for which we had socioeconomic-demographic survey data because of time limits and budget constraints. The survey included questions about recent illnesses for everyone living the surveyed households. A total of 1842 people were covered. Questions were asked about illness or symptoms in the 7 days prior to the survey, including: chronic cough, acute respiratory infection, diarrhea, fever, skin infection, and other acute illnesses. Questions were also asked about risk factors, including source of water, type of toilet facilities, sources

TABLE I
Demographic characteristics of the surveyed communities

| | Type of community | | | | | | | |
| | LOWLAND | | | HIGHLAND | | | | |
	Town	Suburban	Rural North-ern Thai	Rural Skaw Karen	Skaw Karen	Po Karen	Lua'	Hmong
A. Surveyed Population								
Total population of communities surveyed in 1981, 1982 or 1984	1326	7876	670	1158	3054	1031	1563	562
Population of communities in 1984 Morbidity Survey	n.a.	418	718	n.a.	n.a.	n.a.	341	365
Mean household size in 1984 Morbidity Survey	n.a.	4.7	4.0	n.a.	n.a.	n.a.	5.9	12.6
B. Vital Rates per 1000[a]								
Crude birth rate	12.8	24.6	19.4	23.3	39.3	40.5	29.4	49.8
Crude death rate	4.5	3.8	4.5	2.6	4.3	13.5	19.2	8.9
Death rate standardized to "Town" age distribution	4.5	4.2	4.2	2.1	3.3	9.0	13.7	3.8
Crude natural increase	8.3	20.8	14.9	20.7	35.0	27.0	10.2	40.9
C. Age Composition								
Percent under age 15	25.1	33.2	30.0	40.5	45.9	40.9	44.5	54.8
Percent age 65 and over	5.4	3.6	3.6	3.0	2.4	2.8	2.9	1.1
Dependency[b]	43.8	58.3	50.6	77.1	93.3	77.4	90.2	126.6
Median age (years)	25	21	22	18	16	19	17	12

[a] Vital rates were calculated by dividing the number of vital events reported in 12 months prior to survey by the number of the surveyed population at date of survey.

[b] Dependency $= \dfrac{(\text{Number of people under age 15}) + (\text{Number of people age 65 and over})}{(\text{Number of people age 15-64})} \times 100.$

of air pollution in the home, age at first use and frequency and quantity of use of tobacco, betel, alcohol, opium, and other narcotics and stimulants.

LIMITATIONS OF THE METHODS

By most anthropological standards this is a very large study, but the population base is small in comparison with those on which vital and health statistics are usually based. We have tried to compensate for the small size of the subgroups in the surveyed population by collecting historical data, in the form of reproductive histories. This allowed us to analyse a large population (of children) over a long time span, so as to increase the number of person-years at risk on which to base estimates of some of the rates. Nonetheless, we recognize limitations inherent in the methods, including comparisons of rates based on relatively small numbers.

Questionnaires rely on respondents' memories, their ability to respond in categories which are meaningful for analysis, and their willingness to speak about the events which they remember. These limitations apply to all survey methods, not just epidemiological or demographic studies, but the limitations are particularly important because we have relied on the memories of informants going back as much as 50 years, because we are asking for information which is interpreted in a scheme of analysis (e.g., scientifically derived cause of death) which is generally foreign to the respondents' concepts of causality and may be of no particular interest among the population being studied, and because some of the events about which we ask may be surrounded by stigma (e.g., use of narcotics, deaths due to suicide, and in some of the groups, childlessness or inability to rear children to maturity). We believe we were able to get useful information despite these potential problems.

It is conventionally assumed that the completeness of memory declines with the length of time from the event in question, and that births of children who were stillborn or died at a very young age are forgotten more easily than births and deaths of children who lived to a relatively old age or which happened recently. Our experience, both in interviewing and in analysing the results, suggests that these were not important limitations. In general the cohort survival rates shown in Table III indicate that survival rates were lower in earlier years, and have increased for more recent cohorts. This is contrary to what would be expected if deaths in the more remote past were systematically forgotten. Interviews with women of various ages were successful for the most part in determining what seem to have been reasonably complete reproductive histories, except for those from very old women who were in poor health. Interviews were carried out in the household, and it was usually possible to get supplementary or supporting information from other relatives. The fact that these societies are still largely kin-based makes it likely that memories related to children are relatively complete.

In order to check on the quality of the data we compared the stillbirth rate (stillbirths per 1000 livebirths) for various periods (Table III). For births more recent than about 1931 (50 years prior to the earliest survey) we found no consistent trends such as we would expect if earlier stillbirths were forgotten more frequently than recent ones. Stillbirth ratios did not appear to be lower in the past, and annual variation in the most recent five years is generally as great as the variation in the earlier cohorts. We believe that if loss of memory distorts the data, the distortion is relatively small and does not account for reported variation over time, nor between groups.

Diagnosis of cause of an event, such as death, is subject to interpretation, depending on beliefs concerning causality and the amount of information available to and understood by the person reporting the event. Because only a small proportion of those who died were attended by a scientifically qualified observer, respondents usually answered questions on cause of death by giving symptoms or circumstances of death, rather than a medical diagnosis of cause. The symptoms or circumstances were generally clear enough to infer a medical cause. Lowlanders were more likely to have received medical workup before death than were highlanders. Many degenerative diseases require laboratory confirmation of diagnosis, and we may have underestimated the number of degenerative diseases as causes in the highland vs. the lowland groups. Because many degenerative diseases (e.g., cancer) are recognized by highlanders we do not think this is a source of serious bias.

Self-reporting of illness may not accurately reveal illnesses in infants and young children who are unable to describe their symptoms. Unless parents are very attentive to the illnesses of their children this may result in under-reporting for the youngest age classes, and may explain lack of congruence between reported morbidity and age-specific mortality as gleaned from reproductive histories. Again, the results of the morbidity studies in general (except for infants) follow the expected U-shaped curve, indicating that young children (whose death rates are high) also have high rates of reported morbidity.

We believe respondents were willing to report honestly on causes of death, even though the cause might be associated with some negative connotation (e.g., suicide, homicide). This probably was the result of our use of community members (who would have known about "notorious" deaths) to conduct the survey. Likewise, we believe that reported use of alcohol, etc. is reasonably accurate for the same reason. Parents know when their children start smoking (and make no effort to control their smoking), and, though not flaunted, use of opium is not concealed in these communities to the extent it is in the U.S.

A limitation of the method of analysis is that it aggregates the experience of people who happen to be living in the same place at the time of the survey, but who did not necessarily spend their lives in the same place or type of place. This may result in a bias as a result of migration into or away from the community prior to the survey. This is not a major concern in the highland or rural lowland communities, which, in general, have low rates of inmigration. Moreover, the migrants to communities of these types over-whelmingly come from very similar environments. Almost all migrants to such communities came from the same type of community over a relatively short distance within northern Thailand. In town and suburbs, however, almost half the residents are lifetime migrants, many of whom came from considerable distances, and often from other types of communities. The suburbs, which contain migrants from highland and lowland communities in northern Thailand, as well as from other rural lowland and urban places elsewhere in Thailand, are the most heterogeneous, both ethnically and in terms of community of origin (Kunstadter 1984c). This problem can be handled by disaggregating by ethnicity and migration history. Analysis of deaths in the year prior to the survey showed that nonmigrants, as opposed to lifetime migrants, had higher death rates in town and suburban communities (Kunstadter 1984b). We have not yet disaggregated by ethnicity, nor have we disaggregated deaths reported in reproductive histories by place of birth and place of death.

Another limitation of the analysis of reproductive history data is that the cohorts do not include all children born during a given period. They contain only children born to mothers who survived to the date of the survey. Since death of children, especially young children, is probably correlated with death of mother, these data may yield an underestimate of mortality, especially for earlier cohorts.

A similar limitation applies to mortality rates. We interviewed surviving members of households in which there was a death. Individuals who were living alone and died in the year prior to census might not be counted in the survey. This is probably not a serious problem, because we attempted to learn about people who had died by asking about the previous inhabitants of empty or abandoned houses as a part of the survey. An additional problem is the general difficulty of learning about people who are absent from the social unit being investigated, as contrasted with those who are present. Some of the death rates we report here appear quite low. It is possible that some deaths in the year prior to census were not reported during the course of the interviews. To the extent that this was a problem, we have no reason to believe there was any difference with respect to the different community types. This suggests that although the rates we determined may be lower than the actual rates, the relative differences between communities are probably accurate.

RESULTS: FERTILITY AND MORTALITY

Fertility is well controlled in town (where decline in fertility apparently preceded availability of modern birth control methods), and is rapidly coming under control in the suburban and rural lowland Northern Thai communities (Table IB). The spread of modern birth control in other types of communities has been slower. Mortality has apparently been low in town for many years, and has declined rapidly in other lowland communities. Demographic consequences of the interaction of fertility and mortality are shown in the age distributions of the various communities (Table IC). Median ages of the populations of the various communities range from a low of 12 years among the high birthrate Hmong, to a high of 25 years in town, where fertility and mortality are quite low.

Data on deaths in the year prior to survey show major differences between different types of communities, both in crude and age standardized rates. Rates are quite low for all lowland communities and for highland Skaw Karen and are intermediate for highland Hmong. Rates are three or four times greater for Po Karen and Lua' (Table IB). The highest rates were for Lua', and in part resulted from an epidemic of measles in two of the surveyed highland Lua' villages. Comparatively high Lua' mortality may also result from higher prevalence of risk factors as compared with other groups (see below).

Results based on death rates in the 12 months prior to survey suggest that the different types of communities have reached different points in the transition from high fluctuating mortality associated with infectious diseases, to low and relatively stable rates associated primarily with other causes. This impression is supported and refined by data on proportions of deaths in the 12 months prior to survey due to various major causes (Table II). There were no deaths due to infectious diseases in town or in the lowland rural Northern Thai community in the year prior to survey. Proportions of deaths due to infectious diseases ranged from 27 percent in the suburban community to 73 percent among highland Po Karen, 82 percent among highland Lua', 83 percent among highland Skaw Karen, and 100 percent in rural lowland Skaw Karen and highland Hmong communities. These results suggest that even though the total crude and age adjusted death rates are low in rural lowland Skaw Karen and highland Skaw Karen and Hmong villages, the mortality transition is still incomplete in those types of communities. Recent information from the highland Lua' villages shows that these communities are still subject to major fluctuations in annual death rates due to immunizable communicable diseases.

Some of the history of mortality changes can be derived from reproductive histories. The summary figures, including deaths of children going back to the early 1900s suggest that proportions of deaths due to infectious diseases were once much higher in town than at time of the survey (Table III). We can reconstruct the overall pattern of mortality change by examining survival of children both at different dates (Table IV), and then looking at changes in causes of death over time (Table V). Most of the transitional changes in

TABLE II

Causes of death at all ages in 12 months prior to survey (percent of classified causes in each type of community)

Reported cause	LOWLAND				HIGHLAND			
	Town	Suburban	Rural Northern Thai	Rural Skaw Karen	Skaw Karen	Po Karen	Lua'	Hmong
INFECTIOUS (total)	0.0	26.9	0.0	100.0	83.3	72.7	82.1	100.0
gastrointestinal	0.0	0.0	0.0	33.1	58.3	54.5	25.0	40.0
malaria	0.0	7.7	0.0	0.0	25.0	9.1	3.6	0.0
respiratory	0.0	7.7	0.0	33.3	0.0	0.0	3.6	20.0
skin	0.0	0.0	0.0	0.0	0.0	0.0	0.0	0.0
other site, systemic	0.0	0.0	0.0	0.0	0.0	0.0	50.0	40.0
probably infectious[a]	0.0	11.5	0.0	33.3	0.0	9.1	0.0	0.0
NEONATAL	0.0	0.0	33.3	0.0	16.7	0.0	10.7	0.0
MATERNAL	0.0	0.0	0.0	0.0	0.0	18.2	0.0	0.0
DEGENERATIVE (total)	60.0	53.9	0.0	0.0	0.0	0.0	7.1	0.0
cancer	20.0	7.7	0.0	0.0	0.0	0.0	0.0	0.0
cardiovasc., cerebrovasc.	20.0	15.4	0.0	0.0	0.0	0.0	0.0	0.0
other degenerative	20.0	30.8	0.0	0.0	0.0	0.0	7.1	0.0
EXTERNAL (total)	40.0	19.2	66.7	0.0	0.0	0.0	0.0	0.0
accident	0.0	15.4	0.0	0.0	0.0	0.0	0.0	0.0
suicide	0.0	0.0	0.0	0.0	0.0	0.0	0.0	0.0
homicide	40.0	3.8	66.7	0.0	0.0	0.0	0.0	0.0
UNCLASSIFIED (total)	20.0	15.4	0.0	0.0	8.3	36.4	7.1	0.0
unclassified symptoms	20.0	15.4	0.0	0.0	8.3	9.1	7.1	0.0
symptoms not reported	0.0	0.0	0.0	0.0	0.0	27.3	0.0	0.0
TOTAL DEATHS (N)	6	30	3	3	13	14	30	5
classified by cause	5	26	3	3	12	11	28	5

[a] Symptoms include fever.

TABLE III

Causes of death of children of all ages ever born to women in the surveyed communities (percent of classified causes in each type of community)

Reported cause	LOWLAND				HIGHLAND			
	Town	Suburban	Rural Northern Thai	Rural Skaw Karen	Skaw Karen	Po Karen	Lua'	Hmong
INFECTIOUS (total)	63.5	87.1	89.4	86.3	83.0	83.8	85.2	82.8
gastrointestinal	17.6	18.1	25.9	27.5	38.5	34.1	26.8	25.0
malaria	6.8	1.5	21.2	8.1	18.4	20.0	5.7	6.3
respiratory	1.4	4.1	7.1	8.1	8.8	4.3	7.4	10.9
skin	0.0	0.4	0.0	1.3	0.7	0.0	1.3	4.7
other site, systemic	6.8	19.5	8.2	3.8	4.1	9.7	16.8	20.3
probably infectious [a]	31.1	34.8	27.1	37.5	12.4	15.7	27.2	15.6
NEONATAL	13.5	8.0	5.9	3.8	12.4	10.8	12.8	7.8
MATERNAL	0.0	0.8	1.2	0.6	0.1	1.6	0.3	1.6
DEGENERATIVE (total)	12.2	6.6	1.2	7.5	1.9	1.1	1.3	0.0
cancer	2.7	0.4	0.0	0.0	0.9	0.0	0.0	0.0
cardiovasc., cerebrovasc.	4.1	1.6	0.0	3.1	0.4	0.0	0.0	0.0
other degenerative	5.4	4.6	1.2	4.4	0.6	1.1	1.3	0.0
EXTERNAL (total)	10.8	6.2	1.2	1.9	2.5	2.7	0.3	6.3
accident	4.1	4.5	1.2	1.9	0.9	1.1	0.3	3.1
suicide	1.4	0.5	0.0	0.0	1.5	1.1	0.0	3.1
homicide	5.4	1.2	1.2	0.0	0.2	0.5	0.0	0.0
UNCLASSIFIED (total)	14.9	17.6	11.8	5.0	7.9	16.8	22.1	14.1
unclassified symptoms	10.8	12.9	11.8	5.0	4.8	5.4	9.7	12.5
symptoms not reported	4.1	4.7	0.0	0.0	3.1	11.4	12.4	1.6
TOTAL DEATHS (N)	85	869	95	168	737	216	364	72
classified by cause	74	739	85	160	683	185	298	64

[a] Symptoms include fever.

TABLE IV

Fetal death rates and proportions of children liveborn in different years surviving to exact age one, five and ten years in different types of communities

LOWLAND COMMUNITIES

Town

Birth date	Number live-born	Fetal death rate[a]	Proportion surviving		
			One year	Five years	Ten years
Before 1931	34	235.3	0.911	0.853	0.853
1931–1940	68	29.4	0.912	0.868	0.868
1941–1950	138	50.7	0.971	0.928	0.928
1951–1955	132	75.8	0.955	0.932	0.924
1956–1960	145	75.9	0.972	0.959	0.952
1961–1965	102	107.8	0.971	0.960	0.951
1966–1970	94	85.1	0.989	0.989	0.957
1971–1975	85	94.1	0.965	0.965	0.965
1976–1980	111	99.1	0.973	—	—

Suburban

Birth date	Number live-born	Fetal death rate[a]	Proportion surviving		
			One year	Five years	Ten years
Before 1931	96	93.8	0.938	0.917	0.885
1931–1940	309	45.3	0.890	0.825	0.796
1941–1950	718	96.1	0.904	0.816	0.787
1951–1955	702	65.5	0.910	0.859	0.843
1956–1960	897	51.3	0.921	0.883	0.870
1961–1965	988	46.6	0.931	0.910	0.899
1966–1970	887	75.5	0.953	0.936	0.923
1971–1975	872	81.4	0.946	0.928	0.923
1976–1980	891	84.2	0.969	—	—

HIGHLAND COMMUNITIES

Highland Skaw Karen

Birth date	Number live-born	Fetal death rate[a]	Proportion surviving		
			One year	Five years	Ten years
Before 1931	54	37.0	0.907	0.741	0.611
1931–1940	144	34.6	0.854	0.806	0.764
1941–1950	298	43.6	0.852	0.725	0.691
1951–1955	277	46.9	0.863	0.733	0.700
1956–1960	361	69.3	0.886	0.762	0.740
1961–1965	458	65.5	0.873	0.786	0.764
1966–1970	518	48.5	0.911	0.837	0.821
1971–1975	535	46.7	0.920	0.849	0.845
1976–1980	537	35.4	0.933	—	—

Po Karen

Birth date	Number live-born	Fetal death rate[a]	Proportion surviving		
			One year	Five years	Ten years
Before 1931	8	0.0	1.000	1.000	1.000
1931–1940	29	172.4	0.897	0.793	0.759
1941–1950	102	107.8	0.922	0.784	0.775
1951–1955	88	34.1	0.852	0.784	0.739
1956–1960	114	52.6	0.904	0.877	0.860
1961–1965	126	23.8	0.873	0.817	0.794
1966–1970	147	34.0	0.871	0.796	0.796
1971–1975	157	12.7	0.887	0.824	0.811
1976–1980	207	38.6	0.884	—	—

[a] Fetal deaths per 1000 livebirths.

Table IV (continued)

Rural Northern Thai

	N				
Before 1931	15	0.0	1.000	0.867	0.800
1931—1940	43	23.3	1.000	0.953	0.907
1941—1950	43	0.0	0.907	0.837	0.837
1951—1955	48	20.8	0.938	0.896	0.854
1956—1960	83	36.1	0.922	0.900	0.844
1961—1965	90	22.2	0.956	0.911	0.911
1966—1970	88	45.5	0.864	0.796	0.773
1971—1975	76	65.8	0.803	0.803	0.803
1976—1980	66	0.0	0.985	—	—

Rural Skaw Karen

	N				
Before 1931	8	0.0	1.000	1.000	0.875
1931—1940	34	88.2	0.853	0.765	0.765
1941—1950	98	51.0	0.847	0.745	0.724
1951—1955	101	59.4	0.772	0.723	0.713
1956—1960	113	70.8	0.903	0.823	0.814
1961—1965	151	33.1	0.894	0.854	0.854
1966—1970	171	23.4	0.936	0.889	0.871
1971—1975	164	42.7	0.927	0.921	0.915
1976—1980	171	35.1	0.953	—	—

Lua'

	N				
Before 1931	55	18.2	0.964	0.836	0.782
1931—1940	72	83.3	0.903	0.792	0.708
1941—1950	150	80.0	0.820	0.667	0.627
1951—1955	112	53.6	0.848	0.777	0.741
1956—1960	146	47.9	0.890	0.836	0.815
1961—1965	183	43.7	0.902	0.842	0.831
1966—1970	234	46.6	0.915	0.850	0.825
1971—1975	285	73.7	0.912	0.821	0.796
1976—1980	301	29.9	0.907	—	—

Hmong

	N				
Before 1931	0	—	—	—	—
1931— —1950	40	50.0	0.900	0.675	0.650
1951— —1960	69	87.0	0.971	0.942	0.928
1961— —1970	138	43.5	0.942	0.899	0.877
1971—1975	98	81.6	0.969	0.918	0.908
1976—1980	144	69.4	0.951	—	—

[a] Fetal deaths per 1000 livebirths.

TABLE V

Number of deaths of children age 0—4 which were classified by cause in different cohorts, and percentage of death due to infectious diseases in these cohorts

Birth Date	LOWLAND				HIGHLAND			
	Town	Suburban	Rural Northern Thai	Rural Skaw Karen	Skaw Karen	Po Karen	Lua'	Hmong
Number of Deaths of Children Age 0—4 Classified by Cause								
Before 1951	24	159	11	31	120	25	58	13
1951—1960	16	177	13	46	149	21	38	3
1961—1970	7	128	21	38	170	42	54	11
1971—1975	2	49	11	12	75	22	46	6
1976—1980	2	23	2	10	38	25	40	9
Percentage of Deaths of Children Age 0—4 Due to Infectious Disease								
Before 1951	83.3	89.9	100.0	93.5	82.5	80.0	96.6	84.6
1951—1960	75.0	80.2	92.3	91.3	82.6	90.5	86.8	66.7
1961—1970	71.4	79.7	95.2	81.6	87.1	78.6	85.2	81.8
1971—1975	0.0	83.7	90.1	100.0	82.7	90.1	80.4	66.7
1976—1980	0.0	73.9	50.0	90.0	76.3	84.0	60.0	88.9

mortality rates, especially the declines in infectious diseases, have their greatest effect at the younger ages, so we can look for trends even among children born in recent years. Results of the analysis of child survival by date of birth and type of community (Table IV) may be summarized as follows:

— Town children have had high survival rates. Survival rates rose steadily at all ages from the earliest to the most recently born cohorts.

— Suburban children have relatively high survival rates, with irregular increases in proportions surviving, especially after 1950. Decline in death rates followed a period of high mortality around the time of World War Two, and the beginning of the malaria control program in the early 1950s.

— Lowland rural Northern Thai infants probably had a lower survival rate than town children in the past. Major improvements in survival apparently did not come until late in the 1970s.

— Lowland rural Skaw Karen children seem to have had lower survival rates than rural Northern Thai children, and survival rates seem to have declined until the mid 1950s. Survival has risen rapidly since that time.

— Highland Skaw Karen children have had low survival rates for all cohorts, and the decline in mortality seems to have taken place at least five years later than the improvement in the lowland rural Skaw Karen communities. In both level of mortality and time of decline in mortality these communities lag 30 years or more behind the children in town.

— Highland Po Karen children, though small in numbers in our study population, appear to have had mortality rates comparable to highland Skaw Karen, but improvement in survival seems slower and more recent for Po Karen children. This is consistent with the greater isolation of the Po communities until about 1965, and with their poverty. Po Karen mortality rates remain higher than the rates in town 50 years ago.

— Highland Lua' children seem to have been exposed to greater fluctuations in mortality rates than have Karen children. The very low survival of the cohort born around the time of the Second World War is consistent with reports of very heavy mortality in highland Lua' villages associated with a smallpox epidemic at the end of the war. Improvement in survival seems to have started in the late 1950s, but has not been sustained. Lua' rates in the 1970s are comparable with town rates before 1931.

— Hmong figures are similar now to those for lowland rural Skaw Karen, but there has apparently been little improvement in survival of Hmong children since the 1950s, when they appear to have been roughly comparable to the rates in town.

The picture we get from this comparison of historical changes in survival rates seems consistent with the history of the study area. The town enjoys an advantage in survival over other lowland communities. Child mortality seems to be more or less a direct function of isolation or distance from town; highland communities are generally the most isolated, and improvement in survival was slower and less regular than in the lowlands. The Second World

War was a time of considerable social disruption. Men from some of the highland villages were corvéed by Japanese for highway labor, and toward the end of the war some of the villages were temporarily abandoned for fear of bombing attacks. A severe smallpox epidemic apparently followed the retreat of the Japanese army out of Burma and across this part of northern Thailand. Government services were strengthened after the war, and major public health measures began with malaria control in the early 1950s. Modern economic development projects began with the construction of an all weather road, completed to the town in 1965. Feeder roads were built to many rural lowland villages, but the major improvements in living conditions in town spread only slowly to the rural areas.

We can get more detailed information on the history of mortality changes by looking at causes of death, and especially at the proportions of deaths of children reported to have been caused by infectious diseases. Gastrointestinal diseases are still important in all communities except town, and malaria was (and in some communities continues to be) an important health problem, especially in some rural communities. Respiratory illnesses are important causes of death, as are diseases which we have classified as "probably infectious". Some clear patterns can be seen in Table V.

Infectious diseases declined, and then disappeared as causes of death of town children, as proportions surviving rose to a high level. Infectious diseases have declined in importance more slowly and more recently among suburban children. Based on very small numbers, it appears that infectious diseases are declining in importance among children of the lowland rural Northern Thai community, but they continue to be important in the lowland rural Skaw Karen communities. The proportion of deaths due to infectious diseases among highland children appears to be high and fluctuating, suggesting that contagious diseases are still important causes of child death (as we know to be the case in Lua' communities). It should be noted that this tabulation is only a rough indication of the child mortality picture. Aside from infectious diseases, many deaths of children in highland communities which could be classified by cause, were due to causes classified as "neonatal", meaning that they occured very shortly after birth, and include such causes as birth injuries, or what might be called "failure to thrive". Some of the neonatal deaths are probably difficult to prevent, but the very low rate of neonatal and infant deaths in town may be a result of the increased use of modern sterile delivery in hospital, rather than delivery by traditional birth attendants, and possibly a higher rate of immunizations, e.g., against tetanus.

RESULTS: MORBIDITY

The general pattern of morbidity in the Mae Sariang study area is indicated in the tabulation of diagnoses of patients seen at the Mae Sariang Christian Hospital (Table VI). This hospital draws most of its patients from a radius of

TABLE VI
Primary diagnosis of outpatients at the Mae Sariang Christian
Hospital, 1981

Diagnosis	Number	Percent
Upper respiratory infections	1985	22.3
Lower respiratory infections	819	9.2
Gastrointestinal infections	125	14.2
Worms	267	3.0
Skin infections	626	7.0
Genito-urinary infections	376	4.2
Genito-urinary, other	422	4.7
Venereal diseases	135	1.5
Influenza, all forms	541	6.1
Measles	598	6.7
Tuberculosis, all forms	197	2.2
Malaria	602	6.8
Leprosy	57	0.6
Hepatitis	26	0.3
Encephalitis	7	0.1
Dengue haemmorhagic fever	4	0.0
Cardiovascular, incl. rheumatic heart disease	209	2.4
Tumors	64	0.7
Diabetes	7	0.1
Nutritional deficiencies	265	0.3
Trauma, burns, bites	421	0.5
Total	8885	

Figures supplied by Dr. Bina Sawyer, Mae Saring Christian Hospital

about 25 km, which includes most of the villages in our study population. As might be expected, these figures show a high proportion of outpatient visits associated with infectious ailments, particularly respiratory and gastrointestinal illnesses. Because these statistics are based on aggregated hospital visits, not broken down in terms of a defined population base, the results cannot be interpreted with regard to any particular group in the population we studied. We have therefore relied in the following discussion on morbidity as revealed in the survey of morbidity conducted in four communities in 1984.

We inquired with regard to every individual in each household about chronic and acute respiratory illnesses (cough, difficulty breathing, cold, etc.), chronic and acute diarrhea, eye, and skin illness, fever in the past seven days, or other illness. As a rough measure of the burden of illness in these communities, we totaled reported illnesses for each individual, and calculated the proportion of individuals reporting none vs. one or more ailments.

Reported morbidity generally follows a U-shaped curve, high in the earliest years of life, declining to a low among teenagers and young adults, and then increasing to a high level in old age (Table VII). With some exceptions this pattern was followed in each of the four communities in which we surveyed morbidity, and for each of the types of illness which we analysed. It was surprising that in every community the proportions of infants for whom illness was reported was lower than the proportion reported among those age 1—4. One possible explanation for this result is that prolonged breast-feeding is common to all groups studied, and breast-feeding may protect infants from some of the major causes of illness (e.g., diarrhea). As indicated above, another possible explanation is under-reporting of the illnesses of infants (who cannot speak for themselves).

Proportions reporting illness generally declined after age 4, but the lowest level, and the age at which the lowest level was reached, varied between the groups. The smallest association of age with proportion reporting illness was found among the highland Lua', who also showed the highest levels at all

TABLE VII

Percentage of persons reporting one or more illness, by community type, age and sex[a]

| Age (years) | Lowland | | | | Highland | | | |
| | Suburban | | Rural | | Lua' | | Hmong | |
	N	%	N	%	N	%	N	%
< 1	14	28.6	14	35.7	5	40.0	10	20.0
1— 4	39	33.3	58	58.6	17	70.6	79	25.3
5— 9	34	14.7	64	43.8	26	46.2	60	8.3
10—14	52	17.3	68	29.4	33	57.6	56	12.5
15—19	45	11.1	90	24.4	22	45.5	50	12.0
20—29	84	17.9	167	24.6	43	69.8	38	10.5
30—39	51	23.5	89	25.8	15	40.0	26	26.9
40—49	43	34.9	67	37.3	31	80.6	19	57.9
50—59	33	21.2	51	43.1	11	81.8	12	58.3
⩾ 60	23	30.4	38	63.2	5	100.0	8	75.0
Total	418	22.0	706	34.6	208	62.5	358	20.9
Total adjusted to "Suburban" age distribution		22.0		35.3		62.9		26.6

[a] N = number of persons in the age group for whom illness was ascertained; % = percentage of persons in age group who reported one or more illnesses, including: chronic cough, difficulty breathing, acute respiratory illness, chronic eye, acute eye, chronic diarrhea, acute diarrhea, chronic skin, acute skin, fever, other illness in the seven days prior to survey.

Total includes only those persons for whom both age and illness reports were recorded, and does not include 11 individuals with incomplete illness reports and 1 without age recorded in the lowland rural community; 131 with incomplete illness reports in the Lua' village, and 3 persons with incomplete illness reports plus 4 without age recorded in the Hmong village.

ages. The apparent lack of relationship between age and morbidity in the group with the highest reported morbidity is not what might be expected on the basis of life tables of high mortality groups, which show a sharp difference in mortality rates at different ages.

There were no major or consistent sex differences in level of reported morbidity in any of the groups.

Overall levels of morbidity vary among the four types of communities, as do the absolute and relative levels of different types of illness. Highland Hmong (with 20.9% of the population reporting one or more illness), and lowland suburb (with 22%), have the lowest proportions; lowland rural is intermediate, and highland Lua' is the highest (62.5% reporting one or more illnesses). These are crude figures, not age-adjusted, but differences in age structure of the populations do not explain the variation when age-specific or age-adjusted rates are examined. Community differences are generally represented among all age groups. The Hmong population has a very high proportion of infants and young children, but the Hmong rates of reported illness among young children are the lowest among the four communities. The low levels of reported illness among Hmong and high levels among Lua' are remarkable. An explanation for some of the differences between these two highland communities may be found in the discussion of risk factors (below).

Respiratory and diarrheal diseases generally accounted for higher proportions of illnesses than did other types of illnesses, but proportions reporting these types of illnesses varied between the communities (Tables VIII and IX). Respiratory illness was particularly important in the Lua' village (59.7% of the people reported one or more respiratory ailment), and the rural lowland Northern Thai (46.2%). Diarrheal disease was particularly important among the Lua' (26.5% reported diarrheal illness). The generally high rank and level of reported respiratory illnesses in these communities is consistent with the emerging recognition of the importance of respiratory illnesses as leading causes of morbidity and mortality in populations of developing countries (Chretien et al. 1984; WHO 1984).

Reported morbidity in the surveyed communities parallels the general pattern in reports of deaths of children in the reproductive histories from the same community types, both in terms of relative levels of infant and child mortality, and in the reported causes of deaths. Results of the morbidity survey support the conclusion that there are major differences in health conditions associated both with ethnic and ecological variables: both lowland communities are predominantly Northern Thai in ethnicity, but the morbidity levels and rank ordering of causes of morbidity are quite different; the highland villages represent different ethnicities (Hmong and Lua'), with different micro-ecologies, and their morbidity and mortality patterns differ from each other and from the lowland groups.

TABLE VIII

Percentage of persons reporting one or more diarrheal illnesses, by community type, age and sex[a]

| Age (years) | Lowland | | | | Highland | | | |
| | Suburban | | Rural | | Lua' | | Hmong | |
	N	%	N	%	N	%	N	%
< 1	14	7.1	14	7.1	6	16.7	10	20.0
1— 4	39	7.7	59	16.9	36	36.1	79	16.5
5— 9	34	0.0	65	7.7	39	12.8	60	5.0
10—14	52	0.0	68	5.9	46	28.3	56	1.8
15—19	55	0.0	90	3.3	39	17.9	50	0.0
20—29	84	0.0	167	7.2	54	33.3	38	5.3
30—39	51	5.9	90	6.7	25	16.0	26	0.0
40—49	43	9.3	67	7.5	39	35.9	19	15.8
50—59	33	12.1	51	9.8	19	36.8	12	16.7
≥ 60	23	4.3	39	7.7	18	16.7	8	12.5
Total	418	3.8	710	7.6	321	26.5	358	7.5
Total adjusted to "suburban" age distribution		3.8		7.8		27.0		7.5

[a] N = number of persons in the age group for whom reported illness was ascertained; % = percentage of persons in age group who reported one or more diarrheal illnesses, including chronic diarrhea and acute diarrhea in the seven days prior to survey.

Total includes only those persons for whom both age and illness reports were recorded, and does not include 7 individuals with incomplete illness reports and 1 without age recorded in the lowland rural community; 28 with incomplete illness reports in the Lua' village, and 3 persons with incomplete illness reports plus 4 without age recorded in the Hmong village.

RESULTS: RISK FACTORS

The risk factors we examined included sanitary facilities for the households and individual consumption of narcotics and stimulants. We have analysed these data only at the community level and have not tried to relate disease within the household to sanitary conditions within the household.

Type of toilet facility is strongly associated with community type. Almost all the households in the suburb use waterseal latrines either in the house (23.7% of households) or outside (67.8%). This contrasts with the lowland rural Northern Thai community (42.6% waterseal, 36.1% pit, 19.7% in the forest). Approximately the same proportion in the Hmong village use waterseal toilets (37.9%), but a much higher proportion go to the forest for defecation (62.1%). Almost every household in the Lua' village has a waterseal latrine, built as a result of a development project, but only one household (1.7% reports using it; two thirds (65.5%) use pit latrines, and one

TABLE IX

Percentage of persons reporting one or more respiratory illnesses, by community type, age and sex[a]

| Age (years) | Lowland | | | | Highland | | | |
| | Suburban | | Rural | | Lua' | | Hmong | |
	N	%	N	%	N	%	N	%
< 1	14	0.0	15	6.7	7	28.6	10	0.0
1— 4	39	2.6	59	33.9	31	45.2	80	3.8
5— 9	34	0.0	65	26.2	38	26.3	60	0.0
10—14	52	1.9	68	14.7	46	28.3	56	3.6
15—19	45	2.2	91	11.0	33	27.3	50	4.0
20—29	84	3.6	170	8.2	50	44.0	39	5.1
30—39	51	2.0	90	14.4	25	20.0	27	14.8
40—49	43	7.0	68	17.6	37	54.1	19	21.1
50—59	33	6.1	51	13.7	19	42.1	12	16.7
≥ 60	23	8.7	40	27.5	17	58.8	10	20.0
Total	418	3.3	717	16.0	303	37.3	361	5.8
Total adjusted to "Suburban" age distribution[b]		3.4 *		16.3		37.2		8.7

[a] N = number of persons in the age group for whom reported illness was ascertained; % = percentage of persons in age group who reported one or more respiratory illnesses including chronic cough, chronic difficulty breathing and acute respiratory illness in the seven days prior to survey.

Total includes only those persons for whom both age and illness reports were recorded, and does not include 1 individual without age recorded in the lowland rural community; 46 with incomplete illness reports in the Lua' village; and 4 without age recorded in the Hmong community.

[b] The difference between total and age-adjusted total is due to rounding.

third (32.8%) used the forest). To the extent that "modern" (waterseal) latrines reduce the spread of water- or fly-borne diarrheas, we would expect a lower prevalence of diarrhea in the suburb than in the other communities.

None of the villages covered by the morbidity survey has a purified piped water supply; most households rely on wells inside or outside the house compound. The exception is the Lua' village, where cisterns were dug and water was piped to taps at several points in the village. Although the cisterns were disinfected when built, the water is not purified at the source, and because the pipes are leaky and most households in all villages must carry the water to and store it in the house, there are many chances for contamination. Without testing the water where it is actually being used, there is no straightforward way to relate source and transport of water to contamination.

Type of cooking facility gives an indication of the amount of indoor air pollution to which the population is exposed. Most households in all communities use wood as their primary fuel. Low-smoke fuels (charcoal, gas, electricity) are used as supplements more frequently in the suburb. Cooking in both lowland communities is usually done outside the main living space, in a separate kitchen, over a "bucket" stove. Lowland houses are not heated. Open fires for both cooking and heating are built within the main living space in the houses of the two highland communities, which are cooler and damper than the lowland communities. These houses generally have no chimneys or venting system (a few of the Hmong households have chimneys attached to some of their stoves, but also have unvented fireplaces). Smoke percolates slowly through the roof or out the door and windows (most of the higland houses have no windows). Hmong houses are generally larger than Lua' houses, so that dilution of the smoke may be greater in Hmong than in Lua' houses.[1] Smokey village houses are familiar to anyone who has visited a rural area in the developing world, but few measurements have been made on the quantity and composition of the smoke to which residents of these houses are exposed. Indoor air pollution is now coming to be recognized as a risk factor especially relating to respiratory diseases (e.g., Douglas et al. 1984), but its role in relation to respiratory disease in the developing countries is not yet fully appreciated (EWC Working Group 1985). Indoor air pollution levels have not been systematically measured in the study communities, but one preliminary observation using monitoring equipment showed that the level of carbon monoxide in a Lua' house at the time a cooking fire was being lit exceeded U.S. safety standards. Monitoring of formaldehyde levels, using passive monitors in the same household, confirmed a very high level of that pollutant as well (Smith and Kunstadter unpublished data).

Use of stimulants and narcotics varies widely among the different kinds of communities in relation to types which are used, rates of use, and amounts and distributions of use. It is widely recognized that smoking tobacco greatly increases risks for a variety of diseases, and the importance of passive smoking is now gaining wider recognition. Most research on the epidemiology of smoking has been done in developed countries; little attention has been paid to the relationship of smoking and passive smoking to illness among rural populations of developing countries such as Thailand.

The proportion of tobacco smokers is higher for men than for women in all surveyed communities, and varies greatly between community types. The highest rate is found among highland Lua' for both sexes; the lowest is among Hmong of both sexes. Among males age $\geq$ 20 the proportion smoking ranges from a low of 27.3% (Hmong) through 83.1% and 87.3% (lowland suburb and lowland rural Northern Thai), to a high of 93.4% (Lua'). The distribution of smoking is similar among women, ranging from a low of 6%

(Hmong) to 46.2% among suburban women and 51.5% among lowland rural Northern Thai to a high of 87.5% among Lua' women.

The form of smoking also varies systematically between sexes and among the communities. Among suburban men, purchased, commercially made cigarettes are the most popular form of smoking (60.5% of all men age ≥ 20). This contrasts with suburban women, among whom the locally made Burmese cigarette (known locally as *ki yo*), rolled in a banana leaf, and containing finely cut bark and bits of wood as well as local tobacco, is the most popular smoke (32.7%). Homemade and purchased cigarettes are equally popular (45.3%) among the rural lowland Northern Thai village men; women in that community (26.8%) favor locally made cigarettes (wrapped in banana leaf or scrap paper, containing locally grown or purchased tobacco), over the Burmese style cigarettes (19.7%). Pipes, generally filled with home grown sun-dried tobacco, are the most popular form of smoking in the Lua' community where 74.3% of the men and 88.5% of the women age ≥ 20 smoke pipes. In recent years, when they could afford it, the Lua' villagers have preferred to buy their tobacco in the market. Hmong men who smoke prefer homemade cigarettes (24.1%), as do the very few Hmong women smokers (4.1%).

Proportion of people who smoke is highest in the Lua' community for both males and females (Table X). Smoking starts earliest among Lua' (54% of the male smokers and 65% of the female smokers started before age 15). Lua' villagers say they have to smoke while they are working in the fields in order to keep the insects away.

TABLE X
Percentage of adults (age ≥ 20) using stimulants and narcotics, by community type and sex

Type of stimulant or narcotic	Lowland suburb		Rural		Highland Lua'		Hmong	
	Male	Female	Male	Female	Male	Female	Male	Female
Smoking tobacco	83.1	46.2	87.3	51.5	93.4	87.5	27.3	6.0
Chewing tobacco	1.5	0.0	0.5	0.5	36.4	2.3	0.0	0.0
Chewing betel	3.1	8.7	5.4	5.1	38.7	46.0	0.0	0.0
Chewing miang	58.5	57.7	52.0	49.5	68.9	65.1	0.0	0.0
Drinking liquor	73.8	6.7	83.3	7.1	84.0	0.0	54.7	0.0
Smoking opium	0.8	0.0	0.9	0.5	24.0	0.0	14.8	2.0
Using other substance	13.1	0.0	0.0	0.0	0.0	0.0	1.9	0.0
Number of persons ≥ 20[a]	130	104	221	198	76	87	55	50

[a] *Note*: Denominator for calculating the percentages of users varied for some types of stimulants or narcotics because of missing observations.

Chewing tobacco is popular only among Lua' men (36.5% of those age ≥ 20). Chewing betel quids (*Catechu areca* nut wrapped in *Piper betel* leaf, plus lime, sometimes with tobacco and other ingrediants) was formerly very wide-spread in the lowlands, but is now found in the lowland communities generally only among older people of both sexes. Betel chewing is still popular with Lua' men (38.7%) and even more popular with Lua' women (46%).

Miang is a variety of fermented tea leaves, chewed or sucked with salt and sometimes with peanuts. This traditional Northern Thai specialty is enjoyed by both men and women, especially as they grow older. In the suburb 58.5% of the men and 58.3% of the women chew miang; 53% of the men and 44.3% of the women in the lowland rural Northern Thai community chew, as do 67.6% of the Lua' men and 66.3 percent of the Lua' women. Steady users say they get headaches when they have no miang to chew. No Hmong men or women report chewing tobacco, betel or miang.

Liquor is popular among the men of all four communities (73.9% of the suburban men, 83.3% of the lowland rural Northern Thai men, 84% of the Lua' men and 54.7% of the Hmong men drink). Alcohol consumption is much lower among women (6% of the suburban women, 6.1% of the rural lowland Northern Thai women, none of the Lua' or Hmong women report drinking). In the lowland communities, several varieties of liquor are available in the market, the most popular of which is probably commercially prepared Mekong, or the product of one of the local licensed distilleries. The most common drink among the Lua' is a *sake*-like home-distilled rice liquor. Hmong distill corn liquor with a very high alcohol content.

Opium is known in all the study communities both as a medicine (especially for diarrhea or coughs) and as a narcotic. When used as a narcotic in this area it is generally smoked in the unrefined form. Use is very low in the lowland communities (0.8% of the suburban men, 0.9% of the rural lowland Northern Thai men), but high in the Hmong village (14.8% of the men), and very high among Lua' men (24%). Only one woman opium user was reported in any of the communities (0.5% of rural lowland Northern Thai women).

These results suggest that despite their reputation as growers and users of opium, Hmong make low use of stimulants and narcotics (tobacco, betel, *miang*, liquor, opium) as compared with the other communities we studied. Lua', in comparison, make relatively high use of all local forms of stimulants and narcotics. This heavy use, along with their relative poverty and poor sanitary conditions, may contribute to their high rate of reported illness, and comparatively high mortality rates. Early and sustained heavy use of tobacco by Lua' probably contributes to their high rate of reported respiratory illnesses, which is two or three times higher than reported for the other groups.

Development projects are providing protected water supplies for many villages in Thailand, starting first in cities and towns, then in the lowland rural areas, and then in the highlands, where there seem to be problems of maintenance as well as delay in construction of the facilities. Cross-sectional mortality data in this study suggest a relationship between protected water supply and low rate of diarrheal diseases in town. This might suggest that this intervention was effective in changing exposure to water-borne pathogens, thereby reducing diarrheal disease. Historical data (from reproductive histories) suggest that the decline in diarrheal diseases occurred in town long before the piped water system was installed there. A piped water system was installed in the Lua' village about five years before the survey, but diarrheal rates there remained high. Diarrhea rates were low in the Hmong village which had no piped water system. These comparisons suggest that a piped water system, by itself, may be neither necessary nor sufficient to reduce diarrheal disease. Observation of living conditions in the highland villages suggest that risk factors in addition to water supply might be involved. To date no effort has been made to develop sanitary storage methods for water which is not piped into homes. The water is carried and stored in unsanitary containers, and in Lua' villages is commonly consumed without boiling. Hmong villagers more often drink boiled water in the form of tea, and seem to eat food promptly after cooking. Lua' villagers frequently save leftovers for the next meal, without the benefit of refrigeration or protection from flies, but Hmong villagers apparently do not do this.

Development efforts have frequently been directed at persuading villagers to install waterseal latrines. In the Lua' village, although latrines were installed, they were rarely used because of shortages of water. No efforts seem to have been directed at reducing the risks of water- or fly-borne diseases from feces deposited in the forest. To the contrary, the Lua' villagers, for example, traditionally used pigs as scavengers of human feces, but development workers have urged these villagers, for the sake of sanitation (to prevent the spread of pig feces around the village) and "modern" appearence to keep their pigs penned underneath their houses at all times. Removal of these traditional scavengers may increase the risk of transmission of human diseases associated with feces.

To date no attention has been paid in this area to reducing exposure of villagers to indoor air pollution from smokey fires, or even from tobacco smoking. In communities close to transportation routes, firewood has sometimes been supplemented with low pollution fuels, but there has been little change of this type in the poorer and more remote communities, except for the substitution of smokey kerosene lamps for wooden torches. Ventilation in traditional highland village houses is poor and may be getting worse as a result of substitution of non-porous corrugated metal for traditional grass or leaf roofs. Corrugated metal roofs are now coming into use in some highland villages because of a shortage of traditional roofing material related to the increase in highland population, and the increase in the highlands of cattle which eat the roofing grass. Metal roofs are fireproof and easier to maintain, but Lua' villagers recognize they increase the problem of smoke pollution in their relatively small, low-roofed houses.

Consumption of tobacco, alcohol and opium are clearly related to a variety of health problems. Betel and possibly miang may be related to mouth cancers, but appear to be less serious problems, and may be declining in use (cf. Mougne, MacLenna and Atsana 1982). Betel was outlawed about 40 years ago because of the unsightly and non-modern appearance of betel chewers. Use of opium has been illegal since 1957, and there are a number of programs to treat addicts as well as to suppress the production, sale and use of opium. Addiction seems to be a more serious problem among Lua' and other groups who do not grow it than among Hmong who seem to have lived with it long enough to learn its dangers, and who may be better able to control the level of use.

Health authorities are only beginning to become aware of the problems of abuse of manufactured drugs. These problems seem to develop earliest in urban areas. Little or no attention is being paid to controlling consumption of tobacco and alcohol. To the contrary, the tendency seems to be to allow encouragement of the use of liquor and tobacco, which are major sources of tax revenue, through advertising. Patterns of tobacco use seem to be changing, with substitution of purchased cigarettes (which may be inhaled more deeply) for the traditional pipes and Burmese cigarettes. This suggests that health problems related to use of stimulants and narcotics may be increasing in these communities.

DISCUSSION AND CONCLUSION

Differences in rates, causes and changes in mortality patterns have been described for different types of communities in northwestern Thailand. Reproductive histories appear to be useful for reconstructing recent trends in mortality rates and causes. The picture that emerges is consistent with the recent history of socioeconomic development of the area, in which the town population benefitted most and soonest from modernization, while the more remote communities, especially those in the highlands, benefitted more slowly and to a lesser extent. Infectious diseases have declined in importance in town, but remain important in more isolated communities. It appears that mortality rates in young, rapidly growing populations, such as those of the highland communities have been somewhat reduced even before infectious diseases are fully controlled. Apparently such declines may result from relatively minor and indirect changes, as well as the control of a few important infectious diseases.

It is important to note that although both Mae Sariang area hospitals are located in suburban communities, child mortality in the suburbs remains higher than in town. Physical distance to a modern medical facility does not, by itself, account for mortality differences. Comparison of mortality rates and trends in Skaw Karen populations in different ecological settings suggests that geographic and possibly social distance from the focus of development does play some part in determining the path of the mortality transition in different types of communities in this area. Comparison of Skaw Karen communities with communities of other ethnic groups in similar environments suggests that ethnic differences or social isolation may also affect the path of mortality changes.

Smallpox was controlled by immunization programs carried out primarily in the lowlands. Highland populations apparently benefitted from "herd immunity" effects, and no fatalities from this cause were reported after about 1950. Malaria, which was a very serious problem primarily in the lowlands, has been effectively controlled in the densely settled valleys, but is now being reported as a cause of death in highland communities. If confirmed serologically, this might suggest that development, in the form of expanded irrigation or increased travel to lowland forests, may be creating environmental conditions suitable for transmission of malaria to highland populations. Immunizable "childhoold" diseases appear to be well controlled in the lowlands but are still occasionally very disruptive in the highlands which have not yet benefitted to the same extent from maternal and child health programs. The apparent decline in gastrointestinal diseases in town long before the installation of a safe water system there, and the continued importance of gastrointestinal illnesses after piped water systems have been introduced in some highland villages suggests that a general level of affluence, education and cleanliness may be important in limiting these diseases. Persistence of high rates of neonatal deaths in remote communities may be a result of traditional birth practices, or may reflect poor socioeconomic conditions. Chances for survival of children born in town are now at the same level as in developed countries; chances for survival of children born in villages a few kilometers away remain much lower. This is a challenge for an integrated approach of social and medical sciences.

Analysis of the data on morbidity reveals a picture which generally parallels that for mortality in terms of rates and causes of illness. Analysis of risk factors in the environments and behavior patterns of the communities suggests that behavioral differences (especially the use of stimulants and narcotics) may be an important factor accounting for differences in disease rates between the different types of communities. The early, widespread and heavy rate of tobacco smoking, coupled with poor environmental sanitation, probably contributes to the relatively high rate of illness and mortality in the Lua' village, despite the appearance of modern sanitary features (e.g., piped water, waterseal latrines, and penned pigs).

The present study was carried out to identify differences in morbidity and mortality rates. Identification of the reasons for the observed differences will require different techniques. In an earlier period of fieldwork we noted that Highland Lua' villages characteristically experience epidemics of infectious diseases (e.g., chickenpox) in which everyone under a certain age becomes ill. This is in contrast with the pattern in neighboring Skaw Karen villages where only the youngest children become ill with chickenpox and similar contagious diseases. Ethnographic observation suggested at least one reason for this epidemiological difference. Karens going to market normally go in complete household groups (including young children), but Lua' ordinarily leave their young children at home when they go to market. Thus non-immune Karen children are more likely to be exposed to contagious diseases at an early age, and the pool of non-immune children will be small, while non-immune Lua' children are unlikely to be exposed until they reach the age when they are allowed to go to market, and the pool of non-immune children will be large (Kunstadter 1972). Discovering relevant behavioral differences between ethnic groups, and testing their epidemiological significance, is a subject for future research.

Ideally, integration of epidemiological and social sciences might require several stages of research to attack problems of the type outlined in this chapter (gross epidemiological differences between identifiable groups within a relatively small geographical area). Social science methods would be used to identify significant population subunits for analysis and describe medically relevant environmental and behavioral differences between them. Quantitative demographic or epidemiological methods would be used to gather data to describe patterns of morbidity and mortality associated with the groups, and to identify leading health problems. The next step would be to search for specific behavioral and environmental risk factors which were associated with the differences in morbidity and mortality. Finally, social science data and techniques would be used to assist in designing and implementing programs to reduce risks and prevent or treat the important diseases.

We have suggested that a combination of social and epidemiological approaches may have wide applications. One example is in morbidity and mortality surveys in relatively remote populations. In such surveys, one problem is collecting statistics where low proportions of deaths are attended by a physician. Without medical certification it is necessary to rely on lay reporting or verbal autopsies for cause of death (e.g., WHO 1978). Use of these techniques is complicated where the local terminologies and concepts of cause of death may have little direct relationship to modern medical diagnostic categories. To be successful the forms designed for lay reporting or verbal autopsies require a good knowledge of local diagnostic categories, and the ability either to translate these categories into medically meaningful terms, or to elicit symptoms which are adequate for assignment of cause.

ACKNOWLEDGEMENTS

Research supported by National-Science Foundation Grant 7914093 et seq. and the East—West Population Institute. This is a revised version of a paper presented at the Annual Meetings of the American Anthropological Association, 19 November 1983, Chicago, Illinois. Assistance of Kae Boe, Khru Booneng, Nai Chalerm, Khru Chit and Nai Saman in collecting the data, and of Ms. Naomi Higa, Khun Sutthita NaChiengmai, and Ms. Nitaya Pickop in data processing is greatfully acknowledged.

NOTE

1. The relatively low rate of respiratory diseases reported in the Hmong community is anomalous. Residential crowding, measured as number of people per household, and numbers of susceptible individuals who are in contact with a source of infection are generally recognized as risk factors for respiratory infections. Large household size presumably increases the risk of transmission of the disease organism among susceptible individuals who are in close contact. Hmong households are very large (well over 10 persons per household, twice the average size found in other groups), and as suggested by the very young age distribution, generally have large numbers of young children who may be more susceptible to respiratory infections than adults. Thus Hmong might be expected to have higher rates of respiratory illness than the other groups. Our failure to find the expected relationship between household size, number or proportion of young children, and prevalence of respiratory illness suggests that some other environmental factor, such as air pollution, may be involved. This is a subject for future research.

REFERENCES CITED

Baker, P.
    1977 Problems and Strategies. *In* Paul Baker (ed.), Human Population Problems in the Biosphere: Some Research Strategies and Designs. MAB Technical Notes 3. Paris: UNESCO, pp. 11—33.
    1982 Human Population Biology: A Viable Transdisciplinary Science. Human Biology 54(2): 203—220.
Chretien, J., W. Holland, P. Macklem, J. Murray, and A. Woolcock
    1984 Acute Respiratory Infections in Children: A Global Public Health Problem. New England Journal of Medicine 310: 982—984.
Coale, Ansley J., Barbara A. Anderson and Erna Harn
    1979 Human Fertility in Russia since the Nineteenth Century. Princeton: Princeton University Press.
Douglas, R. M., V. Kumar, and D. L. Miller, et al.
    1984 A Programme for Controlling Acute Respiratory Infections in Children: Memorandum from a WHO Meeting. Bulletin of the World Health Organization 62: 47—58.
East-West Center Working Group on Health Correlates of Domestic Smoke Exposure
    1985 Domestic Smoke Pollution and Respiratory Illness in Developing Countries: Communique to the Medical and Public Health Communities. Honolulu: East-West Center.

Eggan, F.
    1954 Social Anthropology and the Method of Controlled Comparison. American Anthropologist 56: 743—763.
Kunstadter, P.
    1971 Natality, Mortality and Migration of Upland and Lowland Populations in Northwestern Thailand. *In* S. Polgar (ed.), Culture and Population. Shenkman Publishing Co. and Carolina Population Center.
    1972 Demography, Ecology, Social Structure and Settlement Patterns. *In* A. Boyce and G. Harrison (eds.), The Structure of Human Populations, Oxford: Clarendon Press.
    1984a Cultural Ideals, Socioeconomic Change, and Household Composition: Karen, Lua', Hmong and Thai in Northwestern Thailand. Ch. 12 *in* Robert McC. Netting, Richard Wilk and Eric J. Arnould, (eds.). Households: Comparative and Historical Studies of the Domestic Group, Berkeley: University of California Press, pp. 299—329.
    1984b Lifetime Migration and Mortality in a Northwestern Thailand Town. *In* Malcolm A. Fernando (ed.), Human Population Movements and Their Impact on Tropical Disease Transmission and Control. Peradeniya, Sri Lanka: Faculty of Medicine, University of Peradeniya, pp. 69—83.
    1984c Demographic Differentials in a Rapidly Changing Mixed Ethnic Population in Northwestern Thailand. NUPRI Research Paper Series No. 19. Tokyo. Nihon University Population Research Institute.
Mougne, C., R. Maclennan, and S. Atsana
    1982 Chewing and Drinking in Ban Pong, Northern Thailand. Social Science and Medicine 16(1): 99—106.
Smith, K. and P. Kunstadter
    n.d. Unpublished data from field trip to Northwestern Thailand, January 1984. Honolulu: East-West Center.
Syme, S. L., M. G. Marmot, A. Kagan, H. Kato and George Rhoads
    1975 Epidemiologic Studies of Coronary Heart Diseases and Stroke in Japanese Men Living in Japan, Hawaii and California: Introduction. American Journal of Epidemiology 10(6): 477—480.
Sawyer, B.
    1982 Personal Communication. Statistics of the Mae Sariang Christian Hospital, based on hospital records. Mae Sariang, Thailand.
United Nations Economic Commission for Asia and the Far East [ECAFE]
    1973 Comparative Study of Mortality Trends in ECAFE Countries. Asian Population Studies Series, 14. Bangkok: ECAFE.
World Health Organization
    1977 International Classification of Diseases, 9th Revision. Geneva: World Health Organization.
    1978 Lay Reporting of Health Information. Geneva: World Health Organization.
    1984 WHO Annual Statistics Reveals Major Public Health Killers (press release WHO/8). Geneva: World Health Organization.

E. MICHAEL GORMAN

THE AIDS EPIDEMIC IN SAN FRANCISCO: EPIDEMIOLOGICAL AND ANTHROPOLOGICAL PERSPECTIVES

Acquired immune-deficiency syndrome, commonly termed AIDS, has been called perhaps the most serious public health menace of the 20th century. Such pronouncements are made not on the basis of public misunderstanding or hysteria, but on sound scientific grounds. First, although the agent believed to cause the disease has been isolated in the laboratory, it is of a group of poorly understood viruses, termed *retroviruses*. An effective vaccine is not expected for some time. Second, AIDS affects the immune system, one of the most complex systems of human physiology. Third, AIDS has primarily affected a somewhat invisible and stigmatized subculture of American society, a fact that renders matters of health policy and prevention sensitive. This final characteristic of the epidemic means that primary and secondary prevention efforts — for the forseeable future the most effective means of controlling AIDS — are likely to be fraught with fundamental social and ethical issues, including patient confidentiality, stigma, and civil rights.

Because effective biomedical means for treating or controlling the disease are not immediately available, effective prevention policy must incorporate a thorough understanding of the individual behavior that places people at risk for the disease, and the social and cultural factors that influence this behavior. Owing to the increasing sophistication of medical anthropology in understanding disease contexts and identifying the determinants of health behavior, the area of prevention provides a relevant domain for converting epidemiologic understandings of risk into sensible, sensitive, and comprehensive methods for reducing exposure to the disease agent.

The primary purpose of this article is to describe epidemiological and anthropological aspects of the AIDS outbreak in San Francisco. This discussion will be limited to consideration of the highest risk population in that city: gay (i.e., homosexual/bisexual) men. The emphasis will be on two interrelated facets of the epidemiology of AIDS that are social in nature and thus amenable to anthropological analysis. These are first, the effect of AIDS on gay subcultures, involving issues such as stigma, death and dying, contagion, and sexuality; and second, the determinants of behavior that place individuals at risk for the disease. The importance of medical anthropology, and the medical anthropologist for converting epidemiological knowledge of risk into prevention strategies, will form the focus of the discussion throughout.

BACKGROUND: THE EPIDEMIOLOGY OF AIDS

As of January, 1986, over 16,000 cases of the acquired immune deficiency

Craig R. Janes et al. (eds.), Anthropology and Epidemiology, 157—172.
© 1986 *by D. Reidel Publishing Company.*

syndrome had been reported in the United States by the Centers for Disease Control. AIDS is currently thought to be caused by a virus called LAV (Lymphadenopathy Associated Virus) by French researchers, or HTLV-III (Human T-Cell Lymphotrophic Virus, Class III) by American investigators (Barre-Sinoussi et al. 1983: 868—871; Gallo et al. 1984: 500—503).

One of the most curious aspects of the epidemiology of AIDS in the United States is its presentation in seemingly disparate populations: gay and bisexual men, intravenous drug users, Haitians, Central Africans, hemophiliacs, recipients of blood transfusions, and in some cases the sexual partners of these groups (Centers for Disease Control 1981a, 1981b, 1982a, 1982b, 1982c, 1982d). Gay and bisexual men represent by far the largest percentage of the cases (73%), although some 12% of the total are both bisexual and intravenous drug users. 17% of intravenous drug users who have the disease are heterosexual. 1.5% of all cases occurred in individuals with no other risk factor than having received a transfusion of whole blood or a blood product within five years of diágnosis, and 0.7% are individuals with hemophilia who had received clotting factor concentrates. 1% of AIDS cases were the heterosexual partners of the high risk groups identified above. Of all diagnosed AIDS cases, including individuals from the high-risk areas of Haiti and Central Africa, 6.4% exhibited no identifiable risk factors (Curran et al. 1985: 1352—1357).

Outside of the United States, cases have been reported in Canada, Australia, Western Europe, Africa, Asia, the Caribbean, and Latin America. In Australia, Canada, and Western Europe the distribution and behavioral characteristics of cases resembles that of the United States. In Europe there are also a number of cases of African origin. In Africa cases have been reported in over 20 countries, and are more likely to be heterosexual. The male/female ratio of AIDS cases in Africa is approximately 1.1 to 1, in contrast to the United States and other developed nations where the ratio is 9 to 1 (Curran 1985).

AIDS is generally a fatal disease; few individuals live as long as three years after clinical diagnosis. By January, 1986, there had been some 8,000 AIDS-related deaths. Once diagnosed, typical course of the disease includes one or several life-threatening opportunistic infections (including cancer), eventually resulting in death. As of the end of 1985 it was estimated by the Centers for Disease Control that between 500,000 and 1,000,000 Americans had been infected (Curran et al. 1985: 1354). The incubation period between infection and clinical manifestation of the disease averages three years for sexual transmission, and 4.5 years for transfusion transmitted AIDS. Not all individuals infected with the disease go on to develop AIDS; at present the Centers for Disease Control estimates that between 1 and 2% of all those infected will be diagnosed with AIDS in a single year. Given the large population of infected individuals, and the fact that this population will likely increase significantly in the months and years to come, the AIDS epidemic will pose a serious challenge to the American health care system. The economic costs alone are staggering; at present the cost per patient for treatment averages $140,000.

In addition to those who develop clinical AIDS, a large number of individuals manifest lesser symptoms of the disease: swollen lymph glands, occasional and persistent fever, fatigue, diarrhea, various chronic skin infections and oral thrush (candidiasis). Some patients with this syndrome, called AIDS-related complex (ARC), become quite ill, and some, between 6 and 20%, go on to develop one of the life-threatening opportunistic infections or cancers characteristic of clinical AIDS. The long-term effects on the general health and well-being of those individuals who do not develop AIDS or ARC and yet who are antibody positive are, as yet, unknown.

EPIDEMIOLOGY, ANTHROPOLOGY, AND THE STUDY OF AIDS

The determinants and distribution of disease in human populations represent the focus of epidemiological inquiry. Initial epidemiological investigations usually focus on person, time, and place, and relate these variables to disease or health risk and to health maintenance (Lillienfeld 1980). In recent years epidemiologists have become increasingly interested in behavior as it relates to health and the roles it plays in elucidating the features of person, place, and time that define the determinants and distribution of disease. Such interests have led to the development of a subfield of behavioral or social epidemiology. Behaviorial epidemiology may usefully apply anthropological methodologies in documenting behaviors and the meaning of these behaviors in given institutional and cultural contexts as well as identifying their role in causing or preventing dsiease. The anthropologist's skill at gaining entry to the population(s) at risk, in identifying and gaining the confidence of key informants and serving as culture brokers between professional and lay communities can be vital to developing epidemiological research. This is particularly true in the case of AIDS, given the fear and stigma attached to the disease, and the marginality that characterizes the populations at risk. Study of the populations at risk in clinical settings is difficult or impossible.

To date a sufficient baseline of epidemiological data on AIDS has accumulated to provide a broad understanding of the etiology of the disease. However, examination from a social anthropological perspective of the impact of AIDS on individuals, small groups, communities, and institutions is only beginning. This paper aims to integrate these perspectives in order to provide a more comprehensive understanding of the AIDS epidemic.

THE SOCIAL HISTORY OF AN EPIDEMIC

Like all epidemics, which are social processes by definition, AIDS did not happen by chance. Why it occurred at the time it did and in the populations that it has, remain key questions which cannot be answered apart from the wider contexts of these populations: technological changes such as improvements in chemotherapies for hemophilia such as Factor VIII concentrate, increases in numbers of blood transfusions and blood donations, dramatic increases in international travel and migration to the U.S. from continents other than Europe, and changes in sexual mores. The etiologic agent may be identified, but how this agent became widespread in disparate high risk populations as well as how the disease can be prevented are of more than passing anthropological interest (Darrow and Gorman 1980).

The first cases of AIDS in the United States probably developed in the mid-1970s among gay men in New York City. Transmission among Haitian migrants to the U.S. was probably beginning about this time as well. Among the first victims were those who developed lesions that were subsequently identified as an uncommon form of soft-tissue cancer called Kaposi's sarcoma. Kaposi's sarcoma had been a rare disease among North American and Western European populations and historically took an indolent course. In young American homosexual men, however, the disease turned out to be very aggressive, and death usually occurred within two to three years (Safai 1981).

THE SOCIAL CONTEXT OF THE AIDS EPIDEMIC AMONG GAY MEN

The 1960s and 1970s saw dramatic changes in the dynamics of American society, notably the Black civil rights movement, the women's movement, and the gay civil rights movement. It is the last movement that is of relevance to the AIDS epidemic. Although the roots of the gay movement in the United States go back to the 1920s, it was not until well into the 1960s that it gained enough momentum to attract significant public attention. A focal point in this development was the Stonewall Riots of June 28, 1969. This event, a riot at a gay tavern in New York's Greenwich Village, in which gays rebelled against police harassment, was celebrated throughout the country by gay people. It represented the first widely publicized attack by gay individuals on commonplace police actions (such as arrest) intended to limit the rights of gay people to assemble politically. The following year a national gay conference was held in San Francisco that attracted a wide range of gay political, social, and religious organizations. Subsequently, regional meetings were held throughout the country and the gay civil rights movement gathered further momentum, often taking direction from the Black and women's movements. Large cities such as New York, Los Angeles, San Francisco, Boston, and Philadelphia became the centers of much of this political activity, and many of these cities led the way in establishing some measure of legal protection for gay people in employment and housing.

Of the respective civil rights movements, the least analyzed from an anthropological perspective has been the gay movement (Read 1980). On one level all of these processes were concerned with the construction of identity, and with the emergence of a consciousness or sense of self constructed both at individual and collective levels, articulated about a set of symbols and actualized and focussed in a political context. Although time and space limit detailed consideration of this phenomenon here, it is worth noting that significant cultural shifts were occurring in American society which permitted the emergence of a gay social movement and for the public articulation of a set of symbols and institutions uniquely identifiable as gay.[1] Some of these shifts had to do with changes in traditional sex roles and the increasing separation of the cultural realms of biological reproduction from those of sexuality. Some of these changes included advancements in birth control technology, the availability of abortion on demand, and the development of a labor market in which biological differences were of decreasing importance. Further, the gradual emergence of at least a nominal ideology of egalitarianism and non-discrimination based on sex also contributed to the freeing of women, at least those women so interested, from traditional female roles.

The same technological changes that had allowed for the liberation of women from the home and from traditional roles also facilitated the ability of homosexual individuals to establish a lifestyle for themselves. As with women, gay individuals benefitted from the losening of the cultural imperative to procreate, the blurring of the sex role/occupation differentiation, as well as from the general *zeitgeist* of the period that emphasized values of independence and non-traditional lifeways. Gay people took advantage of these sociocultural changes, and, in the larger cities, congregated in territorial communities, often called "gay ghettos" (Levine 1979). Institutions and businesses that met such disparate needs within the gay male community as roomate services, real estate and banking, clothing, and even laundry and cleaning services flourished as these new urban villages became established and defined. A distinctive gay argot evolved too, along with other aspects of a distinctively gay symbolic universe, e.g., identifiable clothing and hair styles, literature with gay themes, art, and films. The notion of a distinctively gay identity and of a "gay person" evolved in tandem with the establishment of the gay ghettos. Homosexual men and women "came out of the closet" — the common metaphor for the secrecy that had characterized homosexual life historically — in great numbers and in the process created new cultural worlds.

On a larger scale, part of this gay cultural emergence resulted from the migration of gay people to "magnet" cities, may of them coastal cities where the tolerance of non-traditional lifestyles was greater. In the 1970s, propelled by the baby boom, a new wave of migration of gays swept into three cities in particular: New York, Los Angeles, and San Francisco. Of the three, perhaps the city most culturally gay, and certainly the city that became the most proportionately and politically gay, was San Francisco.

San Francisco in many ways was paradigmatic of the social, economic, and political changes of the post-Stonewall era, if representing a particularly unique configuration of those processes. Historically a city of toleration, home of the "flower children" of the 1960s, and a center of the anti-war movement, San Francisco was to become a national center for the gay movement by the 1970s. Like other cities, San Francisco developed a number of neighborhoods in which openly gay men and lesbians were frequently seen. But it was the Castro district which was to become a major focal point, cultural center and "main street" of gay life in San Francisco. With the migration of many gay young adults to the Castro district, the construction of a new community began. Older homes were purchased and upgraded, businesses opened that catered to the needs of newcomers, gay professional and social networks were formed, religious organizations were established in the neighborhood and political organizations evolved. Upon the establishment of city supervisorial elections on a district basis, the Castro district elected the first openly gay individual (Harvey Milk) to public office in the United States.

One of the most salient aspects of the social changes of the 1970s was the sexual revolution and the development of singles and open-relationship lifestyles that included sexual experimentation, including experimentation with different partners. This revolution occurred among both heterosexuals and homosexuals.

Changes in norms of sexual behavior were reflected in the health problems of sexually active individuals. During this period, the incidence of venereal infections such as herpes, venereal warts, amebiasis and giardiasis significantly increased, and incidence rates for gonorrhea and syphilis skyrocketed. Gay men were part of this sexual revolution and suffered at least their share of the new diseases. Several diseases, in particular, became endemic among the sexually active homosexual male population, e.g., hepatitis B, syphilis, venereal warts and, in the mid-1970s, amebiasis, giardiasis and shigellosis. The health problems, and indirectly the social and sexual contexts that spawned them, were reflected biologically in antibodies developed by exposure to venereal infections. Once an individual was exposed to syphilis, cytomegalovirus, Epstein-Barr virus, hepatitis A or B, these became etched in the template of his immunological memory. Thus, the social and behavioral changes of the period came to be reflected at the individual, immunological level.

The cultural changes that permitted gay culture to flourish in some cities did not affect all who participated in the gay sexual world. Many married and bisexual men, and those who chose to keep their homosexual behavior hidden, were less touched by the ethos of gay liberation, yet were also at risk for venereal disease. Further, not all gay men, however liberated, experimented sexually with different partners; many entered monogamous relationships soon after declaring their homosexuality. However, for those sexually active with numerous sexual partners — whether "closeted" or "out" — the 1970s were marked by small epidemics of hepatitis A and B, infectious syphilis, and venereal warts. Later in the decade, enteric infections such as amebiasis and giardiasis were to become serious health problems for many gay men. In short, a sexual ecology emerged that provided many opportunities for the contraction of infectious disease. However, in the era of antibiotics these conditions were viewed more as nuisances, the inevitable hazards of a busy sexual lifestyle.

THE AIDS EPIDEMIC IN SAN FRANCISCO: A CASE STUDY

Retrospective epidemiologic investigation revealed that the first cases of AIDS appeared in the San Francisco Bay area in 1979 and were manifested in gay men as Kaposi's sarcoma. Similar to the situation in New York, these cases were initially considered unrelated epidemiologically to each other. By late 1980 it had become evident that a new epidemic was underway. By June of 1981 it was also apparent that the problem had become a national one. Concerted efforts to treat the syndrome in San Francisco began with the opening of the Kaposi's Sarcoma Clinic at the University of California, San Francisco (UCSF) in late 1981.

During the summer of 1982, a group at UCSF representing various health science specialties began working together to develop a major research project to study the disease. The team included an epidemiologist, a statistician, a program manager, support staff, and a medical anthropologist (myself) who had training in epidemiology and infectious diesease, and who had extensive experience working with the city's gay community on health-related issues. Still, at the time the initial numbers of cases were low and concerns both in San Francisco's gay community and the city generally were not very great. As the behavioral epidemiologist on the team, I was assigned a variety of tasks, including contributing to the development of the questionnaire, assisting in the hiring and training of interviewers, piloting the research instrument, and participating in proposal writing.

Before this time, two other AIDS studies had been done in the United States, one under the auspices of the Centers for Disease Control (CDC) on the first 50 American cases, and the other by researchers at New York University (Marmor et al. 1982). The CDC study was selected as a model upon which to build the San Francisco study, although we believed that it could be tailored to the specific setting of San Francisco's gay community. We included questions of demography, medical history, sexual history, social factors, alcohol and drug usage, and sexual contacts. The sexual history represented a particular challenge because it required knowledge of and sensitivity to various aspects of gay male sexual behavior as well as the cultural themes espoused by the many gay subcultures. As part of this initial process of protocol design the investigators undertook an extensive field investigation of the gay community.

An important aspect of this investigation was the obtaining of support of the gay community, without which the study could not have been conducted. Every effort was made to meet with community leaders. A gay scientific advisory panel was established, and the Bay Area Physicians for Human Rights, an organization of gay-sensitive physicians, was sought out for its support. Not all elements in the gay community were enthusiastic. Some did not see the need for so much investigation of what was considered a rare disease. Others feared divulging too much information about some of the heretofore hidden aspects of gay sexuality, fearing that such information could possibly be used against the gay community and might make it vulnerable to the effects of further stigmatization and consequent political repression. However, the study received enough substantial support that it was able to proceed.

After many revisions the questionnaire was piloted on a sample of approximately 50 gay men. Volunteers were obtained from advertisements in gay newspapers, bars, baths, organizations, and through friendship networks. Although this sample was an opportunistic one, our feeling was that this group represented as much of a cross-section of the demographic profile of gay men in San Francisco as was possible to achieve without resorting to expensive area probability sampling techniques.

In addition to the daily involvement with the operation of the project, the team was also involved in some prelimiary efforts at prevention and health education based on what was known of the disease at that time. From our contacts with people in the community, reading gay periodicals, and our interactions with various community leaders, it became all too apparent that there was considerable misinformation about the disease. Views on the seriousness of the problem varied widely, but a commonly voiced opinion was that "everyone has already been exposed". Conversely, the view was also expressed that the disease was so rare that there was no reason to worry. In either case these attitudes made any sort of risk-reduction education difficult. Most gay men in San Francisco at that time — January, 1983 — did not conceive of this epidemic as a threat to their own lives, especially given the fact that there were only about 100 cases in the city. From our perspective as epidemiologists we were aware that the caseload was doubling approximately every six months and that the epidemic curve appeared to be paralleling that of New York, although with approximately a one year lag. The long incubation period contributed to the perception that the problem was not large scale or serious. A related historical and sociological problem was the fact that this generation had had no prior or similar experience of illness which posed such threats to the public health. Infectious diseases in the United States during the last quarter of the twentieth century had not posed serious health threats and were assumed to be amenable to technological innovation and prevention. One of the most difficult and challenging tasks was to convince men in the gay community that a very serious epidemic was underway.

To document the true extent of the epidemic we undertook an analysis of the incidence of those cases occurring between the perceived inception of the epidemic and January, 1983. The result of this analysis demonstrated a concentration of cases by place of residence and time of diagnosis — called "clustering" in epidemiologic terminology — in seventeen census tracts in the very heart of San Francisco and which centered in the Castro district.

Using the 1980 census we attempted to estimate the number of gay men in San Francisco for the purposes of determining a denominator to estimate the prevalence and incidence of AIDS among gay men living in the city. Previously, no accurate census figures of the numbers of gay men existed. The number of never-married males between the ages of 18 and 34 in those census tracts where most of the AIDS cases resided was used as a highly conservative approximation of the population of gay men in San Francisco. This figure was probably an underestimation of the number of gay men in the city since it would not take into account the gay men who had been married earlier in their lives, or gay men who did not reside in the 17 census tracts where the AIDS epidemic was centered.

The most startling epidemiologic finding to come out of this analysis was the discovery of a high prevalence rate of AIDS among gay men in the 17 census tracts under investigation (Moss et al. 1983). By January 1983, approximately one in 350 gay men in that part of the city had already been diagnosed as having AIDS under the strict CDC diagnostic criteria. When the cases were plotted on a curve based on the incidence of the disease to that time, indications were that this figure was likely to double in the succeeding six months.

To disseminate this information, meetings were held with leaders of the gay community. We also decided to publish the information in a major medical journal (Moss et al. 1983). Reaction to the publication of this information was divided in the gay community. On the one side were leaders who wanted to publicize the results more openly and to sound the alarm, even to urge the closing of such institutions as the baths.[2] Some of these individuals were physicians and gay health care workers, others were political leaders who had lost friends or lovers to the epidemic. On the other side were gay political leaders who saw in the publication of these statistics a threat to the political and economic welfare of the gay community. They also argued that such information would cause panic within and outside of the gay community.

The early stages of the AIDS epidemic afforded many unusual opportunities for the medical anthropologist, and anthropological methodologies and point of view were of great relevance in many respects. Epidemiologic inquiry focuses primarily on the determinants of disease in human populations. In this context anthropological knowledge assisted in the more precise delineation of the epidemiological variables of interest: person, time, and place. Specific knowledge of the population at risk and familiarity with the cultural context also aided in the process of investigating the epidemic. Experience with the community and understanding its mores and history likewise facilitated the research process and brought community needs such as health education, risk reduction information, and prevention generally to the attention of the investigators.

THE ANTHROPOLOGY OF AIDS

Issues of anthropological interest raised by the AIDS epidemic in San Francisco include but are not limited to those of stigma, sexuality, confidentiality, contagion, death and dying, and the impact of disease on the emergence of new cultures. Furthermore, resolution of the methodological issues raised by the combination of the role of behavioral epidemiologist and anthropologist is relevant to the further development of medical anthropology.

Perhaps the foremost of these issues is that of stigma, for the epidemic in this population represented an opportunity to encounter stigma and its aspects in very basic terms, as Goffman has described (Goffman 1963). Even in San Francisco, where the gay community had become a potent political force in the city, the scars of discrimination remained and the AIDS issue heightened acts of anti-gay violence. The epidemic brought with it the fear of losing hard-won civil rights, to say nothing of the fear of losing one's life. There was also, of course, the great potential for an anti-gay backlash in the political arena. And clinically, with its disfigurement and its debilitation, the disease represented a terrible embodiment of societal fears of homosexuality itself, and a metaphor for contagion and pollution. Kaposi's sarcoma, referred to by some as the "gay leprosy", imprinted on those it afflicted a stigmata that signified homosexuality. Healthy gay men (the "worried well") spoke with dread of the disease and the question of "why us?" pervaded conversations daily.

A related and equally important issue was that of confidentiality. Confidentiality became a hallmark for several issues related to the epidemic both in the epidemiologic study itself as well as in regard to the larger question of the place of homosexuals in American society. On one level, personal identity had to be protected so that those with a diagnosis of AIDS did not lose employment or housing, which was said to be occurring with increasing regularity in San Francisco. For those participating in epidemiologic studies, protection also had to be accorded due to the stigmatized nature of homosexuality as well as the investigation of illegal activities (e.g., drug use) thought to be implicated in the etiology of AIDS.

Contagion emerged early on as an issue in the epidemic. There was great fear on the part of the larger society of catching the disease through transfusion as well as casual contact. Although there were a few transfusion-associated AIDS cases in San Francisco, and the overwhelming majority of cases were sexually transmitted, fears of exposure to a "gay disease" among the general population remained. San Francisco's public transportation system received telephone calls from irate citizenry demanding protection from exposure to gay males also using the transit system. But there was also fear in the gay community itself; stories circulated throughout the community of some AIDS victims released from hospitals only to find themselves evicted by gay roommates and abandoned by lovers. A few straight and gay individuals perceived the gay community as one doomed by promiscuity. In the medical realm, gloves and masks were not infrequently donned when dealing with AIDS patients. Signs outside AIDS patients' hospital room doors warned about precautions to be taken. All of these symbolized the estrangement and alienation of the AIDS patient.

A major effect of the epidemic was the politicization of those diagnosed with AIDS. Perhaps at no time in medical history has a group of afflicted people so rejected the role of being the sick and helpless victim. They called themselves "persons with AIDS" or "PWAS" — a reference to being political prisoners. Some saw the cause of their disease in social rather than biological terms. They argued that discrimination against gay and other marginal people had actually created the conditions for the epidemic.

This epidemic also marked a new frontier in the evolution of the self-definition of those experiencing illness and being labeled by society as terminally ill. In their rejection of the powerlessness of roles of victim and patient, these people challenged society's notion of how they were to behave and feel about themselves and how they should articulate their final *rite de passage*. Feisty as patients, these individuals revealed great strength of character and resilience against tremendous odds.

An important issue of applied anthropological concern is that of prevention. In the absence of a vaccine, the only effective intervention is preventive education and the development of risk reduction strategies that include the communities at risk in a fundamental role. Anthropologists can contribute in important ways to the design and implementation of successful prevention programs directed to the various high-risk populations. These contributions can be framed in terms of primary, secondary, and tertiary levels of prevention.

Primary prevention refers to all measures that prevent disease from occurring, either by reducing exposure to the agent, or by altering the susceptibility of the individual at risk. Secondary prevention is usually thought of as the detection and diagnosis of disease through screening procedures. Tertiary prevention aims to improve the clinical condition through treatment or cure. Additionally, it may seek to readjust the patient into his or her social setting (Ratcliffe et al. 1984: 56-57).

Because in the case of AIDS there is no cure, the development of tertiary prevention schemes (palliative efforts) represents a significant challenge to the medical community. While most tertiary prevention would be assumed to be clinical (as in the application of antiviral chemotherapy) given the nature of the disease, sensitivity to patient needs in treatment is crucial, particularly in regard to handling lifestyle issues. The establishment of AIDS clinical centers like the San Francisco General Hospice ward provides one model for compassionate care in which attention can be given to the particular needs of gay patients.

Screening procedures, the most important dimension of secondary prevention, likewise represents a complex set of issues given the current state of technology. By January, 1986, the primary serological test available for screening blood donations was the Elisa HTLV-III antibody test. However, this test can only detect exposure of the AIDS virus and not actual infection (although exposure is thought to be highly correlated with at least a transient infection). Issues surrounding who should be screened, who should not, and who should conduct such screenings are problematic given the uncertainty over what the test actually measures. Many questions still remain concerning who should have access to information concerning the identities of those who are antibody positive. Many states have passed statutes protecting the confidentiality of those so tested, given the stigma attached to a positive test result and even the test itself. Until the development of an accurate screening device — one that detects the virus and which can identify those who are likely to go on to develop clinical AIDS — the issues surrounding secondary prevention will remain problematic. Anthropologists can assist by clarifying the issues and the positions of both public health officers and the communities that these health officers attempt to serve. This role of culture-broker is one anthropologists have manipulated with some success in the context of disease control and prevention (e.g., Paul 1955).

It is really under the rubric of primary prevention that the utilization of anthropological skills and expertise is most appropriate. In the absence of a vaccine, education is without a doubt the most effective intervention and risk reduction modality available. Yet programs in development need to be carefully tailored to the needs of the various high risk populations. Whether the population of interest is gay, intravenous drug users, prostitutes, Haitians, or hemophiliacs; and whether the providers include physicians, public health nurses, or social workers; culturally appropriate materials for education prevention are needed. Likewise, culturally sensitive individuals require training in order to communicate public health messages effectively.

A spectre behind the AIDS epidemic is death itself, the meaning of death in our society, and particularly for those diagnosed with the disease and those close to them. Not only does AIDS represent an infectious agent to be dealt with on clinical terms, but one that kills young, active, and vital people in the prime of their lives. The experience of so many tragic deaths is all the more overwhelming given the poignancy of related issues of stigma. For many individuals, diagnosis with AIDS also means having to disclose a stigmatized identity — in this case being gay — to their family of origin. Often there is a double burden for the families of having to deal with a terminal illness and the fact that their son or relative is also gay. Additionally, for cities like San Francisco with large populations of young adults, the experience of this epidemic and death as a social fact has been unprecedented. The manner in which death has been addressed as a social process and rite of passage and to which institutions such as the Shanti Project, an agency providing hospice services to AIDS patients, and others that have evolved to meet these needs, is remarkable.

Finally, the study of the AIDS epidemic is of relevance to the anthropological study of how diseases shape cultural development. As this paper has argued, the past 15 years have seen the development of a distinctive gay lifestyle in most urban areas. In many respects gay people — both men and women — have taken on characteristics of certain ethnic communities, in that their social lives often become centered in distinct "urban villages", with a distinctive argot and symbolic system, an ongoing struggle for full civil rights has been undertaken, and social and economic institutions such as churches, banks, and political clubs have been established to meet the needs of that community. The onset of the AIDS epidemic, however, has dealt a tremendous blow to the self-identity of this emerging community, and has forced substantial changes in sexual behavior. In the future changes can be expected not only in the affective and symbolic meanings of sexual contact, but also in broader, non-sexual areas of gay life. Whether and how such changes might occur is a legitimate focus of anthropological inquiry regarding how disease affects culture change. Investigation of the changes wrought within the gay community as a result of this epidemic can be used as one case study for this theoretical focus.

CONCLUSIONS

The public health crisis that attended the AIDS epidemic represents unique opportunities for the application of social scientific perspectives in epidemiology. Due to the combination of biological, technological, social and behavioral phenomena encompassed by AIDS, rarely has a health crisis represented such a unique nexus of disease and culture. AIDS as yet remains a puzzle whose pieces are only slowly being identified and pieced together. Anthropology has contributed and will continue to assist in the assembling of these pieces.

AIDS represents a unique opportunity to investigate what appears to be a new disease with fundamentally important implications for immunology, virology, and the role infectious diseases play in the etiology of cancer. In particular, the social origins of the disease and the behavioral dimensions are important and unexplored areas of investigation. The role of behavior and culture in infectious disease has been insufficiently investigated, and important infectious diseases, hepatitis B among them, have been understudied from this point of view. AIDS may provide an incentive to develop more fully behavioral epidemiology as a subdiscipline with a particular emphasis that draws on medical anthropology.

AIDS also brings to the fore issues of stigma and marginality in American society, issues to which anthropologists have contributed theoretical as well as practical understanding. All the high risk populations — homosexuals, hemophiliacs, intravenous drug users, and others — suffer from societal ostracism.

The AIDS epidemic offers opportunities to learn about sexuality and especially homosexuality. With few exceptions anthropologists have been reluctant to investigate sexual issues, all the more so homosexual ones (Read 1980). It is time that this area of behavior and culture received the increased attention of researchers.

AIDS carries important political implications. It has been a catalyst for an explosion of information about the major risk groups as well as for political activity. In no small part, impetus for AIDS research funding has resulted from political pressure from these groups. Concomitantly, the epidemic has raised central public policy issues about concerns over confidentiality and protection of human subjects, as well as how best to protect the nation's blood supply. On another level the epidemic has provided opportunities for individuals of quite disparate backgrounds to work together and put biases and labels aside. In many instances, clinicians, researchers, and community representatives have for the first time discussed issues in an even-handed manner.

Another area of public health endeavor for which AIDS has been a catalyst has been health eduction for prevention and risk reduction activities. Even with the announcement of the discovery of the putative agent in May, 1984, it was apparent that a vaccine was several years away. The only intervention strategy likely to succeed in the interim is preventive education. This would entail identifying the high risk behaviors implicated in the transmission of the disease as well as the identification of "baseline" male homosexual behaviors against which to measure behavioral change. Given the scale of the epidemic, community-wide interventions need to be developed quickly and the specific educational needs of the respective communities and their resources identified. Anthropologists can and should play key roles in this process.

Finally, the AIDS epidemic has raised important ethical issues. From the beginning of the epidemic there have been concerns about confidentiality and the protection of human subjects. Homosexuals, illegal Haitian immigrants, and intravenous drug users all have reasons to fear disclosure of their respective identities. This has made epidemiological work all the more difficult; it has required great sensitivity to the populations at risk and the development of trust between the investigating institutions and these communities. This has not always been accomplished, in part because of lack of understanding of the cultures of these communities. Anthropologists have historically provided important contributions in precisely these kinds of problem areas (Gussow 1968; Sigerist 1977; Paul 1977; Dunn 1984). Hopefully, in this epidemic too, anthropologists, particularly those with training in public health and epidemiology, can contribute to the understanding of the natural history of the disease, provide insight into the complex biocultural processes at work, and facilitate the development of effective public health interventions.

ACKNOWLEDGEMENTS

The author gratefully acknowledges the assistance of Andrea Sankar, Richard Herrel, Richard Needle, and Sheryl Ruzek, all of whom read drafts of this paper and offered suggestions; the secretarial assistance provided by Amelia Bass is likewise gratefully acknowledged.

NOTES

1. For further discussion of the notion of identity in terms of culture theory, see Gorman (1980).
2. Gay bathhouses were closed by the San Francisco Health Department in the fall of 1984, but were allowed to reopen with strict compliance to "safe sex" guidelines.

REFERENCES

Barre-Sinoussi R., J. C. Chermann, and F. Rey et al.
    1983 Isolation of a T-lymphotrophic Retrovirus from a Patient at Risk of Acquired Immune Deficiency Syndrome (AIDS). Science 220: 868—871.
Curran, J. W. et al.
    1985 The Epidemiology of AIDS: Current Status and Future Prospects. Science 229: 1352—1357.
Centers for Disease Control
    1981a Pneumocystis Pneumonia — Los Angeles. Morbidity and Mortality Weekly Report 30: 250—252.
    1981b Kaposi's Sarcoma and Pneumocystic Pneumonia among Homosexual Men — New York City and California. Morbidity and Mortality Weekly Report 30: 305—308.
    1982a Update on Kaposi's Sarcoma and Opportunistic Infections in Previously Healthy Persons — United States. Morbidity and Mortality Weekly Report 31: 294, 300—301.
    1982b Opportunistic Infections and Kaposi's Sarcoma Among Haitians in the United States. Morbidity and Mortality Weekly Report 31: 353—354, 360—361.

1982c Pneumocystis Carinii Pneumonia Among Persons with Hemophilia A. Morbidity and Mortality Weekly Report 31: 365—367.

1982d Possible Transfusion-Associated Acquired Immune Deficiency Syndrome (AIDS) — California. Morbidity and Mortality Weekly Report 31: 652—654.

Darrow, W. D. and E. M. Gorman
1985 The Social Origins of AIDS. *In* T. Johnson and D. Feldman (eds.) Social Science and AIDS. New York: Praeger.

Dunn, F. L.
1984 Social Determinants in Tropical Disease. *In* K. S. Warren and A. A. F. Mahmoud (eds.), Tropical and Geographical Medicine. New York: McGraw-Hill.

Gallo, R. C., S. Z. Salahuddin, and M. Popovic et al.
1984 Frequent Detection and Isolation of Cytopathic Retroviruses (HTL-III) From Patients With AIDS and at Risk for AIDS. Science 224: 500—503.

Goffman, E.
1963 Stigma: Notes on the Management of a Spoiled Identity. Englewood Cliffs, NJ: Prentice-Hall.

Gorman, E. M.
1980 A New Light on Zion. Ph.D. Dissertation in Anthropology. University of Chicago.

Gussow, Z, and G. Tracy
1977 Status, Ideology, and Adaptation to Stigmatized Illness: A Study of Leprosy. *In* D. Landy (ed.), Culture, Disease, and Healing. New York: Macmillan.

Levine, Michael D.
1979 Gay Ghetto. *In* M. P. Levine (ed.), Gay Men: The Sociology of Male Homosexuality. New York: Harper and Row.

Lillienfeld, A
1980 Foundations of Epidemiology. New York: Oxford University Press.

Marmor, M., A. E. Friedman-Kien, and L. Laubenstein et al.
1982 Risk Factors for Kaposi's Sarcoma in Homosexual Men. Lancet (8281), 1083—1086.

Moss, A., P. Bachetti, and E. M. Gorman
1983 AIDS in 'Gay' San Francisco Neighborhoods. Lancet (8330): 923—924.

Paul, B. (ed.)
1955 Health, Culture, and Community: Case Studies of Public Reactions to Health Programs. New York: Russell Sage Foundation.

1977 The Role of Beliefs and Customs in Sanitation Programs. *In* D. Landy (ed.), Culture, Disease, and Healing. New York: Macmillan.

Ratcliffe, J., L. Wallack, and F. Fagnani et al.
1984 Perspectives on Prevention: Health Promotion Versus Health Protection. *In* J. de Kervasdoue, J. R. Kimberly, and V. G. Rodwin (eds.), The End of An Illusion: The Future of Health Policy in Western Industrialized Nations. Berkeley: University of California Press.

Read, K.
1980 Appendix 1 — Observations on the Current State of Anthropological Research on Homosexual Behavior. *In* Other Voices: The Style of a Male Homosexual Tavern. Novato, CA: Chandler and Sharp.

Safai, B and R. S. Good
1981 Kaposi's Sarcoma: A Review and Recent Developments. Cancer 31: 2—12.

Schneider, D.
1968 American Kinship: A Cultural Account. Englewood Cliffs, NJ: Prentice-Hall.

Sigerist, H.
1977 The Special Position of the Sick. *In* D. Landy (ed.), Culture, Disease, and Healing. New York: Macmillan.

SECTION III

NON-INFECTIOUS DISEASES

CRAIG R. JANES

MIGRATION AND HYPERTENSION:
AN ETHNOGRAPHY OF DISEASE RISK IN
AN URBAN SAMOAN COMMUNITY

Migration is one of the major demographic processes affecting world populations today. However, knowledge of how social and cultural discontinuity affect health remains poorly developed. One reason for this lack of understanding has been the persistence of artificial disciplinary boundaries between the behavioral and health sciences. Social scientists have for some time been interested in the adaptation of migrant *groups* to complex urban settings, yet have not until very recently extended research to consider the physiological consequences of such adaptation for *individual* migrants. Similarly, health scientists — particularly epidemiologists — have treated the social and cultural dimensions of migration in a superficial manner when studying health among migrating populations. The major problem in bridging these disciplinary perspectives lies in creating operational definitions of such explanatory concepts as "Westernization", "acculturation", and "stress" that adequately encompass the full complexities of adaptation to new environments. Thus, there is a need for developing an approach to understanding the health consequences of migration that integrates social scientific and epidemiologic perspectives.

The research discussed in this article represents an effort to integrate anthropological and epidemiological approaches in analyzing the relationship of migration to hypertension. The research population is that of Samoans, a Pacific Island group of Polynesian descent who in the past three decades have been migrating in substantial numbers to California. In previous publications we have examined obesity, mortality, blood pressure, blood glucose levels, and patterns of health behavior in this group (Pawson and Janes 1981, 1982; Janes and Pawson 1986). In this paper I consider the particular social and cultural changes that accompany migration, and how these are related to blood pressure. In addition to this primary agenda, I also hope to illustrate through a particular case study how the generally descriptive methods of anthropology are relevant for considering an epidemiological problem.

The methodological approach used to distinguish the particular characteristics of Samoan migration is that well-known to anthropologists: ethnography. An ethnographic approach to disease, which will be discussed more fully in a later section, involves two essential elements: (a) holistic depiction of the group being studied that leads to an understanding of the interrelated social and cultural processes that affect health; and (b) identification of specific variables and methods for further epidemiological analyses that are firmly grounded in the particular socio-cultural context of interest. Ethnog-

175

Craig R. Janes et al. (eds.), Anthropology and Epidemiology, 175—211.
© 1986 *by D. Reidel Publishing Company.*

raphy permits a greater understanding of how risks to health are manifested and patterned in a community, and hence provides data that are of direct relevance to minimizing risks through public health education and prevention programs.

In the next section I develop the specific methodological and theoretical perspective that guided the research from its inception. I examine the various conceptual models used in the area of stress research and suggest an alternative theoretical strategy for understanding stress that views migration and adaptation as a problem in human ecology. This model is then extended to explain the role of migration and adaptation in contributing to cardio-vascular morbidity among Samoan migrants to California.

MIGRATION AND HEALTH: AN ECOLOGICAL PERSPECTIVE

The Stress of Change

It has been observed for some time that migrants from rural, non-Western cultures to Western urban centers experience, within a generation, striking increases in the incidence of a number of non-infectious diseases, hyper-tension being one of the major health threats (Antonovsky 1979; Cassel 1975; Fleming and Prior 1981; Haenszel 1970; Henry and Cassel 1969; Hull 1979; Prior 1979; Wessen 1971). For this reason the study of migrants has provided a context for isolating and defining the interaction of environ-mental, social, cultural, and psychological factors related to the increase in the incidence of non-infectious diseases. Several methodological strategies have been used to study the health effects of migration. These range from comparing the vital statistics of migrant populations with those of the home and host populations to examining the particular life experiences of individual migrants. Of these strategies, only the latter is useful for deter-mining the specific interaction of geographic displacement and health among individuals. Group level comparisons, provocative as they may be, do not lend themselves to revealing more than general patterns, and certainly do not permit the analysis of the mechanisms, often as not based on individual behaviors, that underlie patterns of disease rates (c.f. Robinson 1950).

In studies of migrants, health scientists have been interested generally in how specific health-related behaviors change with migration. For example, significant alterations in nutrition and exercise patterns have been observed to occur subsequent to migration, and these changes have been shown in epidemiologic studies to constitute risks for disease (e.g. Prior 1979; Fleming and Prior 1981; Wessen 1971). However, beginning in the 1960s there has been an increasing interest in how the socio-psychological ramifications of migrant adaptation affect disease risk. Many studies have yielded results that suggest that "acculturative stress", encountered as a consequence of migration to an alien social environment, is an important factor in the epidemiology of hypertension (e.g., Beaglehole et al. 1977; Cassel 1975; Hackenberg et al. 1983; Henry and Cassel 1969; Prior 1979; Scotch 1963; Waldron et al. 1982; Yano et al. 1979).

Before discussing this literature further, it is important to consider just what is meant by the term "stress" and how it is operationalized in medical social science and epidemiologic research. Beginning with the writings of Wolff (1953) and Selye (1956), the concept of stress has been understood to be an outcome state occurring as a result of the individual's psychological appraisal of external events that are somehow threatening or cause a state of tension. These external events can be termed "stressors". In the presence of stressors the individual is assumed to strive to return to a normal state of balance, or "homeostasis" (Dressler 1982). If corrective actions fail, and the psychological effects of stressors persist, the individual is then assumed to be under stress. The fundamental and commonly overlooked part of this equation is that concerning the degree to which persons can mobilize resources to effect positive corrective actions. These resources, consisting of biochemical, physiological, psychological, social or cultural attributes, are termed "resistance resources", and include such psychosocial phenomena as "coping", and "social support" (Antonovsky 1979; Berkman and Syme 1979; Caplan 1974; Kaplan, Cassel, and Gore 1977; Lazarus 1966; Levine and Scotch 1970; Pilisuk and Froland 1978).

It is possible to collapse research on the stress process in contexts of social change into three broad, though often overlapping, categories. First, it has been suggested that personal experiences with cultural differences, often termed "cultural incongruity", causes stress. This postulate has been phrased in many ways, but the primary operative assumption is that change is bad; and the kind of sudden change migrants experience is severe enough to have serious physiological consequences. For example, Cassel (1975) has argued that migration to a society with different value systems leads to situations where previously sanctioned behaviors, especially those the individual acquired during critical learning periods, can no longer be used to express normal behavioral "urges". This in turn creates repeated autonomic nervous system arousal that may lead to high blood pressure, probably atherosclerosis, and possibly several other diseases. Other expressions of this idea have tended to emphasize the individual experience of disjuncture between the cultural values or social skills they possess and the statuses they desire to occupy or situations with which they must cope in the new environment (Beiser et al. 1976; Cassel and Tyroler 1961; Hackenberg et al. 1983; Henry and Cassel 1969; Scotch 1963; Syme et al. 1966; Tyroler and Cassel 1964).

The concept of disjuncture has been refined and applied specifically to contexts of *in situ* social change. In this second model, stress is hypothesized to stem from "status inconsistency". The assumption here is the same as above — that change places persons in circumstances for which they are unprepared. However, two more precise hypotheses have been advanced. First, it is suggested that if a person occupies a status with which he or she has no experience or knowledge, they will be unable to fulfill others' expectations, and will experience stress. Secondly, it is hypothesized that if status positions a person desires become available, but access to these positions is blocked, or difficult to maintain, stress will result (Dressler 1982: 43—45). Researchers have observed that social change creates situations where new statuses become available, but where the resources necessary for achieving and sustaining these statuses are scarce (e.g., Merton 1949). Dressler (1982, 1985), for example, suggests that status inconsistency is a common attribute of many contexts of culture change where people are exposed to European and American behaviors, and thus become aware of the high status that accrues to individuals who can emulate these behaviors. Migration might also be expected to create such potentially incongruous situations. Status inconsistency has been significantly correlated with a higher prevalence of coronary heart disease and hypertension (Antonovsky 1979; Dressler 1982; Lehr et al. 1973; Syme et al. 1964).

Lastly, it has been found that exposure to acute life changes or difficulties leads to a greater prevalence of disease. The term used most often in the literature to describe such difficult circumstances is that of "stressful life events" (Dohrenwend and Dohrenwend 1974; Rahe 1974; Theorell 1976). Events considered stressful are those that cause the individual a significant change in lifestyle, role, or status. The hypothesis used to explain the importance of such events is: the greater the number of such life changes a person faces, and the greater the perceived impact of such changes, the greater the risk for disease. Although the results of this line of inquiry have not been particularly striking, and have been rather soundly criticized (Young 1980), life events research continues to be ubiquitous to medical social science, and has been conducted in a variety of cultural contexts.

Although the foregoing discussion does not do justice to what is a large and complex field of study, it is sufficient to illustrate the explanatory models now in use and general differences in the way stress is conceptualized. First, although stress is generally assumed to be primarily a psychological phenomenon, there is a tendency to either measure it only in terms of individual perception, or conversely, measure the behavioral, social, and cultural concomitants of individual experiences of stress. Thus, life events researchers are more interested in the perception of acute personal experiences while those interested in status inconsistency emphasize the degree to which prevailing social conditions place groups and individuals in situations that are potentially stressful. It has not been until recently, in fact, that researchers have attempted to integrate socio-cultural and phenomenological models of stress, particularly in contexts of migration or social change (Dressler 1982, 1985; O'Neil, this volume). The success of these studies suggests the need for continuing efforts to integrate various perspectives on stress and social change. As Caudill (1958) argued, stress should be conceived as arising from the interaction of three open systems: the physiological, psychological, and sociological. Stress occurring in any one system is likely to "spill over" and affect changes in another.

It was this ecological conceptualization of stress that guided the design and implementation of the research project I report here. In the following section I will discuss ecological models of disease in greater depth, emphasizing in particular those areas where medical ecology and contemporary epidemiology differ.

Ecological Perspectives on Urban Adaptation and Health

Medical ecology, which developed as a specific area of interest within human ecology, is now a significant theoretical specialty in medical anthropology (Foster and Anderson 1978; Wellin 1977). The basic tenet of medical ecology is that health and disease are interrelated with culture, biology, and environment (Alland 1970; Montgomery 1973). In studying specific diseases, the usual emphasis is on the effectiveness with which communities, groups, or sub-groups adapt to their environment, or to rapid environmental change (Lieban 1973).

It is noteworthy that the major feature of ecological models is not so much a unique methodological approach, but a theoretical model of disease and disease-related behavioral phenomena that is significantly more complex, and potentially more comprehensive, than typical linear models of risk and disease characteristic of epidemiology. While medical ecologists may employ methods that are based on linear relationships between variables, the theoretical impetus of such research is to add to the store of knowledge on how human-environmental systems function. The same cannot be said of the majority of current epidemiological research, even though textbooks of epidemiology claim an ecological foundation (e.g., Mausner and Bahn 1974: pp. 26—40).[1]

A medical-ecological perspective on disease entails several important conceptual sequalae. First, assemblages of cause and effect are considerably broadened in systems-models of disease (Audy and Dunn 1974; Dunn 1984; Montgomery 1973). This represents a significant departure from general epidemiological research in the way the determinants of disease in human groups, termed risk factors, are understood and formulated. Epidemiologists generally refer to observed correlates or determinants of disease as comprising "risks". Simply stated, risks are factors whose presence is associated with an increased likelihood that disease will develop at a later time. Risks are measured as attributes of individuals; e.g., age, sex, income, ethnicity, smoking, exercise level, exposure to a pathogen, and so forth. However, risk factors arise in unique communities rather than population aggregates, they are embedded in a cultural context, and they often occur in clusters or configurations within well-defined human groups, such as families, house-holds, kin groups, churches and schools. This is particularly critical if the interest is prevention, in which the *primary* target of efforts must be those things that effect health related human behavior. Health related behavior (both deliberate and non-deliberate) may be related to variables such as: social status and roles, attitudes, economic practices, and cultural values. To date the best evidence of the utility of ecological approach is found in infectious disease research (see Nations, this volume; also Dunn 1979, 1984).

Second, as the above comments suggest, the methods of medical ecology typically require an in-depth study of a specific group, in most cases a unique culture. Epidemiology, on the other hand, is a survey-based field that has as one of its major focuses an emphasis on population aggregates rather than single, well-defined human communities. Such an approach is essentially incompatible with research conceived to examine health from an ecological perspective, which generally emphasizes the interrelationship of social, behavioral, and psychological processes within a single community or geo-graphic area.

Third, an ecological perspective tends to shift analytic interest to a critical *process*: adaptation.[2] The basis of a health-oriented view of human adapta-tion is concerned with asking whether human groups, through the instrument of culture, are capable of adjusting to environmental alterations. And, conversely, it is equally important to examine the causes and nature of environmental alterations, for some environmental insults — such as extreme poverty or social marginality — may not permit reasonable or "healthy" adaptation. Operationally then, analysis of adaptation and health involves assessing the adaptability of values, beliefs, and social institutions — the flexibility with which people can meet and effectively respond to change — and the nature of the change itself. Models of adaptation are effective tools for conceptualizing the potentially negative health effects of migration, since adaptability refers to the full range of responses people are capable of employing in order to fit themselves and their institutions to a particular environment.

Significant attempts have been made to develop a theoretical approach that combines the ecological concept of adaptation with the more standard epidemiological approach of measuring individual attributes as they are patterned in large population aggregates (cf. Cassel 1976; Cassel et al. 1960; Caudill 1958; A. Leighton 1959; D. Leighton et al. 1963; D. Leighton 1978). The unifying concept in these works is that disease arises when the adaptive processes triggered by environmental change leave the needs of some individuals unsatisfied. Leighton (1978) argues, for example, that all people can be seen as having needs that either they alone, or in cooperation with others in their families and society, must satisfy. These are: physical needs for food, shelter, and clothing; psychological needs for love, recogni-tion, and a sense that one is esteemed and valued; and socio-cultural needs to feel they are part of a well-defined group that subscribes to a coherent set of values regarding right and wrong. Where environments are stable, humans develop institutions that function to satisfy these needs — for example kinship systems, technological traditions, religious rituals, and so on. When environments change rapidly, these institutions may break down, or fail to provide reliable avenues to satisfy basic needs for all members. Thus, in the case of migration a critical factor may be how existing institutions serve to meet the needs of individuals, whether these resources are available to all individuals, and the degree to which the host society may place members of a group in situations where needs cannot be met. Leighton suggests that where basic needs are not met, and people cannot find alternate solutions, mental or physical breakdown may result. Stress is thus thought to occur when basic needs are not met and people can find no alternate solutions. In this scheme, there is an equal focus on "adaptive capacities" as well as on specific environmental stresses. This approach serves to integrate the three models of stress and disease described earlier, insofar as the adaptive capacities to which Leighton refers are defined as the psychological, physical, social, and cultural characteristics of people and the groups to which they belong.

The idea in these conceptualizations of stress is that there are basic prerequisites for proper social functioning (see Aberle et al. 1950 for a similar argument). Although it may be argued that such a conceptualization is an essentially static and reductionist view, it does provide an effective vehicle for organizing research questions designed to evaluate success and failure in migrant adaptation. It is critical, however, to insure that such research questions take measure of historical factors as well as individual variation in healthy adaptation (see O'Neil, this volume; Young 1980).

Based on such an adaptation model, the important research questions to ask here are: (1) what are the nature of the changes with which Samoans must cope? (2) to what degree are existing characteristics of the migrants — e.g., technological skills, religious rituals, and political institutions — capable of serving the needs of all members of the group? and (3) what are the past patterns of change against which the contemporary picture of adaptation can be described and evaluated?

METHODS

The Research Population: Samoans in California

The islands of Samoa straddle the latitude of 14 degrees in the Pacific Ocean, approximately midway between the Hawaiian islands and New Zealand. The easternmost islands of the Samoan archipelago, Tutuila and the Manua group, comprise American Samoa; the major islands to the west, Upolu and Savaii, are the independent state of Western Samoa. American

Samoa is an unincorporated territory acquired by the United States through treaty in 1899. Because American Samoans are considered American "nationals", with the right of free entry into the United States, they constitute the largest percentage of Samoan migrants to Hawaii and California. However, a substantial proportion of the Samoan population of the United States is from Western Samoa, having obtained entry through normal immigration channels, or by establishing American Samoan citizenship.

The migration of Samoans to the American mainland was initiated in the post-World War II decade when the U.S. Navy terminated operations in Pago Pago and transferred its civilian Samoan employees and enlisted men, including their dependents, stateside. These first families served as magnets for prospective migrants who desired to achieve more education, find better employment, or to join the U.S. military forces. The extent of the migration has made California the major population center for American Samoans, followed closely by Hawaii. Together, Hawaii and California can be estimated in 1985 to have a Samoan population of 60,000 persons (Northwest Regional Educational Laboratory 1984). The Samoan population of California in 1985 probably numbers 30,000, of which 10,000 live in the San Francisco Bay Area.

Because of the important role of the military in stimulating and supporting Samoan migration, the first Samoan settlements, and the largest today, are associated with major West Coast military bases. The San Francisco Bay area not only possesses a major Navy port, but until the early 1970s maintained large shipbuilding and repair facilities at various locations. The Army also maintains a very large base, Fort Ord, near Monterey, and the smaller Presidio within San Francisco itself. These military facilities played a central role in bringing Samoans to northern California. In addition to the city of San Francisco, substantial settlements of Samoans can be found in the cities of South San Francisco, Daly City, San Mateo, Oakland, San Leandro, East Palo Alto, San Jose, and Milpitas. In southern California settlements have been established in Oceanside, National City, San Diego, and Long Beach.

In the San Francisco area, Samoans tended to move into areas of the city where housing was inexpensive and available. The typical pattern was for migrants to live with relatives until financially able to rent or buy their own home. Most commonly, modest accomodations were sought in public housing developments, or in adjacent areas where rents were most affordable. Members of the first migrant cohort were often able to purchase their own homes within a few years after arriving. However, faced with rising housing costs and rents, many of those migrating since the mid-1970s have been forced to remain in subsidized public housing.

Social organization in Samoa is based on a localized cognatic descent group, termed the 'aiga. At the head of each 'aiga is a matai, or "chief", who exercises authority over 'aiga land and property, the ceremonial distribution of goods, and the actions of 'aiga members. An individual potentially belongs to several local 'aiga, and is often involved in the affairs of cognates living elsewhere. Affiliation with a particular 'aiga is usually based on individual perceptions of political opportunity, residential propinquity, and the desires of other close family members.[3]

The process of kin-linked chain migration that has characterized Samoan mobility from its beginnings has permitted the partial reconstitution of kinship groups. The 'aiga has retained some of its function as a cooperative economic institution, though the nature of economic transactions, forms of mutual aid, and internal authority have changed significantly in response to the demands of a monetary economy. The migrant 'aiga is no longer a residential group, but a network of kinship ties uniting dispersed urban households. It is useful to think of the urban 'aiga as representing three overlapping units of social organization. The smallest unit is that of the household, generally based on a single conjugal relationship, though it is somewhat common for siblings and their families to establish joint house-holds. Series of households are linked by close consanguineal relationships; the most important in economic and psychological terms being those with siblings and siblings' children. This group represents the core kinship network for migrant Samoans.

Beyond the central household network is that diffuse kinship network that ties together individuals and households in other parts of California, Hawaii, and Samoa. This network, termed the *kindred*, represents often latent relationships that are activated in family crises or rites of passage, called *fa'alavelave*. These kindred network relationships primarily represent obliga-tions for the individual migrant. For example, patterns of economic exchange in these far-flung kindred networks have been intensified with migration, and represent a significant drain on the individual with little opportunity for immediate reciprocity (Janes 1984; Rolff 1978).

An important consequence of chain migration is variation in the structure of families in urban California. Families may be large or small, well-organized or loosely affiliated. Individual household heads may decide they no longer wish to share their resources and opt instead for American material success at the cost of their membership in the Samoan community. Some families may function more as supportive and cooperative institutions than others. Social support is not equally available to every Samoan migrant despite a continuing emphasis on traditional family relationships.[4]

Outside of the kin group, the organizational unit of utmost importance to Samoans is the church congregation. Samoans have been devoutly Christian for more than a century, and religion has been integrated into nearly every area of daily life. Inevitably, when and wherever possible, groups of migrants established exclusive Samoan church congregations. Churches are a focus of social activity, and function today as urban villages for the majority of migrants (Ablon 1971a, b).

Though in many ways the reestablishment of traditional social structures in urban California is "adaptive", there are increasingly telling signs that such adaptiveness has limits (Franco 1978). The economic conditions in northern California have worsened over the past decade, causing a rapid erosion of the resources on which Samoan communities depend, placing growing stresses on the cooperative mutual aid functions of family households, and making financial obligations more difficult to fulfil. Given the economic trend in California away from heavy industry and toward high technology, the Samoans' economic situation is likely to worsen. For the near future, economic hardship, scarcity of housing, and poor job prospects will plague the Samoan community and together constitute major deleterious influences on health — in terms of stress, poor diet, and restricted access to adequate medical care. It is to this topic I now turn.

Sample

My work with Samoan migrants dates from the summer of 1979 when I became a research assistant for a project designed to survey the health status of the Samoan community of Northern California (Pawson and Janes 1981, 1982). As part of this work, the research team visited several churches where approximately 300 adults were briefly interviewed and examined. The research was designed to maximize the gathering of both medical and demographic data. Contact with most participants was thus brief and highly formal; in no way could this phase of the research be considered ethnographic. While such brief and superfluous contacts were decidedly frustrating, the large amount of basic health data we gathered served to suggest several hypotheses which necessitated more in-depth studies. Hereafter I refer to this initial project as Phase I of the study of Samoans in northern California.

There is an important lesson here for medical anthropologists interested in working in areas where the primary concern is with disease etiology. Because the methods of anthropology typically emphasize depth over breadth, we cannot approach the large sample sizes considered appropriate to epidemiological investigations. Thus, where medical anthropologists wish to take an ethnographic approach, as I advocate here, they must often rely on prior extensive research that, at minimum, helps define the problem and refine research questions that can then be subject to in-depth, often qualitative, scrutiny. In this context, I was fortunate enough to have access to such work gathered in the course of many related investigations by professionals and students from Pennsylvania State University, the University of California, San Francisco, and the University of Hawaii. Collectively, these studies have been called 'The Samoan Migration Project' (Baker and Hanna 1981).

These data suggested the central role of social and cultural factors in determining the distribution of hypertension in the California Samoan subpopulation (Pawson and Janes 1982). To ascertain the exact nature of these relationships, I designed a two-stage research project designed to collect basic descriptive and ethnographic data on Samoan migrant culture, and to address the hypothesis that certain social and cultural aspects of the urban adaptation process were implicated in the etiology of Samoan hypertension. The first stage involved selecting a representative community, observing group events and social behaviors, interviewing community members in an unstructured or informal manner, and in general trying to accomplish an insider's — or "emic" — perspective on stateside Samoan culture. The second stage involved selecting and interviewing a representative sample of 115 Samoan adults.[5] In this report I present quantitative data from 104 interviews, 47 women and 57 men. The remaining 11 interviews were not coded for this analysis due primarily to seriously insufficient or incomplete data.[6] Table I summarizes the demographic characteristics of the formal sample.

TABLE I
Demographic characteristics of sample

Characteristics	Men		Women	
	%	N	%	N
Number interviewed:	54.8	57	45.2	47
Age:				
30—40	22.8	13	38.3	18
41—54	43.9	25	25.5	12
55—64	22.8	13	29.8	14
65 +	10.5	6	6.3	3
Cohort of migration:				
1945—1959	31.6	18	23.4	11
1960—1969	40.4	23	38.3	18
1970—1982[a]	28.1	16	38.3	18
Age left Samoa:				
< 22	12.3	7	21.3	10
22—30	45.6	26	29.8	14
31—40	21.0	12	19.1	9
41—50	14.1	8	12.8	6
51 +	7.0	4	17.0	8

[a] All respondents had lived in California at least one year at the time of the interview.

The concept of community is often a difficult one to define in complex urban settings, but in this context such definitional problems do not exist. Samoans have shaped their religious organizations, primarily Protestant Christian churches, to constitute, in effect, their urban villages — a fact that

Samoans explicitly recognize (Tofaeono 1978). My ethnographic work took place primarily, but not exclusively, within one large, well-established church. The formal sample referred to above was subsequently chosen from the church membership rosters of this church plus another branch of the same church in another city. In addition, I recruited individuals from other religious denominations in order to have members of different church communities represented.

The formal interview instrument consisted of a range of questions regarding background, migration history, kinship, social network exchange and helping patterns, church participation, social status, attitudes toward Samoan and American culture, stressful life events, and health. It generally took from one and one-half to two hours to complete an interview. The interview was administered in English if possible, and in a combination of English and Samoan, either with or without a translator, if the respondent did not speak English well enough to understand the questions. Blood pressure measurements were taken three times: once before the interview began, and then twice at the conclusion of the interview. The lowest reading was recorded and was that used in subsequent analyses. Blood pressures were taken using standard methods with a mercury sphygmomanometer and a variety of cuffs to accommodate different arm sizes.

RESULTS AND DISCUSSION

Previous studies of Pacific Island peoples have shown that the expected consequences of migration and urbanization include increased weight, elevated blood pressure, a higher prevalence of diabetes, and generally higher levels of known cardiovascular risks (Fleming and Prior 1981; McGarvey and Baker 1979; Hanna and Baker 1979; Prior 1974, 1979; Taylor and Zimmet 1981; Zimmet et al. 1980; Zimmet and Whitehouse 1980; Zimmet et al. 1978). Some changes appear to be especially pronounced among Samoans; in particular, massive weight gain among Samoans living in the main port area of American Samoa (Pago Pago), Hawaii, and northern California compared to those living in rural villages in Samoa (Pawson and Janes 1981, 1982; Baker and Hanna 1981; Hanna and Baker 1979; McGarvey and Baker 1979).

Studies of Samoan migrants to Hawaii suggest that weight increase is linked to an overall rise in blood pressure, especially among adult males aged 30 to 50, and to a significant rise in the prevalence of hypertension (as defined by the World Health Organization standard of systolic pressure in excess of 165 mm Hg, or diastolic pressure in excess of 95 mm Hg). However, the relationship of weight gain and higher blood pressure to urbanization is not a direct one. In Hawaii, blood pressure among Samoans living in the city of Honolulu appears to be lower than among those living in rural areas on the island of Oahu (Hanna and Baker 1979; McGarvey and

Baker 1979). In our Phase 1 study of Samoans in the San Francisco Bay area of Northern California, both mean blood pressure and weight by age are the highest of any of the other subpopulations, however, the relationship of weight to blood pressure in individuals is complex. Among men there is a moderate positive correlation of body mass with blood pressure, and among women the greatest predictor is age. This is somewhat unexpected, since in white European populations body mass and age are the most significant risk factors for hypertension among both men and women. However, the Samoan data appear similar to that collected from Black Americans in the Evans County study (Tyroler et al. 1975).

These findings suggest two things. First, environmental change resulting from migration appears to be strongly associated with observed patterns of weight and blood pressure changes. Secondly, such links are apparently quite complex; the factors often invoked by epidemiologists to explain blood pressure changes in migrants — diet and increases in body weight — account for only a minor proportion of the variation. One might hypothesize that some of the socio-cultural "risk" factors identified as contributing to cardio-vascular disease, for example "psychosocial stress" caused by environmental and cultural discontinuity, occupies an important etiologic role.

Because age and body mass (weight/height^2 × 100) are important risk factors in the epidemiology of hypertension, and weight gain is such a distinguishing characteristic of Samoans, it is necessary to examine first the role of these variables in explaining variation among the sample I describe here. Table II presents a correlation of age and body mass with systolic and diastolic blood pressure. Unlike the other subpopulations of Samoans described above, the age range in this sample was smaller: 30 to 70 years of age.

These data indicate a different pattern of blood pressure variation by age and body mass than that suggested by previous studies. The only statistically

TABLE II
Correlation of age and body mass[c] with blood pressure

	Age	Body mass
Men; $N = 57$		
Systolic	0.19	0.28[a]
Diastolic	−0.08	0.17
Women; $N = 47$		
Systolic	0.53[b]	0.10
Diastolic	0.29[a]	0.14

[a] $p < 0.05$.
[b] $p < 0.01$.
[c] Weight/Height^2 × 100.

significant correlate of blood pressure in men is body mass. In women, age is the most important variable by far, alone accounting for over 25% of the variance in systolic blood pressure. Body mass is relatively unimportant. Because age and body mass are important factors for both sexes, however, in subsequent analyses their effects on blood pressure will be statistically controlled, except where noted.

Migration and Stress

The most abrupt change Samoans experience in migrating to urban California is a shift in economic subsistence from one based on cooperative agriculture, fishing, and animal husbandry to one that is wholly monetary. While the last decade has seen the disruption of the subsistence agricultural system of American Samoa, due primarily to the availability of wage-earning opportunities, individuals there know that in times of shortage their lands are usually available. Land has not been alienated from the local descent group, and this fact more than any other gives Samoans a measure of security. This sense of security is often lost by migrants who commit themselves to life on the mainland. Even though they may be familiar with a cash economy, the loss of the security of having available family lands means that there is little recourse should one lose cash income. Although most migrants have access to lands should they return to Samoa, economic hardship and ties to family members established on the mainland may make a return impossible. Most important is the degree people are committed to working toward those goals they set for themselves when they left Samoa. Migrants come seeking education for themselves and their children, employment, and for a brighter future. In so doing they place themselves at risk of economic problems created largely by factors beyond their control. This is where the greatest difficulties in adaptation for Samoans now lie: there is a growing cleavage between the need for economic resources to sustain family and community activities and access to these very resources.

The first Samoans to arrive in the United States had had sufficient experience with Americans and American institutions to know where to look for employment and housing. They helped later arrivals as much as they could, which was enough as long as there was ready access to the American economy (cf. Ablon 1971a, b). As noted previously however, in the past several years fewer opportunities, combined with burgeoning numbers of immigrants, have begun to overtax existing helping networks. Jobs are simply not available in the same number for individuals possessing minimal language, education, and employment skills.

The most problematic consequence of worsening economic conditions is the introduction of significant economic heterogeneity into the structure of stateside Samoan society. Two aspects of economic differentiation directly affect processes of social and cultural adaptation. First, a growing population of economically disadvantaged constitutes an added burden on existing Samoan resources. Established relatives must provide housing and sustenance. Although this system, supplemented where needed by welfare and subsidized housing, still functions to provide most Samoans with some measure of economic security, it represents a serious burden to all involved. Those who do have the resources resent providing for those who do not, and yet their position within the church and kin group depends on demonstrated generosity. Secondly, and on the other side of the issue, those with sparse resources have fewer avenues to positions of status and prestige, which in the stateside context requires expensive participation in church and kindred activities. For those with little money, life is simply more difficult.

The degree to which Samoan institutions have become monetized is an important consequence of their development on the mainland. The most visible and remarkable of these affairs is the *fa'alavelave* or life crisis event. Funerals and weddings are the two most important fa'alavelave. In Samoa these events are occasions for competitive exchange, feasting, and oration. The goods exchanged are not used to defray expenses of the event, but are redistributed to those in attendance. The exchange itself is a mechanism for showing generosity, demonstrating oratorical skill, and accruing prestige. In the American context, life crisis events involve considerable direct expense: burial plots, caskets, rental of a hall for a wedding, and food for a feast. These are all things that must be purchased. In this way cash has become the item of greatest importance in ceremonial exchange. Moreover, the basic status and prestige functions of the exchange have persisted. The infusion of cash into what was originally a competitive institution has resulted in a tradition of overgive, of ostentatious presentation not unlike the potlatch (Rolff 1978). This overgive has grown to represent the strong cultural values placed on generosity in giving that commodity which is most dear. Prestige in the American sense has come to represent a person's ability to amass cash, and therefore, ironically, becomes modeled upon American cultural symbols of economic success.

The monetization of prestige is also apparent within the church. Churches have held a central role in Samoan society since the 19th century, and their development in migrant society has followed the island pattern. Like everything else in the American context, a church is an expensive institution to maintain: land and buildings are needed, bills must be paid, and the minister and his family must be housed and fed. Consequently, to be a member in good standing of one's community — the Samoan church — one must be active in giving to the church and participating in its affairs. The church represents, perhaps, an even greater pressure for conformity in giving, for unlike economic exchange within the kin group, church giving is more of an individual affair. For kin group events one can often give as a member of a group, a branch of a kindred. There is always the possibility that one can go to others for help in making a contribution. However in the eyes of a church, ones gives for oneself and one's household. The pressure on the individual to give is therefore much greater and is made more severe by very strong cultural values regarding the support of religious activities. For those with few resources who decide that immediate family needs must come first, marginalization or alienation from the church community may result.

For these individuals, the situation is made more serious by the fact that the church and kin group function in the urban setting to meet a number of important needs. The 'aiga provides one with at least short-term economic support, and if an important life crisis event comes up in the context of the immediate family, one can count on substantial assistance. Within the kindred small clusters of cooperating households, often based on sibling or close bilateral kin ties actualized in the migration process, share a number of important activities. This group is potentially a secure "haven" for veteran and recent migrants alike. The church, usually comprised of a few primary kindred groups, has arisen as a focus of community interaction, cultural revitalization, and Samoan identity. The church has become the urban Samoan village. Persons locate themselves in the framework of Samoan culture by identifying their 'aiga history and the church congregation to which they belong. As a center for social and cultural activity, the church permits the redevelopment of Samoan systems of leadership, but blends this with the more functional need for leaders who are knowledgeable of American ways. Socially, the church binds together members of dispersed households into a functioning village-like social structure. Culturally, the church unites members into a single moral community possessing a unified set of beliefs and practices. Together people can enjoy the events, rituals, and feasts that represent what they like about *fa'asamoa* — the Samoan way. Psychologically, participation in church affairs offers members a sense of belonging, a strong sense of personal identity, value and importance.

There is a paradox here. On one hand, active participation in church and 'aiga affairs sustains strong community values and provides individuals avenues to satisfying the needs discussed above. On the other hand, because involvement is expensive, active participation in both institutions is a potential stressor. The root of this paradox lies not in the nature of the institutions themselves, but in the nature of the urban economic system in which they have developed and are now embedded. In situations of plenty, access to participation is not limited. In circumstances of poverty, some may either be barred access, or more commonly, struggle to both maintain their positive identification with their 'aiga and church, while satisfying their own and immediate family's needs.

The tension between status or community involvement and economic resources has been found to be a common consequence of social change cross-culturally. Dressler (1982) suggests that the monetization of social status that accompanies social change, particularly when it results in a localization of resources in the hands of a few, creates situations where people are caught between the desire for a new and apparently superior way of life, and their abilities to pay for it. The change of migration is somewhat similar, only more disruptive. In the Samoan situation individuals have not come to espouse American economic or soical goals, yet ironically pathways to Samoan status within the urban community have become somewhat Americanized. Situations are thus created where lack of resources blocks access to social participation at a desired level. Alternatively, such participation leads to a tension between satisfying individual's physical, emotional, and social needs met through social participation.

The struggle of maintaining an unrealistic status, or having access to desired statuses blocked, termed "status inconsistency", has been correlated with hypertension, hypertension-related mortality, and coronary heart disease. Operationally, status inconsistency can be defined as a significant difference between any two pairs of status continua (Dressler 1982). As noted for Samoans, two interrelated status dimensions are primary: economic status, and status in the church or 'aiga. Most researchers consider that any status inconsistency will cause stress. However as discussed earlier, it was expected that the most severe stress would occur where individuals are of relatively high status in the community, but have limited access to the resources necessary for demonstrating one's rank and accruing prestige. To test this hypotheses, three separate status scales were constructed.[7] The first consisted of rank of per capita income. The second was a leadership scale, consisting of different items for men and women. Thirdly, a scale of kindred involvement was constructed that reflected financial commitment to maintaining obligations in contexts of kindred fa'alavelave. Each of these three scales was divided at the median into high and low categories. Two pairs of status dimensions — economic resources/leadership, and economic resources/kindred involvement — were cross-tabulated. Mean systolic and diastolic blood pressures were calculated for the individuals within each of the cells in the resulting 2 × 2 tables. The results are presented in Tables III and IV.

TABLE III

Mean systolic/diastolic blood pressure by category of per capita income and leadership status

		Leadership status	
		Low	High
Per capita income	Low	138.0/89.5 $N = 33$	143.3/92.3 $N = 19$
	High	138.3/88.1 $N = 30$	135.2/88.0 $N = 21$

TABLE IV

Mean systolic/diastolic blood pressure by category of per capita income and involvement in
Fa'alavelave

		Involvement	
		Low	High
Economic resources	Low	139.0/92.0 $N = 19$	140.6[a]/90.1 $N = 30$
	High	139.4/87.6 $N = 23$	131.1[a]/88.0 $N = 27$

[a] High income/high involvement compared with low income/high involvement (systolic), $t = 1.81$; $p < 0.05$.

Although only the difference between the high and low income category in the high kindred commitment cells is statistically significant, the data suggest that inconsistency is an important stressor. There is a fairly substantial difference between the "consistent" and "inconsistent" groups in the high leadership and family involvement categories. Most interesting is the degree to which those in the status consistent categories of high economic status have much lower blood pressures than those in the other three categories. I believe this not only reflects the lower level of stress experienced by those who have the means to sustain a high level of family and church involvement, but also the positive aspects of high status in the Samoan community. Those who possess the resources to participate fully in their society and at a fairly high level do not have to struggle to achieve what Leighton (1978) describes as a fundamental human need for recognition. In general, these results support the hypothesis that relative poverty results in higher blood pressure, and that whatever stress this causes in the individual is exacerbated by his or her attempts to maintain obligations to family and church. For those more fortunate, the basic adaptive functions of church and 'aiga appear protective in regard to blood pressure.

Further analysis of these data revealed that the effects of status inconsistency were notably stronger for women than for men. Two reasons come to mind to explain such gender differences in this cultural context. First, women's status and roles are often based on those of their husbands'. For example, a woman may be ascribed a leadership position in the church women's group subsequent to her husband's achievement of a parallel status in the men's leadership hierarchy. A similar sort of thing happens in the context of the extended family: a woman is given a status complementary to that of her husband. Further, while in the urban context men receive the public rewards of status achievement, women bear the majority of both public and private responsibility for maintaining the achievement. Therefore, it might be hypothesized that for women leadership represents less of a desired status and offers fewer fruits, especially where concerns for family welfare may take precedence. Women may experience the day-to-day pressures of poverty with greater intensity; poverty that is exacerbated by her and her husband's commitment to the exigencies of Samoan family and church involvement and leadership.

To role of poverty in contributing to stress can be further demonstrated by examining the relationship of blood pressure to exposure to chronic and difficult situations entailed by urban life. In the literature these troublesome events are generally called "life events stresses", and a sophisticated methodology has arisen to measure both the occurrence of a specific "stressful" situation and the meaning it has for the individual concerned (Dohrenwend and Dohrenwend 1974; Rahe 1974; Theorell 1976). This line of research suffers on two logical grounds: it emphasizes the relationship of acute, ahistorical factors to chronic diseases or disorders; and it is based on putative assumptions about the nature of psychological stress that is probably more a part of white, middle-class conceptions of stress than any "objective reality". Because of these fallacies, research that depends on the *a priori*, and acultural identification of stressful life events has been soundly criticized (Young 1980). To avoid these logical problems, I chose in this research to focus on difficult situations of some chronicity that are embodied in Samoans' adaptation to urban life, and which are culturally salient. I term these "situational stresses".

Based on my earlier ethnographic research, a list of 15 potentially stressful situations was compiled. Individuals interviewed in the epidemiologic portion of the study were asked to indicate the frequency in the past year that they experienced each situation. For this paper six items reflecting the difficulties of urban adaptation and exhibiting acceptable variation across the sample were selected for analysis: (1) frequency running short of money, (2) troubles on the job, (3) death in the family, (4) troubles or worries about the welfare of children, (5) moving to a new home, and (6) problems with the present housing situation. Scores on these questions were combined into a scale, and analyzed in relation to blood pressure.[8] The results are presented in Table V.

The correlation of situational stress with blood pressure in the full sample

TABLE V
Partial correlation of situational stresses with blood pressure[a]

	Total sample	Men	Women
Systolic B.P.	0.22[b]	0.17	0.33[b]
Diastolic B.P.	0.24[b]	0.23	0.32[b]

[a] $p < 0.05$.
[b] Controlling for the effects of age and body mass (weight/height^2 × 100).

is statistically significant. Tabulated separately for men and women this measure continues to show an association with blood pressure in each group, although the strength of the association is greater among women than men. As hypothesized in foregoing discussion of status inconsistency, it is possible that situational stresses are more salient for women, particularly those that affect the day-to-day functioning of the household.

Social Resources

The degree to which social and cultural stressors affect blood pressure is ultimately dependent on the psychological and social resources individuals possess that enable them to cope. These are termed "resistance resources". In situations of poverty, for example, if individuals have a large group of close relatives and friends to whom they can turn in times of need, a modicum of economic security is assured. The psychological dimensions of social support are more difficult to measure but are at least as important. This kind of support is believed to reassure individuals that their psychological needs are being met; that they are esteemed, loved, and respected (Antonovsky 1979; Cobb 1976). I have not differentiated in my analysis between emotional and instrumental support, and it is probable that the two are inextricable dimensions of any important relationship. The critical component in the measurement of social support is rather to distinguish relationships that are of social and cultural significance. It is in the identification of psychologically meaningful relationships that an ethnographic approach is most useful.

For example, it is sometimes assumed that social support is a synonym of social integration; that is, where people are involved in large and culturally meaningful social networks, they are thought to be receiving the psycho-logical benefits of such membership (e.g., James and Kleinbaum 1976; Neser et al. 1971; Harburg et al. 1973). However, such assumptions are based on studies of American groups where many individuals are found to be com-paratively isolated from others, or are subject to significant social instability. In groups that retain strong values regarding the role of kinship in organizing social behavior, immersion in social networks may represent a significant cost in both psychological and material terms. Social support may be difficult to distinguish at first glance form social obligation. Samoan kinship is bilateral and extends far beyond the nuclear family. Thus, each Samoan is well-integrated into a large network of kin to which he or she may turn from time to time as a source of information about jobs and housing, a place to stay perhaps, and as a source of money when family events require it. However, reliance on kin entails obligations to attend family ceremonies and provide money and goods for such functions, to honor and respect the position of family chiefs and elders, to provide housing if asked, and in general to behave properly to such kin in order to maintain one's reputation as properly fulfilling kin obligations with aplomb and *alofa* (loving concern).

Anthropologists have observed the high price migrant Samoans pay in both economic and psychological terms for heavy involvement in their large, traditional kinship networks (e.g., Graves et al. 1983; Rolff 1978).

The fieldwork reported here, in addition to writings on Samoan culture in general, suggests that for Samoans the most supportive relationships are those found in the nuclear family, within the close bilateral circle, and with certain close friends. The most important of these are probably the relationships individuals maintain with siblings, among whom intimacy and economic interdependence is often striking (Janes 1984; Shore 1982). People have a number of other relatives outside this group, and with whom they will interact from time to time, but these are not truly supportive in the sense used here. Such kin are simply those with whom one is bound in a cultural context of mutual obligation.

Individuals were asked to number the siblings they had in the area, the number of other relatives they visited regularly and with whom they were involved in frequent interaction and cooperation, and the number of friends with whom they felt they were especially close. I call this group the "core social network". In Table VI I present a ranking of the total. One can see a substantial variation in the size of these networks, and hence, the availability of social support.

TABLE VI
Core social networks by sex

Number of persons	Men		Women	
	%	N	%	N
Two or less	5.7	3	21.4	9
Three to five	28.8	15	26.2	11
Six to eight	34.6	18	31.0	13
More than nine	30.8	16	21.4	9
Total	100.0	52 [a]	100.0	42 [a]

[a] I was unable to obtain this information from some individuals, hence the N will total less than 104.

The determinants of this variation were found to consist of a combination of four important factors. First, variability in the migration process, combined with demographic realities, may have resulted in some people migrating with little help from relatives, having few relatives in the area, or having these relatives die or move elsewhere. Secondly, some persons have chosen to pursue a more self-reliant strategy of adaptation and have purposely not developed close mutual aid relationships with relatives and friends (cf. Graves and

Graves 1980). Thirdly, there are some generational differences in the degree to which people become involved with relatives to the exclusion of friends, or vice-versa. Younger people (aged 30—40) in my sample were more concerned with maintaining friendships and were involved to a comparatively greater extent in informal mutual aid networks comprised of friends. Older people, on the other hand, were comparatively more committed to relatives, and named fewer friends. Lastly, personality factors undoubtedly play a role in the size of a person's network; some individuals are more adept at social relationships, and others may prefer more isolation.

Table VII presents a correlation of the size of core social networks with blood pressure. The direct effects of social network size on blood pressure are quite striking, supporting the hypothesis that social support is important for helping individuals cope with the stresses embodied in urbanization.

TABLE VII

Partial correlation of core social networks with blood pressure[a]

	Total sample	Men	Women
Systolic B.P.	-0.24^b	-0.31^b	-0.29^b
Diastolic B.P.	-0.17^b	-0.28^b	-0.16

[a] Controlling for the effects of age and body mass (weight/height^2 × 100).
[b] $p < 0.05$.

In addition to the size of one's core social networks, church participation and kin group involvement may offer support, though in a more subtle way: providing a sense of identity or social solidarity, a setting to interact with others and perhaps make friends, and a place where one can observe and participate in important cultural rituals (Walsh 1980). To test the strength of such support in conjunction with the support provided by significant individuals, I constructed a composite social resources measure that was based on church participation, size of social networks, and frequency of weekly visiting with relatives.[9] Table VIII shows the correlation of social resources with blood pressure, and Table IX presents a crosstabulation of blood pressure by category of social resources.

The relationship of social resources to blood pressure is a very strong and direct one. It is interesting to note, however, that the relationship between social resources and blood pressure is much stronger in men than it is in women. The data I collected do not explain this, however it may be hypothesized that social support functions differently and carries unique meanings for each gender. This represents an area that requires further cross-cultural scrutiny.

TABLE VIII
Partial correlation of social resources with blood pressure[a]

	Total ($N = 94$)	Men ($N = 52$)	Women ($N = 42$)
Systolic B.P.	−0.24[c]	−0.40[c]	−0.24[b]
Diastolic B.P.	−0.20[b]	−0.39[c]	−0.15

[a] Controlling for the effects of age and body mass (weight/height^2 × 100).
[b] $p < 0.05$.
[c] $p < 0.01$.

TABLE IX
Mean systolic and diastolic blood pressure by category of available social resources

Social resources	Total sys/dias	Men sys/dias	Women sys/dias
High	133.6[a]/86.5 $N = 28$	136.3/88.3 $N = 14$	130.9/84.8 $N = 14$
Medium	137.3/89.3 $N = 32$	136.6/89.3 $N = 16$	138.1/89.4 $N = 16$
Low	141.5[a]/91.1 $N = 34$	140.7/93.7 $N = 20$	142.7/87.4 $N = 14$

[a] High level of resources compared with low level of resources (systolic), $t = 1.71$; $p < 0.05$.

Stress, Resistance Resources, and Blood Pressure: Combined Effects

Although the foregoing and separate considerations of status inconsistency, situational stress, and social resources are each of substantive interest to understanding the health consequences of migration, it is perhaps of greater importance to examine how these independent variables combine and interact in explaining variance in blood pressure. Three analytic questions are important to address in this context: (1) how do the independent and dependent variables intercorrelate? (2) what is the combined power of the independent variables in predicting blood pressure? and (3) are there synergistic effects or interdependencies between pairs of independent variables that shed light on how sociocultural factors affect blood pressure?

Table X shows zero-order correlations of the variables considered in this paper. The variable of status inconsistency was constructed from the analysis reported earlier; individuals were assigned scores based on their membership in consistent or inconsistent categories.[10] Status inconsistency shows only a minor relationship to blood pressure in men, but a fairly substantial relation-

TABLE X
Zero-order correlations of selected variables by sex

MEN (N = 57):

	(1)	(2)	(3)	(4)	(5)	(6)	(7)
(1) Systolic blood pressure	1.0						
(2) Diastolic blood pressure	0.81	1.0					
(3) Age	0.19	−0.08	1.0				
(4) Body mass index[a]	0.28	0.17	−0.15	1.0			
(5) Situational stresses	0.15	0.22	0.01	−0.03	1.0		
(6) Status inconsistency[b]	0.10	0.12	−0.07	−0.08	0.23	1.0	
(7) Social resources	−0.29	−0.33	0.07	0.19	0.24	0.10	1.0

WOMEN (N = 47):

	(1)	(2)	(3)	(4)	(5)	(6)	(7)
(1) Systolic blood pressure	1.0						
(2) Diastolic blood pressure	0.78	1.0					
(3) Age	0.54	0.29	1.0				
(4) Body mass index[a]	0.10	0.14	−0.14	1.0			
(5) Situational stresses	0.15	0.22	0.01	−0.03	1.0		
(6) Status inconsistency[b]	0.29	0.21	−0.11	0.26	0.28	1.0	
(7) Social resources	−0.22	−0.17	0.02	−0.09	−0.16	−0.12	1.0

[a] Weight/height^2 × 100.
[b] Membership in one or more inconsistent categories as described in Note 10.

ship to blood pressure in women. Further analysis of the status inconsistency measure suggests that it is also correlated with situational stress, a measure that is in turn related to economic deprivation.

To assess the power of the sociocultural variables, both singly and in combination, for explaining total variation in blood pressure, a multiple regression model was constructed. To summarize systolic and diastolic blood pressure readings into a single measure, I used Dressler's (1985) method for calculating "Mean Arterial Pressure" [((systolic pressure) + 2(diastolic pressure))/3]. Estimated coefficients, significance of the coefficients, and multiple R and R^2 for the full sample and by sex are shown in Table XI.

It is apparent from this table that the distribution of blood pressure and its correlates differs markedly by sex. For women, age is by far the strongest predictor of blood pressure, followed by situational stress. For men, conversely, social resources, body mass, and situational stress all contribute significantly to explaining variance in blood pressure, with social resources being the best predictor. Status inconsistency is not a predictive factor in these models for either men or women. This is perhaps not surprising given the fact that the situational stress variable may in fact be a more detailed measure of the class of phenomena represented by the structural charac-

TABLE XI

Regression of mean arterial pressure[a] on age, body mass index, and selected sociocultural variables: full sample and by sex

Variable	Total (N = 104)[b]		Men (N = 57)		Women (N = 47)	
	Beta	T	Beta	T	Beta	T
Sex	−0.120	−1.29				
Age	0.272	3.07[f]	0.116	0.96	0.452	3.59[e]
Body mass index[c]	0.255	2.67[f]	0.340	2.76[f]	0.193	1.42
Situational stresses	0.273	2.98[f]	0.295	2.36[e]	0.273	1.98
Status inconsistency[d]	0.099	1.09	0.115	0.94	0.154	1.11
Social resources	−0.287	−3.28[f]	−0.446	−3.56[f]	−0.135	−1.06
Multiple R:	0.513[f]		0.532[f]		0.606[f]	
Multiple R²:	0.264		0.283		0.367	

[a] Mean arterial pressure = ((systolic pressure) + 2(diastolic pressure))/3 (from Dressler 1985).
[b] Missing values recorded to the mean for each independent variable.
[c] Weight/height^2 × 100.
[d] Membership in one or more inconsistent categories as described in Note 10.
[e] $p < 0.05$.
[f] $p < 0.01$.

teristic of status inconsistency — viz., stressful situations either caused by or made more difficult by economic deprivation.

The significant main effect of social resources on blood pressure in men is striking. It has been suggested that the relationship of social resources to blood pressure is dependent upon the existence of some stress which it would serve to "buffer" (e.g., Cobb 1976; Dressler 1982). The important role of social resources in explaining blood pressure among men in this sample may indicate the existence of a constant and diffuse stress or set of stresses that is part of the migration and urbanization process. Given this constant stress, social resources will show a marked and direct effect on blood pressure.

Such striking gender differences are difficult to explain given the scope and design of this phase of the study. Based on an interpretation of ethnographic data, however, it can be noted that age is an important status marker in the Samoan cultural context. Among urban Samoan women, increasing age often brings more responsibility for extended family well-being, and thus perhaps a heightened sensitivity to family troubles or problematic situations. Conversely, for Samoan men the responsibility entailed by age status appears more likely to bring equivalent rewards in terms of leadership and prestige. For women, therefore, age may reflect some degree of stress that was not captured in the present study, or conversely, the relationship between stress or social resources and blood pressure may vary as a function of age.

One method for scrutinizing such complex interdependencies in the context of a multivariate analysis is to add "interaction effects" to the existing model. The conventional method for doing this is to add the product of two independent variables into the equation after the main effects have been entered (Cohen and Cohen 1975). Any significant amount of variation explained by the interaction term is thought to reflect an interdependent relationship between the independent variables under consideration and the dependent variable. As discussed above, it was hypothesized that the relationship between social resources, stress, and blood pressure in women may vary as a function of age. Also, based on the current thinking about the stress process and resistance resources, it was hypothesized that in addition to the main effects of the social resources measure noted in Table XI, social resources would also serve to buffer the effects of measured stresses. In other words, I suggest that the relationship between stress and blood pressure varies as a function of available social resources. In this context, stress was defined rather broadly to include body mass (a physiological stress), situational stress, and status inconsistency.

A stepwise procedure was utilized to construct a hierarchical regression model. The 5 independent variables listed in Table XI were forced into the model first, and then the interaction terms were allowed to enter on a stepwise basis (alpha to remove and enter = 0.15). Table XII shows the resulting model for men, and Table XIII shows the resulting model for

TABLE XII

Stepwise multiple regression analysis of mean arterial pressure with age, body mass, sociocultural variables, and interaction effects[a]: men

Variable	Beta	Cumulative R^2
Age	0.072	0.001
Body mass index[b]	0.308[d]	0.054
Situational stresses	0.284[d]	0.099
Status inconsistency[c]	0.123	0.105
Social resources	1.023	0.283
Social resources × body mass index	−1.486[d]	$R^2 = 0.361$[e]
		$R = 0.601$

[a] Main effects were forced into model first; interaction terms were permitted to enter stepwise (alpha-to-enter and alpha-to-remove = 0.15). Coefficients were estimated from a full non-hierarchical multiple regression model of blood pressure on independent variables plus interaction effects.

[b] Weight/height^2 × 100.

[c] Membership in one or more inconsistent categories as described in Note 10.

[d] $p < 0.05$.

[e] $p < 0.01$.

TABLE XIII

Stepwise multiple regression analysis of mean arterial pressure with age, body mass, sociocultural variables, and interaction effects[a]: women

Variable	Beta	Cumulative R^2
Age	−0.443	0.175
Body mass index[b]	0.223	0.210
Situational stresses	−0.784	0.329
Status inconsistency[c]	0.142	0.349
Social resources	−0.191	0.367
Situational stresses × age	1.438[d]	$R^2 = 0.416$
		$R = 0.645$[e]

[a] Main effects were forced into model first; interaction terms were permitted to enter stepwise (alpha-to-enter and alpha-to-remove = 0.15). Coefficients were estimated from a full non-hierarchical multiple regression model of blood pressure on independent variables plus interaction effects.

[b] Weight/height^2 × 100.

[c] Membership in one or more inconsistent categories as described in Note 10.

[d] $p < 0.05$.

[e] $p < 0.01$.

women. Beta was estimated from a full, non-hierarchical model, because stepwise techniques are somewhat prone to error in estimating coefficients. The cumulative R^2 to the right of the table, from which R^2 change can be easily calculated, shows the incremental addition of explained variance to the model with the addition of each set of variables.

The interaction of body mass and social resources in men is significant, explaining an additional 8% of variance in blood pressure. Further analysis of this interaction suggests a curvilinear relationship where at the lower levels of social support, the partial correlation of body mass with blood pressure is highly significant. By contrast, at high levels of social support the relationship between body mass and blood pressure is a weak one (Janes 1984). In women, the interaction of age with situational stress is significant, explaining an additional 5% of the variance. This latter result adds credence to the hypothesis that leadership and family responsibilities for migrant Samoan women, accrued with increasing age, are more stressful than they are for migrant Samoan men.

The significant interaction effects noted here can also be said to support the theory that an ecological approach is the most relevant one for elucidating etiological factors in hypertension. An examination of the relationship of socio-cultural and physiological concomitants of the migration process to blood pressure demonstrates this with some clarity. Stress, social resources, age, and body mass are found to be differentially interrelated by gender in their correlation to blood pressure. Undoubtedly there are other risks or resistance resources one could add to this identified complex that would explain more variation in blood pressure: sodium intake, exercise, genetic predisposition, perceived stress, and coping. I would argue that based on the findings presented here, additional variables implicated in hypertension etiology would be interrelated with socio-cultural stressors, age, social resources, and level of obesity. This research also indicates a need, especially in this population, for further ecologically-oriented studies in order to build more factors into this model, while simultaneously examining the causal linkages between them.

CONCLUSIONS

Toward an Anthropology of Disease Etiology

The study described here was originally designed to take a social epidemiologic approach to hypertension among a culturally unique migrant population. It soon became apparent, however, that the basic knowledge required to understand the epidemiologic concepts of stress and social support required pursuing what in many ways was a conventional ethnographic analysis. The need to derive carefully and make context-specific such variables as stress and social support has therefore resulted in more of an anthropology than an epidemiology of hypertension. I have termed this approach an "ethnography" of disease risk, and believe it to be an important means for examining diseases where a number of important risk factors are behavioral in nature. It also represents a method by which epidemiologic problems and concepts can be tailored to specific social and cultural contexts.

Ethnography is the process of deriving the data of cultural anthropology. Ultimately it is a process based on the naturalistic observation of behavior, and the correlation of these observations to material culture, technology, religious and symbolic systems, and so on. There are two characteristics of this approach that make it unique. First, the manner by which data are gathered and interpreted is typically qualitative; that is, not subject to treatment by statistical analysis, though most anthropologists do employ quantitative methods when and where they are seen do the most good. Second, ethnographic analyses are not usually designed to test hypotheses that are conceived in linear fashion; for example the relationship of independent to dependent variable(s). Rather, the interest is in constructing an holistic account of a particular culture. Research problems are conceived and analyzed in the context of all other systems of culture with which they are interrelated. A "systems" or ecological model is, implicitly at least, the underlying methodological framework for most ethnographic research.

Though this brief description is necessarily general, it does serve to highlight some of the basic methodological differences between the more formal science of epidemiology, and perhaps what some would call the "craft" of anthropology. The terms that serve to emphasize the most fundamental differences between the two disciplines are those of "naturalistic" and "holistic". Whereas anthropologists undertake a process of very direct, close, and intense involvement with the subjects of their investigations, epidemiologists usually do not. Whereas anthropologists attempt to attain a basic understanding of the relatedness of cultural phenomena, epidemiologists strive to examine the statistical relationships between discrete and quantifiable risk factors and a specific disease. Even in the case of social epidemiology, which focuses on the role of behavioral factors in explaining the distribution of a disease, the emphasis is on factors that can be lumped into discrete measurable categories, for example, acculturation, cultural incongruity, and so forth. Social scientists have thus usually been involved in the enterprise of epidemiology only as providers of hypotheses (Cassel 1964).

Admittedly, this role is more valuable than none at all. Yet I believe there is a much more fundamental level on which social science, in this case anthropology, can contribute significantly to the understanding of disease. This involves, in a sense, constructing a "topsy-turvy" epidemiology. Before I explain the meaning of this statement, let me first define that area where anthropology and epidemiology take a similar approach to behavioral phenomena.

Commonly applied epidemiological models of diseases, such as the "wheel" or "web of causation", represent attempts to depict, holistically, man-environment relationships:

The wheel consists of a hub (the host or man), which has genetic makeup as its core. Surrounding man is the environment, schematically divided into . . . three sectors . . . biological, social, and physical . . . the model of the wheel implies a need to identify multiple etiologic factors of disease without specifying the agent of disease (Mausner and Bahn 1974: 35).

The reader will immediately note the congruence between this model and the ecological "stress" model I have applied throughout this paper. And it is precisely at this level where the practice of anthropology potentially has the greatest relevance for epidemiology. As I see it, an anthropology of disease is an elucidation of those causal mechanisms and interrelationships that may then be examined in the context of conventional epidemiologic analyses. There are two reasons why anthropology is particularly suited to this purpose. First, a multicausal model of disease is the underlying framework of most ethnographic analyses. An ethnographic analysis of disease risk involves determining which factors are important and then examining their interrelationships with all other aspects of culture. For epidemiology, however, attention given to the interrelationships of risk factors, or to the understanding of host-environment interactions in a unique social or cultural group is typically emphasized to a lesser degree than explicitly analyzing the distribution of a disease.

This brings us back to the idea I proposed of a "topsy-turvy" epidemiology. I would argue that we need to reassess the goals and methods of social

epidemiology. One often gets the impression that the use of socio-cultural data is an afterthought, factors considered after all the other "relevant" issues are addressed. This has certainly been the case in cardiovascular disease epidemiology. I call this the "top-down" method. The problem is considered before the community, the design constructed before the actual appropriateness of measures to the group being studied is evaluated. I would argue that a method that still employs basic epidemiologic methods and yet incorporates the elucidation of causal assemblages, is that of the "bottom-up" approach. In this method an understanding of risk is derived from the naturalistic observation of data and its interrelationships. What is then supplied for epidemiologic investigation are a set of potentially significant factors that reflect processes meaningful to the individuals or population examined. Hence, an anthropology of disease is a topsy-turvy epidemiology, a method of deriving quantitative measures from qualitative analyses.
qualitative analyses.

In this study I examined social and cultural processes that occur as a consequence of migration and which place some individuals into potentially stressful situations. From my direct observation of and contact with Samoans, I was able to derive a range of potentially important factors which I then subjected to quantitative analysis. While this analysis illustrated that the overall hypothesis was true — that social factors did affect blood pressure — perhaps a more important result was an understanding of how these factors took on meaning in the Samoan cultural context.

No one study of this type is ever complete: the findings I have presented here point to two additional tasks. First, it is important that the role of social factors in the etiology of hypertension and other diseases be examined in the context of larger samples of Samoans. I have tried to lay a firm groundwork here upon which these later studies can be based. Second, it is imperative that we search for ways to remedy the particular situations that cause people stress.

ACKNOWLEDGEMENTS

The research reported here was supported in part by a grant from the National Science Foundation (BNS-8204572). I gratefully acknowledge Linda Holland, Ron Stall, and Sandra Gifford for offering helpful criticisms on earlier drafts of this paper. I am especially indebted to members of the Samoan community who supported this research, in particular Mr. Vaita Utu and Mrs. Falefasa Tagaloa.

NOTES

1. Ecological "models" should be distinguished from ecological "methods". Ecological

models, as referred to in the text, provide schema for understanding the interaction of humans with their environment. Ecological *methods*, however, are the means by which the attributes of *groups*, rather than the attributes of individuals, are compared. Thus, in terms of migration, an example of an ecological method would be to look at the relationship between mean body mass, gross differences in diet, and cardiovascular disease rates among culturally and genetically similar people living in three different environments. The inferences drawn from this analysis, however, are weak, since it is impossible to determine the relationship between body mass, nutrition, and disease in individuals. The profound experiences of a few may mask the effects of migration on the rest. For a good critique of the ecological method, consult Robinson (1950).

2. It is critical to recognize the basic conceptual differences between the concepts of "adaptation", "adaptedness", and "adaptability". Generally speaking, the verb *adapt* means to adjust to new or different conditions (from the Latin *adaptare*, "to fit to"). Adaptability refers to the capability of individuals, groups, or organisms to respond to change over time, and hence describes the processual dimension of adaptation. Adaptedness describes biological or socio-cultural stability, and thus more of the static dimension of adaptation (cf. Dunn 1976).

3. Several excellent works are currently available on Samoan social organization. The interested reader is encouraged to consult Holmes (1974) for a discussion of American Samoan social and cultural organization; and Shore (1982) for an analysis of politics and social organization in Western Samoa.

4. A considerable anthropological literature exists on the adaptation of Samoans to West Coast cities. Ablon (1971a, b) presents an excellent, though by now somewhat dated, account of urban Samoan institutions. Rolff (1978) presents an insightful analysis of a small Samoan community in California, and Kotchek describes the Samoan community of Seattle. See my other work (Janes 1984) for a detailed analysis of the social structure of a large Samoan community in Northern California.

5. The sample selection process involved the following steps: a list of the church membership of two large church congregations was obtained, numbering about 130 households. From this pool, 60 households were chosen at random. This resulted in 89 interviews with men and women in these households. Where possible, I would interview a couple separately, but typically, I would interview just one member of the household. In addition, with the aid of a Samoan research assistant, who was also a well-known and respected member of the community, I selected a sample of 25 individuals from other religious denominations.

6. The 11 interviews not coded for quantitative analysis were unusable primarily because of either language problems, or the reluctance of the respondent to answer several important questions. Though I did achieve some fluency in Samoan, I was never able to use it effectively except as an aid in conveying simple ideas or clearing up a misunderstood question. An examination of these excluded interviews reveals that they were primarily of older people who had been on the mainland just a short time. It is doubtful that any bias was introduced into the sample by virtue of the exclusion of these individuals, for this subgroup represents a very small proportion of the total population.

7. These scales were constructed as follows: Per capita income was divided at the median; the upper 50% of the sample were placed in the "high" category; the rest in the "low" category. Leadership was measured for men as consisting of the nature of chiefly status, occupation of a position of leadership in the context of the church, and occupation of a leadership role in the kindred or household (regardless of matai status). For women this scale consists of the same variables save for the question regarding chiefly status. Each variable in the leadership scale consisted of three possible ordinal values: no status, minor or limited status, and high status. The sum of these ranks was taken as the leadership score. Kindred commitment was based on percentage of income contributed for fa'alavelave events, and "high" and "low" were figured as with with per'capita income above.

8. Respondents were asked to indicate the frequency with which events happened in the past year, ranging from never, to once a month or more. Events that are very significant in this culture, such as deaths in the family, and that would be expected to happen less frequently than running short of money, for example, were weighted so that more than 1 death in the last year was scored the same as one of the other, less serious events, happening once a month or more. One would normally want to assess the "internal" reliability of a scale such as this; i.e., how well it "hangs together". This is determined by measuring the correlation of each item with the total score. However, because the events considered are are relatively rate occurrences, and are determined by factors largely beyond the person's control, they represent alternative sources of environmental stress rather than different dimensions of a single "syndrome" or psychological state. Consequently, item-total score correlations are not worth reporting. To insure as much instrument reliability as possible, I simply kept those items in the scale in which there was some variation.

9. The construction of the social resources scale was accomplished by assigning individuals one of five ranks for each of the variables used to construct the measure (church participation, size of social networks, and frequency of visiting with relatives), and then summing these ranks. In analyzing the intercorrelation of these variables it was discovered that there was very little variation in the question regarding number of friends among women respondents. It was also generally more difficult to obtain information regarding social relationships from women. This is probably an outcome of the interview process where the presence of a male investigator resulted in a more formal atmosphere and interaction than among men. Thus, for women the question regarding number of friends is not part of the social resources measure. To make the measures comparable, the social resources score was standardized within each gender group.

10. Individuals were first assigned two scores on the basis of their membership in a leadership/economic status inconsistent category, or in a kindred involvement/economic status inconsistent category. Individuals in the hypothesized lowest-stress cell (high income and high involvement or leadership) were assigned a score of 0. Individuals in the presumed highest-stress cell (low income and high involvement or leadership) were assigned a score of 2. Membership in the remaining cells of either table were coded as 1. The two scores were then summed, resulting in a normally-distributed status inconsistency measure with a range of 0—4.

REFERENCES

Aberle, David, et al.
   1950   The Functional Prerequisites of Society. Ethics 32: 100—111.
Ablon, Joan
   1971a The Social Organization of an Urban Samoan Community. Southwestern Journal of
        Anthropology 27: 75—96.
   1971b Retention of Cultural Values and Differential Urban Adaptation: Samoans and
        American Indians in a West Coast City. Social Forces 49: 385—393.
Alland, Alexander
   1970   Adaptation in Cultural Evolution: An Approach to Medical Anthropology. New
        York: Columbia University Press.
Antonovsky, Aaron
   1979   Health, Stress, and Coping. San Francisco: Jossey-Bass.
Audy, J. R. and F. L. Dunn
   1974   Health and Disease and Community Health. In Sargent, F. (ed.), Human Ecology.
        New York: American Elsevier.

Baker, Paul T.
    1981 Migration and Human Adaptation. *In* C. Fleming and I. A. M. Prior (eds.), Migration, Adaptation, and Health in the Pacific. Wellington, New Zealand: Wellington Hospital Epidemiology Unit.
Baker, Paul T. and Joel M. Hanna
    1981 Modernization and the Biological Fitness of Samoans. *In* C. Fleming and I. A. M. Prior (eds.), Migration, Adaptation, and Health in the Pacific. Wellington, New Zealand: Wellington Hospital Epidemiology Unit.
Beaglehole, R. C. et al.
    1977 Blood Pressure and Social Interaction in Tokelau Migrants in New Zealand. Journal of Chronic Diseases 29: 371—380.
Beiser, Morton et al.
    1976 Systemic Blood Pressure Studies Among the Serer of Senegal. Journal of Chronic Diseases 29: 371—380.
Berkman, Lisa and S. Leonard Syme
    1979 Social Networks, Host Resistance, and Mortality: A Nine-Year Follow-up Study of Alameda County Residents. American Journal of Epidemiology 109: 186.
Caplan, Gerald
    1974 Support Systems and Community Mental Health. New York: Behavioral Publications.
Cassel, John
    1964 Social Science Theory as a Source of Hypotheses in Epidemiological Research. American Journal of Public Health 54: 1482.
    1975 Studies of Hypertension in Migrants. *In* O. Paul (ed.), Epidemiology and Control of Hypertension. New York: Stratton.
    1976 The Contribution of the Social Environment to Host Resistance. American Journal of Epidemiology 104: 107—123.
Cassel, John and Herman A. Tyroler
    1961 Epidemiological Studies of Culture Change. I. Health Status and Recency of Industrialization. Archives of Environmental Health 3: 25—33.
Cassel, John, Ralph Patrick, and C. David Jenkins
    1960 Epidemiological Analysis of the Health Implications of Culture Change. Annals of the New York Academy of Sciences 84: 938—949.
Caudill, William
    1958 Effects of Social and Cultural Systems in Reactions to Stress. New York: Social Science Research Council.
Cobb, Sidney
    1976 Social Support as a Moderator of Life Stress. Psychosomatic Medicine 38: 300—314.
Cohen, Jacob and Patricia Cohen
    1975 Applied Multiple Regression/Correlation Analysis for the Behavioral Sciences. New York: Wiley.
Dohrenwend, B. and B. Dohrenwend (eds.)
    1974 Stressful Life Events: Their Nature and Effects. New York: Wiley.
Dressler, William W.
    1982 Hypertension and Culture Change: Acculturation and Disease in the West Indies. South Salem, NY: Redgrave.
    1985 Psychosomatic Symptoms, Stress, and Modernization: A Model. Culture, Medicine, and Psychiatry 9: 257—286.
Dunn, Frederick L.
    1976 Traditional Asian Medicine and Cosmopolitan Medicine as Adaptive Systems. *In* C. Leslie (ed.), Asian Medical Systems: A Comparative Study. Berkeley, CA: University of California Press.

1979 Behavioural Aspects of the Control of Parasitic Diseases. Bulletin of the World Health Organization 57: 499—512.

1984 Social Determinants in Tropical Disease. *In* K. S. Warren and A.A.F. Mahmoud (eds.), Tropical and Geographical Medicine. New York: McGraw-Hill.

Fleming, Cara and Ian A. M. Prior

1981 Migration, Adaptation, and Health in the Pacific. Wellington, New Zealand: Wellington Hospital Epidemiology Unit.

Foster, George and Barbara G. Anderson

1978 Medical Anthropology. New York: Wiley.

Franco, Robert

1978 Samoans in California: The 'Aiga Adapts. *In* C. Macpherson, B. Shore, and R. Franco (eds.), New Neighbors. . . Islanders in Adaptation. Santa Cruz, CA: Center for South Pacific Studies, University of California, Santa Cruz.

Graves, Theodore D. and Nancy B. Graves

1980 Kinship Ties and the Preferrred Adaptive Strategies of Urban Migrants. *In* S. Beckerman and L. Cordell (eds.), The Versatility of Kinship. New York: Academic Press.

Graves, Theodore D., Nancy B. Graves, Vineta Semu, and Iulai Ah Sam

1983 The Price of Ethnic Identity: Maintaining Kin-Ties Among Pacific Islands Immigrants to New Zealand. Paper presented at the XV Pacific Sciences Congress, Dunedin, New Zealand, 1983.

Haenszel, W. (ed.)

1970 Symposium on Cancer in Migratory Populations. J. Chronic Diseases 23: 289—448.

Haenszel, W. and M. Kurihara

1968 Studies of Japanese Migrants. I. Mortality From Cancer and Other Diseases Among Japanese in the United States. J. National Cancer Institute 40: 43—68.

Hackenberg, Robert et al.

1983 Migration, Modernization, and Hypertension: Blood Pressure Levels in Four Philippine Communities. Medical Anthropology 7(1): 45—71.

Hanna, Joel M. and Paul T. Baker

1979 Biocultural Correlates to the Blood Pressure of Samoan Migrants in Hawaii. Human Biology 51: 480.

Harburg, E., J. C. Erfurt, C. Chapel et al.

1973 Socioecological Stressor Areas and Black-White Blood Pressure: Detroit. J. of Chronic Diseases 26: 595—611.

Henry, James P. and John Cassel

1969 Psychosocial Factors in Essential Hypertension. American Journal of Epidemiology 90: 171—200.

Holmes, Lowell D.

1974 Samoan Village. New York: Holt, Rhinehart and Winston.

Hull, Diana

1979 Migration, Adaptation, and Illness: A Review. Social Science and Medicine 13A: 25—36.

James, S. A. and D. G. Kleinbaum

1976 Socioecologic Stress and Hypertension Related Mortality Rates in North Carolina. American Journal of Public Health 67: 634—639.

Janes, Craig R.

1984 Migration and Hypertension: An Ethnography of Disease Risk in an Urban Samoan Community. Ph.D. Dissertation in Medical Anthropology, University of California, Berkeley and San Francisco.

Janes, Craig R. and Ivan G. Pawson

1986 Migration and Biocultural Adaptation: Samoans in California. Forthcoming in Social Science and Medicine 22: 821—834.

Kaplan, Berton H., John Cassel, and Susan Gore
1977 Social Support and Health. Medical Care 15 (supp): 47—58.
Kotchek, Lydia
1975 Adaptive Strategies of an Invisible Ethnic Minority. Ph.D. Dissertation in Anthropology, University of Washington, Seattle, WA.
Lazarus, Richard S.
1966 Psychological Stress and the Coping Process. New York: McGraw-Hill
Lehr, I., H. B. Messinger, and R. Rosenman
1973 A Sociobiological Approach to the Study of Coronary Heart Disease. Journal of Chronic Diseases 26: 13—30.
Leighton, Alexander H.
1959 My Name is Legion. New York: Basic Books.
Leighton, Dorothea, et al.
1963 The Character of Danger. New York: Basic Books.
Leighton, Dorothea
1978 Sociocultural Factors in Physical and Mental Breakdown. Man-Environment Systems 8: 33—37.
Levine, Sol and Norman A. Scotch
1970 Social Stress. Chicago: Aldine.
Lieban, Richard
1973 Medical Anthropology. In J. J. Honigmann (ed.), Handbook of Social and Cultural Anthropology. Chicago: Rand-McNally.
Mead, Margaret
1930 The Social Organization of Manua. Honolulu: Bernice P. Bishop Museum, 6.
Marmot, Michael
n.d. Migrants, Acculturation and Coronary Heart Disease. Unpublished MS, School of Public Health, University of California Berkeley.
Marmot, Michael and S. Leonard Syme
1976 Acculturation and Coronary Heart Disease in Japanese-Americans. American Journal of Epidemiology 104: 225—247.
Mausner, Judith S. and Anita K. Bahn
1974 Epidemiology: An Introductory Text. Philadelphia, PA: W. B. Saunders.
McGarvey, Stephen T.
1980 Modernization and Cardiovascular Disease Among Samoans. Ph.D. Dissertation in Anthropology. Pennsylvania State University.
McGarvey, Stephen T. and Paul T. Baker
1979 The Effects of Modernization and Migration on Samoan Blood Pressures. Human Biology 51: 461—480.
Merton, Robert K.
1949 Social Theory and Social Structure. Glencoe, IL: The Free Press.
Mestrovic, Stjepan and Barry Glassner
1983 A Durkheimian Hypothesis on Stress. Social Science and Medicine 17: 1315—1327.
Montgomery, Edward
1973 Ecological Aspects of Health and Disease in Local Populations. In Bernard J. Siegel, et al. (eds.) Annual Review of Anthropology. Palo Alto, CA: Annual Reviews, Inc. 2: 30—35.
Neser, W. B., H. A. Tyroler, and J. C. Cassel
1971 Social Disorganization and stroke Mortality in the Black Population of North Carolina. American J. Epidemiology 93: 166—175.
Northwest Regional Educational Laboratory
1984 Study of Unemployment, Poverty and Training Needs of American Samoans. Final Report to the U.S. Department of Labor, Employment and Training Administration. Portland, Oregon.

Pawson, Ivan G. and Craig R. Janes
  1981 Massive Obesity in a Migrating Population. American Journal of Public Health 71: 508—513.
  1982 Biocultural Risks in Longevity: Samoans in California. Social Science and Medicine 16: 183—190.
Pilisuk, Marc and Charles Froland
  1978 Kinship, Social Networks, Social Support and Health. Social Science and Medicine 12B: 273—280.
Prior, Ian A. M. et al.
  1974 The Tokelau Island Migrant Study. International Jouranl of Epidemiology 3: 225.
Prior, Ian A. M.
  1979 Hypertension Risk Factors: A Preventive Point of View. In F. Gross and T. Strasser (eds.), Mild Hypertension: Natural History and Management. England: Pitman.
Rahe, Robert H.
  1974 The Pathway Between Subjects' Recent Life Changes and Their Near-Future Illness Reports: Representative Results and Methodological Issues. In B. S. Dohrenwend and B. P. Dohrenwend (eds.), Stressful Life Events: Their Nature and Effects. New York: Wiley.
Robinson, W. S.
  1950 Ecological Correlations and the Behavior of Individuals. American Sociological Review 15: 351—357.
Rolff, Karla
  1978 Fa'asamoa: Tradition in Transition. Ph.D. Dissertation in Anthropology, University of California, Santa Barbara.
Scotch, Norman A.
  1963 Sociocultural Factors in the Epidemiology of Zulu Hypertension. American Journal of Public Health 53: 1205—1213.
Selye, Hans
  1956 The Stress of Life. New York: McGraw-Hill.
Shore, Bradd
  1982 Sala'ilua: A Samoan Mystery. New York: Columbia University Press.
Susser, M.
  1973 Causal Thinking in the Health Sciences: Concepts and Strategies in Epidemiology. New York: Oxford University Press
Syme, S. Leonard and C. P. Torfs
  1978 Epidemiologic Research on Hypertension. Journal of Human Stress 4: 43—48.
Syme, S. Leonard et al.
  1964 Some Social and Cultural Factors Associated with the Occurrence of Coronary Heart Disease. Journal of Chronic Diseases 16: 277—289.
Syme, S. Leonard et al.
  1966 Cultural Mobility and Coronary Heart Disease in an Urban Area. American Journal of Epidemiology 82: 334.
Taylor, Richard J. and Paul Z. Zimmet
  1981 Obesity and Diabetes in Western Samoa. Journal of Obesity 5:367—376.
Theorell, T.
  1976 Selected Illnesses and Somatic Factors in Relation to Two Psychosocial Stress Indices. Journal of Psychosomatic Research 20: 7—20.
Tofaeono, Bert
  1978 The Role of the Church in California Samoan Communities. In Cluny Macpherson, Bradd Shore, and Robert Franco (eds.), New Neighbors. . . Islanders in Adaptation. Santa Cruz, CA: Center for South Pacific Studies, University of California, Santa Cruz.

Tyroler, Herman A. and John Cassel
    1964 Health Consequences of Culture Change. II. The Effect of Urbanization on
        Coronary Heart Disease in Rural Residents. Journal of Chronic Diseases 17: 167.
Tyroler, H. A., S. Heyden, and C. G. Hames
    1975 Weight and Hypertension: Evans County Studies of Blacks and Whites. *In* O. Paul
        (ed.), Epidemiology and Control of Hypertension. New York: Stratton.
Waldron, Ingrid et al.
    1982 Cross-cultural Variation in Blood Pressure: A Quantitative Analysis of the
        Relationships of Blood Pressure to Cultural Characteristics, Salt Consumption, and
        Body Weight. Social Science and Medicine 16: 419—430.
Walsh, Anthony
    1980 The Prophylactic Effect of Religion on Blood Pressure Levels Among a Sample of
        Migrants. Social Science and Medicine 14B: 59—64.
Wellin, Edward
    1977 Theoretical Orientations in Medical Anthropology: Continuity and Change over the
        Past Half Century. *In* David Landy (ed.), Culture, Disease, and Healing. New York:
        Macmillan.
Wershow, H. J. and G. Reinhart
    1974 Life Changes and Hospitalization — A Heretical View. Journal of Psychosomatic
        Research 18: 393—401.
Wessen, A. F.
    1971 The Role of Migrant Studies in Epidemiological Research. Israel J. Medical Science
        7: 1578—1583.
Wolff, H. G.
    1953 Stress and Disease. Springfield, Ill: Charles Thomas.
Yano, K., et al.
    1979 Childhood Cultural Experience and the Incidence of Coronary Heart Disease in
        Hawaii Japanese Men. American Journal of Epidemiology 109: 440—450.
Young, Allan
    1980 The Discourse on Stress and the Reproduction of Conventional Knowledge. Social
        Science and Medicine 14B: 133—146.
Zimmet, P., S. Faaiusu, J. Ainuu et al.
    1981 The Prevalence of Diabetes in the Rural and Urban Polynesian Population of
        Western Samoa. Diabetes 30(1): 45—51.
Zimmet, P., M. Arblaster, and K. Thoma
    1978 The Effect of Westernization on Native Populations. Studies on a Micronesian
        Community With a High Diabetes Prevalence. Australia and New Zealand Journal
        of Medicine 8: 141—146.
Zimmet, P. and S. Whitehouse
    1980 The Price for Modernization in Nauru, Tuvalu, and Western Samoa. *In* H. Trowell
        and D. Burkitt (eds.), Western Diseases. London: Edward Arnold.
Zimmet, P., L. Jackson, S. Whitehouse
    1980 Blood Pressure Studies in Two Pacific Populations with Varying Degrees of
        Modernization. New Zealand Medical Journal 657: 249—252.
Zimmet, P., R. Taylor, L. Jackson et al.
    1980 Blood Pressure Studies in Rural and Urban Western Samoa. Medical Journal of
        Australia 2: 202—205.

SANDRA M. GIFFORD

THE MEANING OF LUMPS: A CASE STUDY OF THE
AMBIGUITIES OF RISK

Molly is 27 years old and dying from breast cancer. She first noticed a lump in her breast when she was 21. Her girlfriend urged her to see a doctor and she did. Her doctor told her not to worry — that it was probably just a cyst. Five years later, in extreme pain and unable to walk, Molly was diagnosed as having breast cancer:

I had this little knot and I thought. "I'm sure it's nothing". But she says (Molly's girlfriend) "You should go get that examined . . . just because it's better to be safe than sorry". So we ventured down to this little hospital and this doctor gave me an exam and said, "Well, I feel something like the size of a pea and it seems like it's a cyst but I don't think it's anything you should be concerned about". And I thought, "Oh really? Well wonderful!" But he didn't explain to me the fact that sometimes you need to keep on these things, like cysts can grow into tumors. So I didn't even think about it at all. In my mind it was OK, it was a cyst. So the years after, every time I went for my physical, I would let the doctor know . . . I always made mention of the fact that I had this cyst and I always made mention of the fact that I had irregular menstrual cycles because I figured the more information they received, the better. But maybe because I didn't have a consistent doctor every year, they never thought much of it . . . . Then I was only 21 or 22 and they probably figured, "Oh, no big deal!" Maybe I didn't take it as seriously . . . especially after I heard it was nothing to be concerned about . . . . But, I think they weren't conscientious enough and that really bugs me because that is what we pay them for. That's what they go to school for. And even if a patient doesn't come in and say, "Well, give me a biopsy", they should say, "Well, a cyst? And how long have you had this. Well, maybe we should take a biopsy just to see." You know, I don't care how young you are or what. That really makes me angry because I think that maybe this could have been prevented.

Molly has none of the classic risk factors for breast cancer. She is young, black, and has no family history of the disease. Benign breast lumps are common in young women, breast cancer is not. Within the six months following her diagnosis, Molly underwent a mastectomy, an ovariectomy, radiotheraphy and chemotheraphy. She does not know how long she has to live.

Fiona is 44 years old and has been diagnosed as having mammary dysplasia — what some consider a serious benign breast condition. She has had several biopsies and is currently under close medical surveillance. Because of Fiona's benign condition, her doctor considers her to be at risk of developing breast cancer. Although Fiona knows her condition is serious, she is uncertain of the implications of her disease. Fiona explains:

Dr. Smith said that there are things, mammary dysplasia for one, which could indicate the possibility of cancer in later years. He talked in Latin and much of what he said I did not understand . . . . I'm still not the hell sure what it is I got . . . . At any rate he has been seeing me now every three months. Now he inevitably finds something. He's found a couple of cysts

Craig R. Janes et al. (eds.), Anthropology and Epidemiology, 213—246.
© 1986 *by D. Reidel Publishing Company.*

in the left breast which he has aspirated. Now today I was up there and he found one in the right breast which he felt was a little bit more of a lump than it should have been . . . that more water should have come out of it than did. But he's going to send what little fluid that he did get to the pathologist again and I won't have their report till Wednesday. It has been an ongoing saga now for two years. As I say, he inevitably finds something. I have very lumpy breasts. I have mammary dysplasia. So it's one of those things. Nobody's sure if it's a disease or what the devil it is! But every time he finds something like he did today, he puts me on pins and needles again until he decides what else . . . I have told myself Sandy, I have told myself, I will not think about this anymore . . . . But it never goes away. It is always there.

Fiona has many risk factors for breast cancer. She is 44 years of age, white, never married, has no children, and has been given a diagnosis of benign breast disease. While Fiona does not have breast cancer, the uncertainty concerning her conditon has resulted in the medicalization of her life.

Molly's and Fiona's experiences represent two extremes of the consequences of the ambiguities and uncertainties about risk, benign breast conditions and breast cancer. While Molly's experiences are the more tragic, one might pause to consider the physical and psychological consequences of Fiona's constant medical surveillance. Molly, Fiona and their doctors all are enmeshed in the dilemmas of medical uncertainty about what is known and what is unknown about the future of possible disease. This essay explores the ambiguities of risk which arise out of its translation from epidemiological findings to clinical knowledge and practice and thus to lay experiences of health and illness.

In both epidemiology and clinical medicine the concept of risk plays a central role in underestandings about the etiology and prevention of chronic disease. For the epidemiologist, the concept of risk expresses a statistical measure of the degree of association between a characteristic and a disease within a defined population (Lilienfeld and Lilienfeld 1980). However, this epidemiologic concept becomes more broadly defined when translated into clinical practice and lay perceptions of health and illnes. Within clinical and lay contexts, it is more appropriate to speak of the "language of risk" in that the term is used to convey a constellation of meanings some of which are intended and some of which remain largely unconscious. The language of risk is about scientific uncertainty concerning causal relationships, and clinical and lay uncertainty concerning the prediction and control of unhealthy outcomes. The popularity of the concept is linked to the inability of epidemiologists and other medical scientists to produce models which adequately explain the etiology and population distribution of chronic diseases, and from the inability of clinical medicine to prevent and cure these diseases.

Currently there is much confusion and debate between epidemiologists and clinicians about how to translate concepts of epidemiologic risk into clinical risk. Part of this confusion arises because contextual differences in the meaning and use of the concept have not been fully recognized. To better understand these contextual differences, I present a model in which risk takes on two distinct dimensions; a technical, objective or *scientific* dimension and a socially experienced or *lived* dimension. The assessment and evaluation of risk with epidemiology is an objective, technical and scientific process but for the lay person it is a subjective, lived experience. Lay assessment and evalution of risk is a social process, not a scientific, technical one. Clinical medicine bridges these two dimensions. Risk for the practitioner may sometimes be objective, sometimes lived, and sometimes both — as the practitioner is faced with the task of translating scientific risk into the treatment of individual patients.

The central argument of this paper is that although epidemiologists speak of risk as being a measured property of a group of people, clinicians speak of risk as a specific property of an individual. Risk becomes something that the patient suffers; a sign of a future disease that the clinician can diagnose, treat and manage. For the patient, risk becomes a lived or experienced state of ill-health and a symptom of future illness. To the patient, risk is rarely an objective concept. Rather, it is internalized and experienced as a state of being. These different dimensions of risk as understood and experienced by epidemiologists, clinicians and lay women — further blur the already am-biguous relationship between health and ill-health. This ambiguity results in the creation of a new state of being healthy and ill; a state that is somewhere between health and disease and that results in the medicalization of a woman's life.

This paper contains five sections. First, I discuss the epistemiological assumptions informing the cultural creation of risk within epidemiology and clinical medicine. In the second, third and fourth sections I develop a model of risk which embodies both scientific and lived dimensions. This model emerges from attempts to understand and explain the results of one and one-half years of fieldwork conducted in the Departments of Epidemiology and Surgery at a major teaching hospital, and a private hospital in California. The goal of this research was to explore the dilemmas that clinicians and women face in the diagnosis and management of benign breast conditions.[1] Results are presented that illustrate how clinicians transform the epidemio-logic concept of risk into a physical entity, a sign of future disease; and how this causes serious dilemmas for women diagnosed as being "at risk". In the fifth section I argue that the medicalization of risk has implications beyond this particular example of benign breast disease and breast cancer and that we should consider the extent to which these understandings can be extended to medical thinking and practice of other chronic, non-infectious diseases.

EPISTEMIOLOGICAL ASSUMPTIONS INFORMING EPIDEMIOLOGICAL
AND CLINICAL CONCEPTS OF RISK

Risk is a concept central to the experiences of modern life. It is a socially constructed concept describing and explaining possibilities of future dangers that are becoming increasingly unpredictable. While the concept of risk has always embodied ideas of danger, it has not always embodied ideas about chance. The etymological meanings of risk derive from the Latin word "resecare" meaning to cut back, cut off short. From the Latin meaning, the concept can be traced to both French and Italian meanings of "peril" and to the Spanish meaning of "to venture into danger". The concept of chance was introduced to the definition of risk more recently. The Concise Oxford Dictionary gives the contemporary meaning of risk: "The chance of injury, damage or loss. A dangerous chance, hazard." Contemporary concepts of risk describe relationships between uncertain knowledge and unwanted outcomes. The language of risk is essential to being able to speak about, understand and live in an increasingly unpredictable world.

Within the health sciences, the rise of the popularity of the concept of risk is linked to changes occurring in both epidemiologic models and clinical modes of thought and practice. Current epistemiological assumptions concerning disease etiology can be traced to the view of science and medicine arising during the scientific revolution in the 16th and 17th centuries, and during French and Industrial Revolution in the latter part of the 18th century.[2] The concept of risk as used within contemporary explanatory models has emerged directly from a growing awareness that traditional models of health and illness are undergoing important conceptual shifts. In this sense, the concept of risk can be understood to stem from shifts in epidemiological and medical thinking and points to anomalies arising in contemporary theories of the etiology of chronic disease.[3]

RISK AND CONCEPTS OF CAUSALITY IN EPIDEMIOLOGY

The emergence of models of multiple-causation and the rise of the concept of risk can be traced to developments in the late 1950s when epidemiologists began to seriously question whether models of infectious disease etiology could be applied to the chronic diseases. To account for the anomalies presented by chronic disease, was a shift in the logic of epidemiologic thinking needed, or rather, was it simply a matter of the need for new knowledge about these diseases? Much of this debate was reported in the major epidemiologic and medical journals and the majority of authors argued for the creation of new knowledge rather than for a shift in epidemiologic thinking (Lilienfeld 1959; Sartwell 1960; Yerushalmy and Palmer 1959). Thus, epidemiologic thinking was directed towards re-defining the concept of cause and creating more complex models of causation rather than questioning the very nature of epidemiologic thinking:[4]

Differences in causal thinking about infectious and noninfectious diseases — the latter being more likely to have multiple causal agents — depend upon the frame of reference within which the investigator operates, and reflect differences in our knowledge of the etiology of these two general categories of disease, rather than differences in logical reasoning. (Lilienfeld and Lilienfeld 1980 : 293)

In contemporary epidemiologic models of noninfectious diseases, we find a re-working of the Henle-Koch hypothesis for establishing causation (Evans 1976; Lilienfeld 1959, 1973; Lilienfeld and Lilienfeld 1980; Sartwell 1960; Susser 1973; Yerushalmy and Palmer 1959). The notion of probability is introduced to describe the given uncertainty concerning suspected relationships and the concept of risk replaces the concept of cause.[5] Instead of thinking about the causal relationship between an agent and a disease, we think about the possible association(s) between one or more factors and a disease outcome. Within this framework, many of the more innovative epidemiologists have attempted to create broader and more holistic approaches which might better explain the many complex relationships between the social-environmental contexts within which people live and health status (Berkman 1981; Berkman and Syme 1979; Lindheim and Syme 1983; Marmot 1976; Najman 1980). However, despite the complexity and elegance of current models of multiple causation, I argue that the unstated assumptions and logic of epidemiologic thought underlying these models continue to be based in the belief of (or perhaps wish for) the doctrine of specific etiology. Thus we find an emerging rhetoric speaking of holistic, multi-causal relationships yet a practice which continues to adopt a reductionistic, mechanistic approach towards understanding and managing disease.

approaches to infectious vs chronic diseases

The points I wish to make are that epidemiologic concepts of risk describe relationships which are objective, depersonalized, quantitative, and scientifically measured.[6] Drawing upon Toulmin's (1976) distinctions between general and particular knowledge within medicine, risk within epidemiology represents scientific knowledge about generalized relationships between possible causes and possible effects. Risk is about states of health which are located outside of any one particular individual; it depersonalizes causes of disease. The epidemiologic language of risk is "detached and descriptive; an onlooker's analytical understanding of collective relationships" (Toulmin 1976: 35). And it is in this regard that risk takes on qualitatively different meanings for both medical practitioners and lay women.

The Epidemiology of Risk: Benign Breast Disease and Breast Cancer

Although epidemiologic risk is a scientifically measured concept, there is much controversy concerning the precise nature and degree of risk associated with a given disease outcome. Thus, there is always an inherent degree of uncertainty concerning the understanding of specific risk factors. The risk factors for breast cancer provide a clear illustration of the complexities of accurately defining epidemiologic risk.

It is estimated that at the present rate, 1 out of every 11 women living in the United States will develop breast cancer in her lifetime. Cancer ranks second to heart disease as the leading killer of American women, and breast cancer kills more women between the ages of 40 to 44 years than any other disease. While the incidence of breast cancer has risen, the survival trends for all stages of breast cancer have remained virtually unchanged since 1950 (SEER 1984). The specific causes of breast cancer remain unknown and as yet, there exists no known method of prevention. Epidemiologists have identified many risk factors thought to be associated with the disease and these include increasing age, a history of bilateral pre-menopausal breast cancer in a first degree relative, a previous diagnosis of breast cancer, residence in North America or Northern Europe as opposed to Asia or Africa, late age at birth of the first child, and a history of fibrocystic breast disease (Kelsey 1979). Epidemiologists and medical scientists have found it difficult to adequately define and measure these risk factors and thus much uncertainty remains concerning the extent to which each contributes to the disease.

Benign breast disease further illustrates the ambiguities of risk. Until recently it was thought that a diagnosis of benign breast disease, or what is also commonly referred to as fibrocystic breast disease, significantly increased a woman's risk for breast cancer. Most studies conducted indicated a two to four fold increase in risk (Kelsey 1979). However, there have been many problems in understanding the extent to which this benign condition actually contributes to the disease.

First, it has been difficult for epidemiologists to obtain accurate case definitions because the clinical and histopathological classification of benign conditions suffer from a lack of standardized criteria and terminology. Ernster (1981) has argued that there are no reliable standards for making a clinical diagnosis and what one clinician may consider normal another may judge to be abnormal. Benign breast disease has been clinically defined as ". . . a condition in which there are palpable lumps in the breast, usually associated with pain and tenderness, that fluctuate with the menstrual cycle and that become progressively worse until menopause" (Scalon 1981 pp: 524). Often the distinction between normal physiologic changes and clinical disease is dependent upon a woman's age, the level of concern and the expertise of the clinician (Ernster 1981). Although the majority of breast changes and conditions are labeled as benign, every lump can represent a possible cancer before diagnosis. And therefore, a more reliable definition is based on a biopsy diagnosis. However, there is also much ambiguity in the histological definition of these conditions. Love et al. (1982) have argued that ". . . valid histologic criteria defining fibrocystic disease as a distinct process do not exist and that microscopic differences between the normal breast and those clinically defined as fibrocystic are differences of degree and not quality" (p 101).

A second problem with understanding the nature of risk that benign breast conditions represent concerns that of selection bias. Studies that show an increased rate of breast cancer among women with fibrocystic disease are based on a biopsy diagnosis. This means that risk has been based not on all women with lumpy breasts but rather only on those who have had a biopsy performed. This is a crucial point because not every women with a lumpy breast is selected for a biopsy. Rather, other risk factors are taken into account, and women who have had breast biopsies tend to be in a higher risk group to begin with. Obviously, one would expect to find a higher incidence of breast cancer among a group of women at high risk. Even among those high risk women whose biopsies were normal, the incidence of breast cancer would be higher. Thus, one could argue that a diagnosis of fibrocystic disease alone does not necessarily raise a woman's risk of breast cancer. Rather, a women who has had a biopsy regardless of whether the results are normal or abnormal is more likely to get breast cancer because she is more likely to be at higher risk in the first place (Love 1984). In a recent review of the literature, Ernster (1981) failed to find a significant relationship between cancer risk factors and benign breast disease risk factors.

These two problems have made it difficult for epidemiologists to estimate accurately the incidence and prevalence of benign breast disease within the population and to establish clear evidence for a causal relationship with breast cancer. Indeed, some studies have estimated that a least 50% of all women have palpably irregular breasts and as many as 90% of women may have some sort of histological changes! This has led some epidemiologists and medical practitioners to argue that many benign conditions simply represent a range of normal variation and that therefore, the condition should not be thought of as a disease entity (Ernster 1982; Love 1984).

Despite the problems inherent in the definition of risk, there does seem to be a general association between benign conditions and breast cancer. However, although epidemiologists have been careful to confine their understandings to populations, and to stick to the caveat that "correlation is not causation", many doctors and women have tended to assume that in some as yet unknown way, benign conditions have the capacity to cause breast cancer. The crux of the problem thus lies in the translation of epidemiologic risk into clinical and individual risk.

Bateson (1979) has argued that there is a great difference between statements about a class and statements about an identified individual. "Such statements are of different logical type, and prediction from one to the other is always unsure" (1979: 42). Bateson argues that although we may develop a certain amount of knowledge about the generic, the specifics will always elude us. Toulmin (1976) applies these ideas to the intrinsic uncertainty of knowledge about the particular in medicine. He argues that, "In any developed natural science, our understanding of general principles will eventually outrun our ability to apply those principles to the detailed facts of particular cases" (1976 : 43). There is always an element of intrinsic uncertainty in the practice of clinical medicine because the practitioner is required to translate generalized knowledge to the treatment of a particular individual. And in these situations, there is always a certain amount of uncertainty which cannot be measured. Risk then, for the clinician, takes on the added dimension of unmeasured uncertainty.

There are thus, two kinds of risk: the first is "measurable uncertainty" represented by the laws of probability; the second is unmeasured uncertainty, where numerical probabilities may not be entirely applicable. Knight (1921) has argued that unmeasured uncertainty prevails where:

... numerical probabilities were inapplicable in situations when the decision maker was ignorant of the statistical frequencies of events relevant to his decision; or when prior calculations were impossible; or when the relevant events were in some sense unique; or when an important, once-and-for-all decision was concerned. (Quoted in Ellsberg 1961: 643).

The concept of measured and unmeasured risk can be applied to understanding the different dimensions of epidemiologic, clinical and lay knowledge of benign breast conditions and breast cancer. What distinguishes the two dimensions is the ambiguity of information. Scientific risk is quantitative, objective and relatively unambiguous. Lived risk is qualitative, subjective and highly ambiguous. Epidemiologists create scientific risk, lay people create and experience lived risk, clinicians mediate between and bridge these two dimensions of risk. It is to the clinical experience of risk to that I now turn.

THE CLINICAL DIAGNOSIS AND MANAGEMENT OF RISK

Epidemiologists have identified certain groups of women who are unquestionably at higher risk for developing breast cancer .... For those of us who practice clinical medicine, it is essential to separate those factors that are significant enough to influence our own practice of medicine from those factors that are perhaps statistically important when dealing with large populations but which are not enough to make us alter the advice we give patients about the frequency of clinical examinations, intervals between mammograms, and so forth .... This then, becomes the crux of this discussion, namely, the clinical implications of these risk factors. Which if any, of the recognized epidemiologically significant risk factors should trigger special treatment or follow-up for women (or men) so affected? By identifying these groups of individuals can we detect breast cancer earlier and thereby alter the course and outcome of the disease? (Schwartz 1982 : 26).

This passage from a recent article in the medical journal 'Breast' clearly articulates the dilemmas facing the clinician in the management of women at risk for breast cancer. As the quotation suggests, the language or risk within clinical medicine is about uncertainty concerning the translation of scientific knowledge into clinical practice. A fundamental difference between clinical and epidemiological risk involves the application of risk knowledge. In contrast to epidemiology, which might be best understood as a science of populations, the practice of medicine can be understood as a science of individuals. While clinical medicine developed from similar historical traditions, and shares with epidemiology basic biomedical assumptions about causality and the nature of health and disease, the application of such knowledge is vastly different. One problem facing the clinician concerns the translation of epidemiologic knowledge about groups into practical knowledge of particular individuals:

> One cannot expect . . . to be able to move from a theoretical knowledge of the relevant laws to a prediction of the particular's behaviour. The history of the law-governed mechanisms and of the particular which is their bearer is, so to speak, an intervening variable which always to some degree elude us. (Gorovitz and MacIntyre 1976 : 57).

The practice of clinical medicine depends on the application of certain knowledge. However, given the importance of diseases of unknown and complex etiology, clinicians are increasingly forced to apply uncertain knowledge. Uncertain knowledge represents clinical risk. Errors in epidemiology have theoretical consequences while errors in medical practice have immediate, and often tragic consequences.[7] Within clinical medicine risk must be understood in relation to the practical application of epidemiological and other scientific knowledge to clinical practice. Clinicians must apply general epidemiological knowledge of risk within populations to specific individuals. Therefore, while on the one hand a clinician may judge a patient to be at risk because she has a number of classic epidemiological risk factors, the clinician knows that this diagnosis of risk does not predict, with any certainty, a disease outcome.

In clinical medicine risk can be best understood as assuming at least two additional meanings. The first meaning results from the translation of epidemiologic risk factors into clinical practice. In this instance, clinicians must infer clinical significance from objective epidemiological data. Risk factors are used to aid in the diagnosis and management of patients, and in determining probable prognoses. In this way risk is transformed into a clinical entity.

A second meaning of risk emerges from clinicians' experiences of uncertainty concerning diagnosis, management and prognosis. This experience is a necessary part of clinical practice because clinicians never have complete knowledge of all the variables which lead to disease states within particular individuals. Thus, "fallibility" is always a part of clinical practice (Gorovitz and MacIntyre 1976). In this context risk represents the clinician's personal experiences of being wrong. However, in a way similar to translations of epidemiologic risk into clinical practice, clinicians may transform the trying experiences of uncertainty into clinical entities. The transformation of epidemiologic and personal risk into a clinical problem, a physical sign of disease, allows clinicians to manage risk by physically removing it from the body.

Clinical understandings of and experiences with applying risk are well illustrated in the dilemmas clinicians face in the management of women with benign breast disease. Recall that although benign conditions are not life threatening and do not constitute cause for concern in and of themselves, the danger is in their association with breast cancer. Benign conditions come to symbolize and represent risks over which the clinician has no control. On the one hand they represent the objective existence of risk factors for breast cancer. On the other hand, benign breast conditions represent the clinician's lived risk of failing to diagnose or predict a cancer. Thus, because it is not clear which kinds of benign conditions might be more pre-malignant than others, and because the presence of lumps can camouflage a small underlying cancer, clinical risk takes on both an objective and a lived, or experiential, dimension. I explore these two dimensions below in regard to my research findings.

The assessment of risk factors plays an important role in helping the practitioner reach a clinical diagnosis. To make a risk assessment, the clinician must interpret epidemiologic risk to have clinical relevance, and this entails two shifts in meaning. First, the clinician must shift from thinking about risk as being a statement about disease rates in a population, to thinking of risk as applied to one patient. Second, risk is thus transformed from a statistical concept to a physical entity. The clinician comes to think about risk within existing modes of clinical thought and practice by trans-forming risk into a sign of a "possible" current or future disease. Thus, objective clinical risk comes to be understood and talked about in the same sense as other objective clinical signs of disease.

This transformation is partially illustrated by examining the diagnostic process that occurs when a women seeks consultation for breast symptoms. At one of the hospitals where this research was conducted, a special breast screening clinic had been established. At a woman's first appointment to the clinic, a medical history is taken. During this process, information regarding risk factors is elicited along with other signs and symptoms. One of the nurses responsible for conducting medical histories explained:

We have on our history form, "significant risk factors". These are the ones that Dr. Jones and Dr. Smith have identified as the most significant . . . but these are not proven yet. The ones we have identified are sex, age, obesity in postmenopausal women only, personal family history of invasive breast cancer, and premalignant conditions . . . . My role when I see a woman for screening is to identify and check off which ones she has. Then it's up to the physician to make the risk assessment and outline a plan of care of the patient.

Here we find that the nurse is speaking of risk factors as properties of the patient. The doctor will assess the meaning of elicited risk factors in the same way that he or she assess the meaning of other signs and symptoms. Although clinicians elicit and assess risk factors, much uncertainty remains concerning their clinical significance. This is due in part to the ambiguity of data on breast cancer risk in epidemiology and medical science. Thus, there is an inherent ambiguity in objective clinical risk. And it is this inherent ambiguity that leads to much uncertainty in the clinical management of risk. One surgeon explained:

The problem is that there are certain accepted statistics for the female population as a whole. Then there are statistics that involve specific populations that seem to contradict the general national accepted cancer study statistics. So I don't know. And what ever the genetic predisposition, the environmental predisposition, whatever, I can't tell them how to eliminate that risk!

Because clinicians are faced with interpreting a confusing array of epidemiologic and scientific knowledge concerning statistical risk, benign lumps become physical risk. Practitioners can do nothing about changing risk factors such as age, the number of children a woman has or family history of breast disease. However, a physical lump in the breast is something that can be felt, seen and treated. And it is in this sense that objective clinical risk becomes central to and symbolic of the medical condition of benign breast disease.

However, the attribution of risk to a physical entity does not necessarily lead to clinical clarity. In fact, it can serve to increase ambiguity and uncertainty. Many of the clinicians interviewed expressed great levels of uncertainty concerning the clinical significance of benign breast conditions. On obstetrician explained:

Doctors don't really know what the relationship of fibrocystic breasts are to cancer. Fibrocystic breasts are very common. No one knows how you preselect from one to the other. We're all groping in risk factors and trying to define the high risk population.

Despite uncertainties about the clinical singificance of benign conditions, clinicians do attempt to bring a sense of certainty to some risk factors. For example, practitioners often create risk profiles for individual patients based on statistical patterns. This is illustrated by the following surgeon's expressed concern over the chances that a benign condition might develop into breast cancer:

Those women who have multiple cysts, and I mean come in with four or five cysts in each breast over a period of a year, in this type of patient, 25% will develop cancer. I have one here who I am a little bit concerned about. She has been coming in since 1976 and each time she comes in she's got another cyst and she's been in seven times so far. I'm getting worried about her. There comes a time when you have to sit down and say, "Well, look, statistically you've got about a 25% chance of developing breast cancer". And you ask them to start thinking a little bit about having a subcutaneous mastectomy.

Considering this example, we might wonder about the clinical understanding of probability. Does this surgeon mean that this type of patient has a 25% chance of developing breast cancer over the next five years or over her lifetime? The concept of probability is poorly understood by clinicians and lay people alike. Faced with these uncertain understandings, this surgeon has translated a population risk into an individual risk and has suggested prophylactic mastectomy as a possible method of removing the risk.

When faced with managment of a "high risk" patient, surgeons have a tendency to treat risk as they would other undesirable physical conditions. Thus, we find that clinicians speak of risk as not only a sign of possible current or future disease, but also as something that resides in a particular part of the body and something from which a patient then suffers. Two surgeons explained:

You really have to say to the woman, "you have this much risk in each breast over the next 25 years". Then they really have to decide how they feel about the risk.

Consider you're at significant risk of developing breast cancer, but I can't tell you that you're going to develop cancer. All I know is that every woman suffers somewhere around a 1 in 11 chance of having breast cancer and your risk is greater than that and you're very young. That means for another 30 or 40 or 50 years, you suffer that risk.

This brings me to my final point about objective clinical risk. In the logic of medical thought and practice, if risk is understood as something from which the patient physically suffers, it then follows that risk is something that can be physically treated. In clinical language, risk is spoken of as if it were a sign of a possible future or current disease, a sign that resides in a particular part of the body and can be observed by the clinician. In the clinical management of risk for breast cancer, surgeons may remove the physical condition that they conceive of as being at risk: biopsies are performed to obtain a more definitive diagnosis and to remove the lump itself. Removal of the lump results in the removal of the risk of a possible pre-malignant condition. For example, a surgeon explains:

I tend to be rather aggressive about doing biopsies and sometimes I get a little guilty about that. But you know, you have a situation that you will feel a little guilty about only to have it pop up to be pathologic! I mean we are legally at risk, emotionally at risk, and physically, the patient is at risk.

This comment is revealing as it introduces the second dimension of clinical risk, the *lived* dimension. Lived clinical risk refers to the clinician's own experience with the risk of being wrong. Lived clinical risk results from uncertainty concerning clinical knowledge and its application in practice. Such risk leads to changes in clinical perceptions of normality. As a result, patients diagnosed at risk fall into a grey zone that is between health and disease. This ambiguous state leads to clinical uncertainty concerning diagnosis, management and prognosis.

Clinical uncertainty has always been inherent to medical practice. The art of a diagnosis consists of bringing order and meaning to a complex series of signs and symptoms. The medical model within which which most clinicians operate is based upon two basic assumptions. The first is that there exists an objective physical reality that medical and scientific knowledge can discover.

Second, signs and symptoms refer to some underlying physiological or chemical change the meaning of which can be established and agreed upon (Feinstein 1973; Mcgehee et al. 1979).[8] In theory, this process is straightforward. However, in reality, it is complicated by the fact that knowledge of states of ill-health is forever changing (Foucault 1975; King 1982). Clinicians are forced to make diagnoses based upon rapidly changing and often contradictory scientific knowledge. In the diagnosis of breast conditions the clinician must draw on the expertise of a number of different scientific and technological specialists which include pathologists, epidemiologists, radiologists, and geneticists. Much uncertainty exists in each of these areas concerning the etiology of both benign and malignant breast conditions. This makes the task of diagnosis particularly problematic as clinicians are faced with translating and integrating uncertain scientific knowledge in order to treat a particular patient.

Although in many cases the clinical assessment of risk helps to bring certainty to the diagnosis and management, the often ambiguous meanings of risk factors can act to increase clinical risk. Because of the uncertainty as to whether or not a woman with a benign condition will develop breast cancer, the condition comes to take on the double meaning of being both normal and premalignant at the same time. Clinicians must make some decision based upon a ambiguous condition of uncertain outcome. Thus, clinicians are at risk for making a wrong prognosis. Doctors are also at risk for failing to detect a small cancer which may be hidden by a benign condition. Benign breast lumps can camouflage the real danger. Clinicians then experience personal risk as uncertainty concerning their ability to prognose a currently benign condition and as uncertainty concerning their ability to diagnose or detect an existing but camouflaged cancer.

The clinicians interviewed in this study spoke clearly about their experiences of these two kinds of lived risk and, as with objective risk, sought to remove the physical condition where risk resided. One surgeon stated:

If she has a dominant lump I remove it. I tell women that one way or the other they have to get rid of it. I'm compulsive . . . . I get rid of all lumps. I don't sit and watch lumps. A lot of people do. I get sent a lot of cases where somebody's been following a lump for 6 months, quote a "cyst" and it's cancer! A lot of people think they can tell a cyst from lumps. I don't think I can. I have to get rid of it. I cut my risk down.

Another surgeon expressed his concern over the problem of being able to detect malignant lumps hidden beneath benign ones. Here, clinicians come fact to face with the lived risk of their failure to detect hidden cancers. The surgeon explained:

Multiple lumps are always a little unnerving because you know that they all aren't cancer but you know that there could be one, sort of hanging around in among the others. And you know you can't biopsy everything that feels lumpy.

Ironically, although clinicians perform biopsies in order to cut down both their own risk as well as the woman's, biopsies can have the effect of increasing future risk. Once a woman has had one biopsy, she is at higher risk for another because she will most likely be under closer surveillance (Love et al. 1982). The scars left from biopsies can have the effect of increasing the clinician's risk of being wrong in the interpretation of future clinical examinations. Multiple biopsies can serve to further camouflage small cancers. An older surgeon with much experience managing breast conditions explained:

Unnecessary biopsies I don't understand . . . . I have seen some patients at age 38 or 42, who have had 17 biopsies and they come in with their 18th breast lump. Now I don't know what the heck is going on because their breasts look like hand grenades went off. They have scars on the outside and they're scarring on the inside, and I just don't know what I'm palpating anymore!

Objective risk and lived risk represent two dimensions of clinical risk experienced by medical practitioners. I have argued that clinicians transform both objective and lived risk into a clinical entity that can then be removed by removing the physical location where the source of such risk resides. An extreme example of the physical removal of risk is illustrated by the controversial procedure of prophylactic mastectomy for women at risk for developing breast cancer. Chronic fibrocystic disease, combined with other risk factors, is becoming an indication for prophylactic mastectomy (McCarty et al. 1981). In 1982 an article appeared in the journal *Preventive Medicine* advocating prophylactic mastectomy to prevent breast cancer in women who have combination of fibrocystic disease and a family history of breast cancer (Mulvihill et al. 1982). The article is revealing for a number of reasons. First, the authors openly acknowledge the inability of clinical medicine to modify risk through non-invasive means, and thus suggest that preventive surgery is one way of removing risk:

The major risk factors — age, prior breast disease, and a family history — can be identified but not changed. Efforts to modify minor risk factors, for example, by avoiding high fat diet, caffeine and oral contraceptives are possible and not harmful in theory but are probably ineffective and surely unproven. Alternatives for control, then, would consist of an aggressive plan of surveillance in the hope of early diagnosis or prophylactic mastectomy (p. 506).

Second, the authors make a number of faulty assumptions about the epidemiologic meanings of risk factors for breast cancer. Concerning the risk factor of prior breast disease, they claim that, "A history of clinical or biopsy-proven fibrocystic disease is three to six times more frequent in breast cancer patients than in controls" (p. 503). They interpret this data to mean that fibrocystic disease is a significant risk factor for breast cancer, yet, as I have argued, the epidemiologic evidence shows that fibrocystic disease is not, in and of itself, a risk factor for breast cancer. The relationship between this condition and breast cancer has yet to be clearly understood. Furthermore, although not explicitly stated, the authors imply that caffeine and oral contraceptive use raise a woman's risk of breast cancer. Yet, there is little evidence to suggest that this might be so.[9] Not only are the risk factors selected difficult to define, but the authors make the assumption that the three risk factors which they select as being most important (age, prior history of fibrocystic breast disease and familial history), will have a multiplicative interaction:

Calculated risk estimates for a woman with several risk factors will differ depending upon whether the factors are additive, multiplicative, synergistic in some other way or even antagnositic. Since few studies address the point we assume a multiplicative interaction of major factors and present the risk as 5-year probabilities. (p. 507).

Here, the authors clearly acknowledge that the current knowledge about how risk factors interact to produce breast cancer, is unknown. Yet they assume a multiplicative interaction without stating the basis upon which this assumption is made. The authors then proceed to present four "typical case reports" of women who elected to have prophylactic mastectomy based upon their calculated personal risks:

Because of fibrocystic disease and family history of breast cancer, 29 year-old patient 9 was advised by an oncologist to have prophylactic mastectomy . . . . Her relative risk was estimated to be 27, and her 5-year probability 3% . . . . On follow-up, 7 months later, the patient was satisfied with the operation; however one breast became so painfully firm due to fibrous contraction that she had to cut a hole in her mattress in order to sleep prone. She finally found a surgeon familiar with this complication which he relieved by closed capsulotomy. (pp. 507—508).

The authors conclude their article with:

Despite areas of ignorance and controversy, a few firm conclusions emerge from this study and the literature: (a) Women are raising question about their personal risk of breast cancer and routes for prevention and control; (b) A small number of demographic and epidemiologic features can account for the largest identifiable fraction of an individual's risk: sex, age, prior breast disease, and family history of histologically verified breast cancer; (c) for carefully counseled patients, prophylatic mastectomy may be appropriate therapy (p. 509).

I have presented this article because it illustrates several crucial points concerning trends in the clinical management of breast cancer risk. While those who advocate prophylactic mastectomy to remove risk take an extreme position, I argue that it represents a general mode of clinical thinking and practice that is becoming increasingly common. The clinicians interviewed in the course of this research all evidenced an interest in the idea of preventive surgery. In fact, one of the more alarming aspects of the clinical management of risk through prophylactic mastectomy is that the procedure is discussed under the guise of prevention. One plastic surgeon explained:

Surgeons who are concerned about breast disease have been trained . . . to handle curative surgery . . . . None of us have been taught in medical school or in residency training about preventive surgery .... There's preventive medicine all over but not preventive surgery. We are immunized against polio ... you're immunized for tetanus. You don't wait until you get tetanus. All of these things are preventive types of procedures to prevent you from getting bad diseases. Well, that's where, from a surgical philosophy, it is really very different. If you take a woman who has breast disease, proven breast disease by pathological tissue biopsy, if you then combine family history, if she's over the age of 40 and has not had children, if she's had mammograms that are changing in a suspicious way, if clinically she has breasts that are dense and difficult to follow, then that woman can be considered a candidate for prophylactic subcutaneous mastectomy.

Another surgeon explained:

I certainly feel that probably anyone with a very risky family history is a candidate (for prophylactic mastectomy) or where you have patients with extremely difficult breasts to follow ... and of course those who have more than one of those factors are definitely candidates.

Both surgeons are speaking about the removal of both clinical objective risk and the lived clinical risk of being unable to detect or predict an early cancer. When surgeons speak of prophylatic mastectomies, they clearly articulate that it is the *risk* which they are removing, risk which resides as a sign of future disease within a particular organ of the body. Two surgeons explained:

I feel that when properly done, you can clean out 95% of the breast tissue and in essence, you're reducing the risk factor by 95%.

I've told maybe 10 women to have subcutaneous mastectomies and I don't do that lightly. But when I get to the point of saying "My god! She's got these lumps all over the place and she's high risk", just get rid of them ... get rid of as much risk as you can!

The subject of when and how to perform a prophylactic mastectomy is a controversial one. Much uncertainty exists over how much breast tissue needs to be removed to reduce the risk significantly. No controlled studies have been done to compare the rate of breast cancer among a group of women at risk who elected not to have the procedure as compared to those who do. Thus, the belief that a reduction in a given percentage of breast tissue results in a similar reduction in risk is based largely upon the assumption that risk is in tissue that is evenly distributed throughout the breast. This assumption remains unproven. One surgeon expressed reservations with the procedure as he explained:

You always wonder if you do an 85% mastectomy, do you get rid of 85% of the risk or do you get rid of none of the risk. I'm not sure that risk factors alone would ever make me do a mastectomy.

As a part of this research I regularly attended case conferences at two hospitals over the period of one year. Each hospital had special services for screening, diagnosis and treatment of women with breast conditions. Special case conferences were held to discuss particularly problematic cases, and the issues of risk and patient management were common topics. The issue of risk and prophylactic mastectomy gave rise to much debate among conference participants, and the following case illustrates many of the dilemmas facing clinicians in the management of risk.

The case of a 36 year old women was presented to conference members because the woman's clinician was uncertain about the clinical and patho-logical meanings of detected breast changes. The woman's surgeon began by saying that the woman had been referred to him for a lump in her left breast. Upon examination he diagnosed the lump as a benign fibroadenoma but also recommended that she have a mammogram. The results of the mammogram had come back "suspicious with three clusters of calcifications". The surgeon then performed a biopsy which was diagnosed by the pathologist as "severe atypia".[10] At this point in the conference the pathologist showed the clini-cians slides of the woman's biopsy and said, "Here's a patient you'd think is a nice benign". He then showed the mammograms and said, "There are two lesions in the left breast, one benign and one less well defined". He then asked the clinicians what their diagnosis would be. "Carcinoma? Fat? Or scar tissue?" The pathologist then said, "What it actually represents is an area of duct hyperplasia". He then proceeded to describe the histories of six women with similar conditions who were seen at this hospital, several of whom (he did not cite the exact number) went on to develop carcinomas. He said, "My own personal feeling is to go after it. It is more likely to represent a carcinoma".

At this point an argument took place between the clinicians as to whether the three calcifications on the mammogram represented further evidence of a possible carcinoma. One clinician cited studies which showed that 50% of all women all have at least one calcification and that three were not enough to warrant a diagnosis of carcinoma. An open debate ensued concerning the controversy of prophylactic mastectomies for women with chronic fibrocystic disease. Various studies were cited in support of differing positions. After approximately ten minutes of argument, the pathologist called for the need for a "management decision to be made". Although no definitive decision was reached concerning the treatment or management of this woman's condition, the pathologist ended the presentation by saying to her surgeon, "Wouldn't you do a subcutaneous mastectomy for her? You won't let that drop will you? There are cases when you would with high risks."

This example illustrates several points. The clinicians all agreed that the present diagnosis was that of a benign condition, not a malignant one. However, it was unclear as to just how benign the condition was. In other words, was it very benign or was it premalignant? In fact, it was considered to be both benign and premalignant at different points throughout the presentation. The meanings of the signs also shifted back and forth from that of a non-disease to that of disease. The ambiguity of the condition was clearly acknowledged and this led the clinicians to search for new knowledge as illustrated by the debate concerning the meaning of calcifications detected on the mammogram and the controversy over prohylactic mastectomy.

However, in the end, the pathologist chose to deal with the ambiguous meaning by recommending removal of the physical condition which gave rise to this ambiguity in the first place. The removal of the breast represents removal of risk, both the objective risk of the probability that the condition will become malignant and the lived risk of clinical uncertainty and error. The result is the clinical creation of a physical condition over which the doctor now has control. Thus, the clinical management of risk can result in the physical manipulation of the body in order to create a more certain physical condition.

LAY PERCEPTIONS OF RISK AND THE STATE OF "NON-HEALTH"

As discussed, a diagnosis of benign breast disease is thought to raise a woman's risk for developing breast cancer. Yet, there exists much uncertainty concerning the clinical and epidemiologic meaning of benign breast conditions, and thus the nature and degree of the risk involved is often unclear. For women, a diagnosis of benign breast disease often changes their perceptions of health and illness. For example, consider the following statements from women who have been diagnosed as having the risk factor of benign breast disease:

I have very lumpy breasts. Nobody's sure if it's a disease or what the devil it is.

I had some discomfort but I'd never had the thought that this was a disease!

You know, one day you're walking down the street feeling wonderful and then all of a sudden somebody tells you that maybe you shouldn't feel so wonderful.

Risk for the lay woman is experienced as a symptom of a hidden or future illness, and thus serves to further blur the already ambiguous distinction between health and illness.[11] Women speak of risk in the same way they speak of experiencing other symptoms of illness. Just as clinicians speak of risk as something that women suffer from, women speak of risk as a state of being. Being at risk is a state somewhere between health and illness. Inherent within lay perceptions of risk is a high degree of unmeasured uncertainty: risk for women is not objective or measured. Lay risk has its own terms of reference and requires a different analytic approach to understand more fully how it is experienced by lay women. Such an approach is that of phenomenology, which is most appropriate because it draws on an interpretative methodology and thereby gives priority to understanding the lived experience of risk. This approach is meaning centered the purpose of which is to ground explanations of ill-health in experience (Kestenbaum 1982).[12]

Kestenbaum (1982) argues that for science, reality is the object as lived. However, in everyday experience, reality is the experiencing of the object. This points to a fundamental gap which exists between a person's *experience* of a given reality and science's *explanation* of that same reality (Rosenkrantz 1976). One cannot assume that epidemiologic and clinical notions of risk can be easily translated into lay notions of risk. A major difference between scientific and lay risk is that the latter involves a good amount of unmeasurable uncertainty. Cassell (1976) argues that, "Rational thought processes, at least as they are communicated, are useful only in handling material that is known and that can be converted into language" (Cassell 1976: 36). Cassell's point is an important one insofar as lay risk involves many factors that cannot be known, cannot be measured and thus cannot always be spoken about. Even when there is much information about individual risk, this information often has a high degree of ambiguity about it. Daniel Ellsberg (1961) has argued that:

Ambiguity may be high (and the confidence in any particular estimate of probabilities low) even where there is ample quantity of information, when there are questions of reliability and relevance of information, and particularly where there is "conflicting" opinion and evidence. This judgement of the ambiguity of one's information, of the over-all credibility of one's composite estimates, of one's confidence in them, cannot be expressed in terms of relative likelihoods or events (if it could, it would simply affect the final, compound probabilities) (1961: 659).

For women, information about their own individual risk will always be highly ambiguous because, (a) there exists much uncertainty within epidemiology concerning the significance of identified risk factors, (b) there exists much uncertainty within both epidemiology and other biomedical sciences concerning relationships between identified risk factors and the mechanisms of disease, (c) it is impossible to accurately translate population risk to individual risk and (d) it is impossible accurately know all the contextual factors and how they interact to determine risk for unique individuals. In sum, it is precisely because individuals are unique that we may be unable to know all of the information needed to accurately predict unique outcomes. Lay risk will always possess an inherent quality of unmeasured ambiguity and uncertainty as a central characteristic. It emerges from an individual's subjective feelings about the meaning of scientific and clinical risk mediated by their social and cultural background, context, and experiences. Lay risk is not objective, cannot be quantified or measured, and is not static. Rather, it must be understood as a dynamic experience of personal uncertainty about one's future.

In clinical medicine and public health in general, lay risk as experienced by lay women is often equated with objective clinical risk and with epidemiologic risk. Health practitioners often believe that if individuals fully understand the risks associated with the development of a particular disease, then they will take actions to reduce their risk. However, there is overwhelming evidence to show that individuals often ignore their risks and do nothing to change their style of life.[13] For example, although much attention has been given to the importance of monthly breast self examinations, few women regularly engage in this practice (American Cancer Society 1973; Magarey et al. 1977). Explanations given for individual's failure to recognize risk include psychological, social and structural factors which inhibit what is communicated or inhibit an individual's ability to understand the significance of information. Decision-making theory and models are common approaches to understanding how and why individuals make the decisions they do concerning risk and choice. However, these explanations are inadequate for understanding lay concepts of risk because they do not account for the fact that the concept of risk as developed in epidemiology and clinical medicine is defined by different terms of reference.[14] Therefore, reasons why individuals often fail to take actions to reduce their risk of disease are because they are acting on a concept of risk that is qualitatively different than that of epidemiologic or clinical risk. That these three types of risk are largely incommensurate often goes unrecognized.

For women, risk represents potential changes in their experience of the relationship between their current and future state of health. In order for risk to have a personal reality, women must transform it from an objective entity to a subjective experience. Risk becomes internalized. One woman explained:

I knew *intellectually* that I was at high risk but I didn't feel it inside. And then my mother died of cancer of the pancreas and that's the same time I turned 30 and as a combination of my mother's death and my turning 30, I started to really be in touch with my own mortality . . . I started to really internalized it, that yes, this could happen to me and I started getting a little bit scared. (emphasis added)

In this research, women did not describe their experiences of risk in the language of objective knowing but rather in the language of the subjective senses (e.g. I sense, I feel, I think . . .) The following quotes illustrate the language of lay or lived risk:

Well, now that I have fibrocystic disease I can't help but *feel* that I must have some sort of predisposition . . . but I don't really *know* if I'm at high risk now, more so than I would be if I didn't have this.

Another woman expressed her feelings about her low risk of breast cancer this way:

I've wondered about the risk of getting breast cancer. The most *part of me* is fairly . . . I hate to say this, cocky is not the right word, positive is a better choice. I *feel* that for some reason, I'm here on this earth and I'm meant to be here . . . . But then there is this tiny part of me that *thinks*, "Kid, it's happened to a lot of people and my God! It just might be you!

Women do not experience risk in terms of objective statistical probabilities. It is therefore useful to consider the concept of subjective probability in order to better understand lay risk. Irving Good (1975) has argued that the notion of subjective or personal probability is important for extending scientific logic into useful everyday systems of reasoning. He argues that subjective probabilities constitute a 'body of beliefs' (1975: 44). Using the metaphor of a "black box theory of probability and rationality", subjective probabilities can never be fully measured or accounted for. Subjective probabilities emerge from the interaction of personal and social values about the costs of uncertain futures.

The concept of subjective probability can be usefully applied to understanding women's experiences of lived risk of benign breast disease and breast cancer. First, women interviewed in this study were well aware of the uncertainty that exists in both epidemiology and clinical medicine concerning the meaning of identified risk factors, and were faced with having to make a subjective decision concerning the meaning of these risk factors within the context of their own lives. While women may discount their risk of getting breast cancer, a diagnosis of benign breast disease can act immediately to bring personal meaning to risk. In this sense, a diagnosis of benign breast disease can serve to make the possibility of future illness a physical reality. When a women is diagnosed with benign breast disease she is thrown into a liminal state of being at risk, of being suddenly neither healthy or ill. The discounting of risk until it becomes symbolically expressed in a physical condition is illustrated with the following quotes:

I read somewhere that women who don't have children before the age of 26 or don't breast feed are more likely to get it (breast cancer) but it doesn't seem like such a big thing . . . . But I think my risks are higher now that I have fibrocystic breast disease.

Now that I have fibrocystic breasts, I can't help but feel that I must have some sort of predisposition.

For women who have developed breast cancer, risk has resulted in certain unwanted and feared futures. What was once risk is now an experienced present. Here, risk loses much of its unmeasured uncertainty. Risk is certain and rather than experiencing "being at risk", women experience "risk" as becoming the illness they feared. In the same sense that women "become ill", the onset of breast cancer can be understood as transforming a woman's experience of "being at risk" to "becoming risk". One woman explained that not only was she at risk for a future cancer but that she had also become a risk statistic:

After five years, if nothing has gone wrong, then you are free (of cancer). Then you don't have nothing to worry about. But I still have fear. The thing I do know is that I'm what you call a statistic and I am a cancer patient.

And another woman expressed similar feelings as she reflected why she had developed cancer:

I had early menarche and late cessation of my menses so my risk is higher statistically. I've had no children and that's another risk factor. I mean we're all just bodies and I'm going to fall into some statistic eventually.

These last two women express what is perhaps most important about lay risk: the issue of control. Currently, there is little women can do to change their risk factors. Many of the women in this study expressed frustration concerning their lack of personal control over risk. For example, when I asked a 26 year old women if the doctors had told her of anything she could do to prevent further breast problems, she said:

Well, you know, no coffee, no tea, no caffeine, none of which I do anyway. Which was a great let down to the doctors, which was another thing that frustrated me because they said, "Well, do you drink a lot of coffee?" I said no. I don't do any of that. And they would sigh, like, "Um, what is going on?" You know, "You really got a problem". So part of my frustration was feeling like I already do everything that I'm suppose to be doing.

Ironically, the search for personal control over risk often leads to further medicalization. Because women often feel helpless to do anything to change their risk, they are left at the hands of medical experts. One woman expressed her own frustrations by explaining:

I always feel that Dr. Smith is more in control than I am. Like I say, he's one of the few people who can intimidate me, and I don't think he does that, certainly not intentionally. But he does. I come out of there shaking all over. Now I have to wait until Wednesday to see if it's . . . . Then we have to wait till the next time to see if that's it. But as he said. "What you have is serious and we have to watch it closely". Now I could walk away from it, sure. I could say, "It's been two years doctor, thank you very much for your help. I don't want to discuss it any more. I don't want to talk about it anymore". And maybe one day I will do that. But I am not ready to do that yet. I just simply am not ready to do that. He keeps asking me if I keep getting my periods. I keep thinking that maybe it's true that once your periods stop some of these lumps go away with it. You know, I have no control over that. Who knows. So for the time being, we will play it his way and see what happens. But if he tells me something I don't want, I don't know what I'll do.

This woman raises several important issues concerning lay risk. While it is clear that she does not have cancer, her doctor has diagnosed her as having a serious benign condition and at risk for cancer. The doctor is not quite certain about the outcome of this condition and the woman is not quite certain if she should consider herself healthy or ill. The doctor deals with his own uncertainty by continuing his surveillance over her condition until it either goes away or becomes cancer. The woman is left thinking that her menopause might cause her lumps to disappear but she has no control over when this might occur and it is not all certain whether this will clear up the problem. Therefore, the woman is left feeling that she has no alternatives but to continue with medical surveillance. Faced with the fear of breast cancer as a possible outcome, knowing that there is no way to prevent the disease and that early diagnosis is a woman's primary tactic for survival, this woman is caught in a bind of being both healthy and of needing medical surveillance until her condition either becomes cancer or goes away. In her current state, can this woman ever walk away from her doctor and declare herself well? In a very real sense, being diagnosed at risk is itself a risk factor. It represents the risk of medicalization and the risk of losing control over the definition of one's own health.

The loss of lay control over risk management stems from medicalization of risk. As I have argued, medical practitioners deal with risk by transforming it into a clinical entity, a sign of a present or future disease. Women are diagnosed as having risk factors in the same way that they are diagnosed with having disease. Within this context, women reconstruct these disease experiences into illness realities. Risk becomes experienced both as a symptom of future illness as well as a current illness. As doctors give risk a physical reality, so also do women transform the unknown into a perception of ill-health:

Since I know that your breasts can be filled with fluid and that it drains through these little lymph nodes, I have an image of everything building up and having no place to go and it makes my body like a waste heap. And if it does drain and I mean, the images are totally stupid! It's like, what I know of when they do mastectomies, that they sometimes have to take out those lymph nodes and so, I feel like it's poison. It's poison building up in my breasts with no place to go! I picture these other women with their great systems that just run the stuff through! And here's me, these strange clogs, you know?

What can women do to control their illness of risk? Some choose to create certainty by denying the existence of risk factors. However, this can sometimes lead to deadly consequences if the denial of risk results in the failure to take control over potential health problems. For example, Molly, quoted in the introduction explained that she was consistently told that her lump represented no danger, yet five years later was diagnosed with a late stage breast cancer. Molly did not have the knowledge to take control over uncertainty. She did not have the power to judge whether or not her doctors were making responsible decisions about her risk of cancer. On the other hand, like clinicians, some women may choose to remove the risk through removal of the physical condition where the risk resides:

I don't know if I should tell this to you but I want to tell it to someone. I had a girlfriend die of breast cancer. It was terrible. Her death was worse than I imagined. The cancer went to her spine and liver. She was only 41 and had 3 little children. She had found the lump 2 years before and her doctor told her it was nothing to worry about and to come back and they would follow it. Well, she came back a year later and it was cancer. It had been cancer all along! With my lump, I was referred to Dr. Jones who I understand is a very good doctor. But he wanted to follow it. I wanted it out! Out of my body! There was no way I could live with that in me. I felt funny 'cause I had to insist on surgery. You normally don't do that. But I wanted it out! Out of there!

And in extreme situations, some women feel that they must control risk through prophylactic mastectomy. This extreme act is very much influenced by the practitioner's attempt to remove clinical risk. In other words, inherent to the construction of lay risk is the clinician's risk of being wrong, of failing to detect or predict a cancer. Lay risk incorporates a woman's experiences with her doctor's uncertainties. Rather than sharing responsibility for the diagnostic uncertainty with the doctor, some women choose to resolve this conflict by allowing the removal of that part of their body which makes the doctor and patient uncertain. But ironically, while the doctor is usually successful in removing his or her risk and regaining control over a physical condition, the woman suffers from the removal of her breast. Thus, while doctors treat risk through physical removal of part of the body, risk for women has been transformed into a new physical state of ill-health.

The following case study illustrates this dilemma. One afternoon, I interviewed Alice, a woman in her late 30s who had elected to have a prophylactic mastectomy for a benign breast condition. Her story as she related it to me is thus: Alice had been seeing Dr. Brown for seven years because of lumpy breasts. Alice explained that she had had multiple lumps, had had five cysts aspirated and two previous biopsies. Dr. Brown had told her that her mammograms and shown some calcification but not enough to suggest a cancer. However, because of her lumpy breasts and suspicious mammogram, Dr. Brown had recommended that she have subcutaneous bilateral mastectomies. Alice said that he told her that she had an 80% chance of developing nothing and a 20% chance of developing cancer. She went home and thought about her chances and decided that she didn't want "that 20% chance hanging over her head", so she went ahead with the operation. Alice explained that she was happy that she had had the mastectomies but that she still suffered from much pain. However, she said that she would rather live with the pain than with the 20% chance of cancer. She explained that after her mastectomy her doctor told her that they had found "a tiny, tiny, the size of a pin, cell that was pre-cancerous." She said that it was good that they had done a mastectomy because the 20% risk had gone up to 50%.

Up to this point Alice had been explaining her experience in a rather detached manner. However, after a long pause, she looked down at her breasts and then close to tears said, "But it's hard getting use to something that is not your own". She went on to explain that she tells her doctor that she still has pain, "But he tells me that that I am fine. For him, the surgery was uncomplicated." She said that since she has been able to resume her normal activities, her doctor considers the operation a success. He tells Alice that he has done a beautiful job. Alice continued:

He does not know what I am feeling! I sit there and he nods his head and says that I am doing well and that I shouldn't worry. I feel like taking him and shaking him and saying "Listen to me!" I asked him if the mastectomy would affect my uterus and he said it would not, that the breasts were up here and the uterus and ovaries were down there and that they were two separate systems. But any woman knows that they are not. Around your period, your breasts hurt and when you are pregnant, your breasts fill up. Any woman knows that they are connected. I asked him if it would affect my periods. He said no but the month after the operation, I skipped a period. I felt miserable but he said that it wasn't connected. Even now my breasts hurt around my period but he said that they shouldn't because he removed most of the tissue. I feel like asking him, "Are you married? Why don't you go ask your wife!" My new breasts feel like stones on my chest, like big weights. But you know, the silicone was light, I held it. Why should it feel so heavy? When I lie down they feel like they're falling to the side but when I look at them, they are not. Why do they feel like that? He tells me that it is normal

but it is not! I have no sensation in them at all but he says it will come back . . . . I went ahead
and did it because Dr. Brown is retiring soon and he has seen me all these years and I wanted
it done before that so that I wouldn't have to worry about it.

How many women like Alice choose to remove their risk in this manner
not knowing the consequences that they must live with? The medical treatment of risk through surgical procedures and the lay acceptance of such
procedures, represents a dangerous trend. In my interviews with surgeons, I
concluded by asking them how they would solve the whole breast health
controversy if they had the power to do so. Only one surgeon spoke of
inventing non-invasive preventive measures while all the others spoke of new
treatment procedures. It is alarming to contrast the following surgeon's
response with Alice's story:

I'd have a crystal ball! I'd look in the crystal ball for each patient to determine whether or not
she's going to get cancer and then if I found that she's going to get cancer, I'd know exactly
what to do. That's real easy, because then I could say, "Don't worry at all, you don't need any
surgery for the rest of your life, 'cause your not going to get cancer." And "Yes, you're going
to get it in 4 years or 2 years and we want to save your life!" Because that's what subcutaneous
mastectomies are all about. If you do it on the right patient, you can prevent her from getting
breast cancer. You can have an effect on their life span! That's what it's all about. Let me tell
you a very interesting thing. Probably the bottom line for you and your study here. Breast
cancer is the most common cancer in the female body. 26% of all carcinomas in the female
body are breast. Over 110 or 115 thousand women every year get breast cancer in the United
States. About 35 thousand women every year die of breast cancer in the United States. Those
are pretty awesome figures. In spite of all the advancement of mammograms and in needle
aspiration and in all the modern techniques of surgery and all these things we've evolved in the
last 15, 20 years, the most interesting thing is that there's still an increase. We're finding more
breast cancer . . . perhaps our diagnostic techniques are improving. But in spite of all the
improvement in technique, the mortality rate for breast cancer over the last 40 years, . . . these
figures are from the National Cancer Institue, the mortality rate has stayed almost flat! Almost
the same! So in other words, even though we're being more aware of it . . . and we have all
kinds of medical research going on, all the various things, we still have not had a significant
effect at lowering the mortality rate. So that's where the concern and perhaps the philosophy if
you will, of subcutaneous mastectomy comes into play. If in fact you can take women that
are at truly, I mean without any question, . . . you eliminate the ones that there is a question
on, truly at high risk, and meet all the criteria, and if you can operate on them and lower their
risk factor from 40% to 2%, then you will have an effect over the long term on the mortality
rate of breast cancer. And that's where subcutaneous mastectomy has its hope!

Perhaps what is most revealing about this surgeon's comments is his
assumption that the development of diagnostic and treatment technologies
should in some way reduce both the incidence of and the mortality from
breast cancer. Since these reductions have not occurred the surgeon dreams
of better prediction technologies that would identify individuals at risk. This
enables the clinician to prescribe treatment before the disease develops. I
argue that the epidemiologic search for risk factors has contributed more to
the clinician's crystal ball than to public health policy aimed at changing
underlying socio-environmental factors that give rise to risk.

It is perhaps most appropriate to conclude this essay by discussing some of the consequences of treating risk in individuals rather than treating risk in the wider contexts in which we live.

DISCUSSION

I have argued that the concept of risk takes on fundamentally different meanings within epidemiology, clinical medicine and lay experiences of health and illness. For the epidemiologist, risk is an objective, scientific concept which describes relationships within large populations. However, for women, risk is an experienced condition of non-health. Women most often experience risk by transforming it into a symptom of a future or current illness. Once risk is experienced as an illness, a woman is at risk for further medicalization. For the medical practitioner, risk is understood as representing a sign of future disease from which a woman suffers, and as clinical uncertainty concerning diagnosis. Risk becomes a physical reality that can be manipulated and controlled by treating the affected individual or physical organ at risk for the disease. The desired clinical outcome is the removal of both clinical and lay risk. This process might be thought of as the medicalization of risk, and it results in greater clinical control over uncertainty by substituting an uncertain disease future with a certain state of ill-health. The medicalization of risk further removes the power to define states of health and illness from the individual. Instead, what is experienced are states of being ill, those individuals with less risk are simply less ill than those with more risk. Within current medical thought and practice one cannot be both healthy and at risk at the same time.

The medicalization of risk has implications not only for breast cancer but for other chronic diseases. Epidemiologic evidence suggests that the etiological factors associated with many chronic diseases are more strongly associated with socio-environmental conditions rather than with factors found within specific individuals (Lindheim and Syme 1983). This would suggest that preventive efforts aimed at reducing risk should primarily be directed towards interventions at a socio-environmental level. Yet solutions directed towards macro-level approaches are difficult, complex, and often politically sensitive. Instead, research and clinical interventions continue to be directed primarily towards individuals. Public health programs screen healthy people for risk factors (signs of future disease) and "preventive" measures are taken to "immunize" people against risk. "Patients" are prescribed special diets, exercise, and in some cases, drugs to prevent disease.[15]

Ratcliffe et al. (1984) have argued that a basic conflict exists between health promotion and health protection. Health promotion is based on educating individuals about how to remove themselves from risk whereas health protection is policy-oriented and aimed at removing risk from the environment. Health promotion is clearly linked to the privatization of medicine and the rise of the medical practitioner as the policy-maker in Western medicine. I have shown that this is true in the case of breast cancer. Serious consideration should also be given to the extent to which similar processes are operating with other chronic diseases. The uncritical acceptance of an objective, scientific meaning of risk as conceptualized within epidemiology has resulted in greater control on the part of the medical profession over the diagnosis and treatment of risk in individuals. It has diverted attention away from translating epidemiologic knowledge into population level interventions and has allowed the focus to be directed towards the medicalization of risk within individuals. The redirection of risk intervention to the socio-environmental contexts requires political and economic solutions.

And here lies an important caveat for medical anthropologists who are working within the discipline of epidemiology. Many of us have been concerned with applying our anthropological understandings to epidemiologically defined social and cultural risk factors. And while our contribution is greatly needed, we should be wary that social and cultural processes do not become reduced to factors which are translated *only* into individual health promotion. Rather, we must ensure that our understandings are more general in application and have relevance to health protection research and health policy issues. It is here that our strength as medical anthropologists lie in that the application of our knowledge needs to be directed primarily towards socio-cultural solutions rather than medical interventions.

In conclusion, there are a number of possible courses for thought and action that might reduce the medicalization of risk for breast cancer and other chronic conditions.

Medical scientists, clinicians, and lay women need to recognize the limits of knowledge. It is important that uncertainty in health science, medical practic and lay health be accepted as legitimate, resulting from knowledge which changes and evolves along with the advances in research.

Clinicians need to recognize the difficulties of translating epidemiologic risk into clinical practice. While epidemiologic studies are invaluable in terms of pointing to specific risk factors strongly associated with the onset of a particular disease, clinicians need to assess the relative importance of these risk factors in the context of each individual patient. Clinicians must understand and accept that the translation of epidemiologic and other scientific knowledge into the management of an individual patient will always be fraught with uncertainty. It is simply not possible to predict with certainty, disease outcomes within individuals.

It is important that women learn to accept that their doctors are unable to diagnose many conditions with any certainty and must themselves accept responsibility for their own state of risk. Often, patients want their doctors to tell them what to do, and an essential part of this relationship consists of the trust the patient must develop with their doctor. The sharing of clinical uncertainty should not be seen to threaten this bond of trust. Rather, the discussion of uncertainty can enhance this bond of trust by allowing patient and doctor achieve a mutual understanding about the limits of knowledge. This mutual understanding legitimizes different kinds of knowing. For example, women's intuitive knowledge about their body and health state can become an important piece information for clinical evaluation. A mutual sharing of uncertainty can result in a more equitable relationship between doctor and patient resulting in greater patient participation for decision making.

Breast cancer kills approximately 30,000 women in the United States each year. While emphasis upon mass screening, self breast examinations, early detection and better treatment procedures is vital, none of these procedures prevent the disease. The problem of breast cancer will not be solved through the development of better detection and treatment techniques. The ultimate solution lies in understanding the etiology of breast cancer. Although more research directed towards understanding how the disease can be prevented is certainly needed, it is unlikely that such research will provide substantial results in the near future. The reality of the situation is that breast cancer is a serious health threat that currently cannot be prevented. Treatment is painful and not always successful. As with many chronic diseases, the underestanding and treatment of breast cancer is fraught with many uncertainties. These uncertainties represent risks. And the dimensions of risk as conceptualized within epidemiology, medical science, clinical practice and lay health are qualitatively different. The interpretation of risk from one dimension to another requires a transformation in meaning, and until the different dimensions of risk are fully recognized and made legitimate clinical control over uncertainty through the medicalization of risk will only increase.

ACKNOWLEDGEMENTS

I would like to thank Anthony Colson, Kimberly Dovey and Ramona Koval for their critiques of earlier drafts of this essay.

NOTES

1. The data presented in this essay are based on research where I was concerned with exploring the translation of scientific knowledge into clinical practice. The focus was on the role ambiguity plays in the shaping of clinical and lay understandings of risk, benign breast disease, and breast cancer. My methodological approach was an interpretative anthropological one well suited to exploring issues of meaning. The data are derived from participant observation over a one and a one half year period at two hospitals in a large city in California, from my own involvement as a research associate on an epidemiologic research study of risk factors related to breast disease and from in-depth, open-ended interviews with women and practitioners. The data presented in this essay are drawn from interviews with 30 women diagnosed as having benign breast disease, 15 women

diagnosed as having breast cancer, and 24 medical practitioners — 2 pathologists, 2 radiologists, 1 oncologist, 3 nurses specializing in breast conditions, 1 geneticist, 2 gynecolgists, and 13 surgeons. All interviews were tape-recorded and later transcribed. Transcribed interviews were thematically coded and analyzed for content and meaning. Analysis was conducted from a hermeneutical perspective.

2. For a brief description of the historical relationships between the rise of scientific thought, biology and medicine see Capra (1982: 97—117).

3. I am basing my arguments concerning paradigm shifts on Khun's ideas of scientific revolutions. Kuhn argues that puzzles that resist solution are seen as anomalies rather than as falsifications of a partifular paradigm, and that the existence of a number of unsolved puzzles does not necessarily lead to a scientific crisis. Scientific revolutions occur when competing paradigms are created and when more and more members of the scientific community adopt the new paradigm. Kuhn compares scientific revolutions to political revolutions in that choices between old and new political institutions or scientific paradigms represent choices between incompatiable modes of community life. Thus, the shift from one paradigm to another is not one based on logical argument, rather it is one based on persuasion. This is why Kuhn argues that competing paradigms are incommensurable. The concept of risk and its use within epidemiology and clinical medicine points to a number of anomalies within the current biomedical paradigm. The concept of risk does not represent a shift to a new paradigm, but rather an attempt to explain emerging anomalies within the current paradigm. For a more in-depth discussion of Kuhn's ideas and the philosophy of science, see Chalmers (1978).

4. Few epidemiologists have openly advocated a shift in epidemiologic thinking itself, nor have they seriously considered the epistemiological assumptions upon which epidemiologic methods rest. Marmot's article, Facts, Opinions and Affaires Du Coeur, published in the American Journal of Epidemiology (1976) represents a notable exception to this trend. Other exceptions to traditional modes of thought can be seen in the implicit assumptions of general susceptibility theory. The advocates of this theory argue that instead of focusing on causes of disease in those who are ill, the emphasis should be on understanding why healthy people do not get sick. Thus, general susceptibility theory seeks to broaden the more narrow causal models. Berkman (1981), Berkman and Syme (1979), and Najman (1980) have presented discussions concerning this new theoretical model.

5. Lilienfeld and Lilienfeld argue that "A causal relationship would be recognized to exist whenever evidence indicated that the factors form a part of the complex of circumstances that increases the probability of the occurrence of disease and that a diminution of one or more of these factors decreases the frequency of that disease" (1980: 295). In their text on the fundamentals of epidemiology, Lilienfeld and Lilienfeld argue that ". . . in diagramming the natural history of a chronic disease, we can replace 'etiological factor' with 'risk factor' " (1980: 259—260).

6. Much has been written on how different kinds of risk are defined and calculated within epidemiology. I am not concerned here with particular kinds of epidemiologic risk but rather with the more general concept of risk. Although epidemiologists have gone to great lengths to define different types of risk (e.g. relative risk, attributable risk) few have considered the theoretical implications of the concept itself. A definition of risk and probability as given in the Dictionary of Epidemiological Concepts gives some interesting insights into the epidemiologic definition. Probability is defined as ". . . a basic concept that may be considered undefinable, expressing 'degree of belief' " (Last 1983: 83). Risk then, expresses the degree of belief we have concerning the probability that an event will occur.

7. Gorovitz and MacIntyre argue that ". . . where there is scientific activity, there is partial ignorance — the ignorance that exists as a precondition for scientific progress . . . . This ignorance of what is not yet known is the permanent state of all science and a source of

error even when all the internal norms of science are fully respected" (1976: 53). Epidemiology shares this quest for unknown knowledge.

8. The use here of the terms signs and symptoms is consistent with the definitions given by Stedman's medical dictionary (1976). A sign is defined as "any abnormality indicative of disease, discoverable by the physician at his examination of the patient; a sign is an objective symptom of a disease: a symptom is a subjective sign of disease". Symptom is defined as "any morbid phenomenon or departure from the normal in function, appearance, or sensation, experienced by the patient and indicative of disease". Disussions concerning the history of the concepts of signs and symptoms are provided by King (1982) and Foucault (1975).

9. Some studies have shown that caffeine is associated with benign breast conditions; however, other studies have not confirmed this relationship. Caffeine has not been shown to be associated with breast cancer. The epidemiologic evidence concerning oral contraceptives is just as equivocal. Oral contraceptives appear to be protective against benign breast conditions, and if one assumes that the risk factors for benign conditions and breast cancer are similar, then oral contraceptives might, in fact, be protective against breast cancer (Ernster 1981; Kelsey 1979).

10. There are many types of benign conditions, some of which are more serious than others. Severe atypia is not a malignant condition but is thought to be strongly associated with the development of breast cancer.

11. I am using the terms illness, as opposed to disease, to distinguish lay from biomedical concepts of states of health. Illness can be understood as ". . . the personal, interpersonal, cultural reactions to disease, the human experience of disease or of ill-health" (Kleinman et al. 1978: 251). Diseases can be defined as ". . . abnormalities in the structure and function of the body organs and systems, the biological or physical malfunctioning of the body" (Kleinman, Eisenberg and Good 1978: 251). Disease then is the biomedical and scientific construction of ill-health while illness represents lay experiences of ill-health. Symptoms and signs of ill-health have corresponding relationships. Symptoms are what the patient suffers, they are the subjective experiences of illness. Signs are what the doctor observes, they are the objective manifestations of disease. Much has been written concerning the different dimensions of lay and biomedical experiences and explanations of ill-health, see for example works by Eisenberg (1977), Engel (1977), Engelhardt (1975, 1982), Good and DelVecchio Good (1981), Kleinman (1980), Kleinman et al. (1979), Rawlinson (1982), Treacher and Wright (1982), and Young (1978).

12. A meaning centered approach draws on both phenomenologic and hermeneutic orientations. Proponents of these orientations argue that an understanding of human experience and behaviour must go beyond empirical science based on verification to the bounds of common meanings that are embedded within social reality (Agar 1980; Gadamer 1976; Husserl 1960; Schutz 1967). The strength of an interpretative approach in understanding ill-health is based on the argument that disease, or pathological changes in the structure and function of the body, are experienced and given meaning by both doctors and patients within a cultural framework. Culture, conceived as a system of meanings, has a major influence upon the ways in which sickness is perceived, understood and experienced. For examples of this approach, see: Comaroff (1982), Comaroff and Maguire (1981), Engelhardt (1982), Foucault (1973), Good and DelVecchio Good (1981), Kestenbaum (1982), O'Neill (1982), Rawlinson (1982) and Treacher and Wright (1982).

13. Examples of individuals failing to acknowledge the seriousness of clinical and epidemiologically determined risk factors is particularly evident in smoking practices and lung cancer has recently surpassed breast cancer as the most common cancer among American women. Another example of risk discounting is seen in the self-management of diabetes. Diabetes, if not well controlled, can result in many complications, including blindness, heart disease and amputations. The management of diabetes requires change in life style including eating patterns and exercise. However, many person with this disease

continue to participate in the same types of life style habits as they did before they were diagnosed.

14. I have drawn on ideas concerning risk assessment and the setting of risk standards from the field of occupational health and safety. In a report concerning the assessment of risk and the protection of workers' health and safety, Mathews argues that the risk assessment and evaluation is a two-stage process. "The first is the stage of conceptual evaluation and measurement and clinical and epidemiological research, culminating in the establishment of quantitative links between exposure and its health effects; i.e. a dose-effect curve. This is the province of the technical experts . . . . The second stage involves evaluating the risk consequence upon any particular level of exposure. The process of evaluation is a social process — it means looking at the likely extent of pain and suffering . . . . The first stage of risk assessment is properly the province of technical experts; the second is properly the province of laypersons, including workers who actually run the risks" (Mathews et al. 1984: 25).

15. For example, some doctors are prescribing the drug Danazol as a hormonal treatment for benign breast disease. The drug has many known and serious side effects and does not prevent breast cancer. As Love (1984) points out, "A version of male hormone known as Danazol can be used, and after a fashion it works. You get no lumps, no pain, no periods — and you may grow hair on you chin. It also costs about $200 a month to take. And when you stop taking it, the lumps and discomfort come back again . . . . A drug treatment for lumpy breasts may well produce more serious consequences than the condition itself" (Love 1984: 4).

REFERENCES

Agar, M.
  1980   Hermeneutics in Anthropology: A Review Essay. Ethos 8: 253—272.
Bateson, G.
  1979   Mind and Nature: A Necessary Unity. New York: E. P. Dutton.
Berkman, L. F.
  1981   Physical Health and the Social Environment: A Social Epidemiological Perspective. *In* L. Eisenberg and A. Kleinman (eds.), The Relevance of Social Science for Medicine. Boston: D. Reidel Publishing Co, pp. 51—76.
Berkman, L. F. and L. Syme
  1979   Social Networks, Host Resistance, and Mortality: A Nine-Year Follow-Up Study of Alameda Country Residents. American Journal of Epidemiology 109: 186—204.
Capra, F.
  1982   The Turning Point: Science, Society and the Rising of Culture. London: Wildwood House.
Cassel, E.
  1976   The Organ's Disease, the Man's Illness and the Healer's Art. Hastings Center Report 6 (April 1976).
Chalmers, A. F.
  1978   What is This Thing Called Science? St. Lucia: University of Queensland Press.
Comaroff, J.
  1982   Medicine: Symbol and Ideology. *In* P. Wright and A. Treacher (eds.), The Problem of Medical Knowledge: Examining the Social Construction of Medicine. Edinburgh: Edinburgh University Press.
Comaroff, J. and P. Maguire
  1981   Ambiguity and the Search for Meaning: Childhood Leukaemia in the Modern Clinical Context. Social Science and Medicine 15B: 115—123.

Eisenberg, L.
  1977 Disease and Illness: Distinctions between Professional and Popular Ideas of Sick-
        ness. Culture, Medicine and Psychiatry 1: 9—23.
Ellsberg, D.
  1961 Risk, Ambiguity and the Savage Axioms. Quarterly Journal of Economics 75: 43—
        49.
Engel, G.
  1977 A Unified Concept of Health and Disease. Perspectives in Biology and Medicine 3:
        459—485.
Engelhardt, T. H. Jr.
  1975 The Concepts of Health and Disease. In T. H. Engelhardt and S. F. Spicker (eds.),
        Evaluation and Explanation in the Biomedical Sciences. Boston: D. Reidel, pp.
        126—141.
  1982 Illness, Diseases, and Sicknesses. In V. Kestenbaum (ed.), The Humanity of the Ill:
        Phenomenological Perspectives. Knoxville: The University of Tennessee Press, pp.
        142—156.
Ernster, V.
  1981 The Epidemiology of Benign Breast Disease. Epidemiologic Reviews 3. The Johns
        Hopkins University School of Hygiene and Public Health, pp. 184—202.
  1982 Personal Communication.
Evans, A.
  1976 Causation and Disease: The Henle-Koch Postulates Re-visited. Yale Journal of
        Biology and Medicine 49: 175—195.
Feinstein, A.
  1973 An Analysis of Diagnostic Reasoning. Parts I and II. Yale Journal of Biology and
        Medicine 46: 212—232, 264—283.
Foucault, M.
  1973 The Birth of the Clinic: An Archaeology of Medical Perception. New York: Vintage
        Books.
Gadamer, H.
  1976 Philosophical Hermeneutics. Translated and Edited by D. Linge. Berkeley: Univer-
        sity of California Press.
Good, B. and M. DelVecchio Good
  1981 The Meaning of Symptoms: A Cultural Hermeneutic Model for Clinical Practice. In
        L. Eisenberg and A. Kleinman (eds.), The Relevance of Social Science for Medicine.
        London: D. Reidel Publishing Company, pp. 165—196.
Good, I.
  1975 Explicativity, Corroboration, and the Relative Odds Hypothesis. Syntheses 30:
        30—73.
Gorovitz, S. and A. MacIntyre
  1976 Toward a Theory of Medical Fallibility. Journal of Medicine and Philosophy 1:
        51—71.
Husserl, E.
  1960 Cartesian Meditations: An Introduction to Phenomenology. The Netherlands:
        Martinus Nijhoff.
Kelsey, J.
  1979 A Review of the Epidemiology of Human Breast Cancer. Epidemiologic Reviews,
        Vol. 1. The Johns Hopkins University of School of Hygiene and Public Health, pp.
        74—109.
Kestenbaum, V
  1982 The Experience of Illness. In V. Kestenbaum (ed.), Humanity of the Ill: Phenomeno-
        logical Perspectives. Knoxville: The University of Tennesse Press, pp. 3—38.

King L. S.
  1982 Medical Thinking: A Historical Preface. New Jersey: Princeton University Press.
Kleinman, A.
  1980 Patients and Healers in the Context of Culture. Berkeley: University of California Press.
Kleinman, A., L. Eisenberg, and B. Good
  1978 Culture, Illness and Care. Annals of Internal Medicine 88: 251—188.
Knight,
  1921 Risk, Uncertainty and Profit. Boston: Houghton Miffin.
Last, M. (ed.)
  1983 A Dictionary of Epidemiology. New York: Oxford University Press.
Lilienfeld, A. M.
  1959 On the Methodology of Investigations of Etiologic Factors in Chronic Diseases: Some Comments. Journal of Chronic Disease 10: 41—46.
  1973 Epidemiology of Infectious and Non-infectious disease: Some Comparisons. American Journal of Epidemiology 97: 135—147.
Lilienfeld, A. and D. E. Lilienfeld
  1980 Foundations of Epidemiology. New York: Oxford University Press.
Lindheim, R. and L. Syme
  1983 Environments, People, and Health. Annual Review of Public Health 4: 335—59.
Love, S. M.
  1984 Lumpy Breasts. The Harvard Medical School Health Letter X: 3—5.
Love, S. M., R. S. Gelman, and W. Silen
  1982 Fibrocystic "Disease" of the Breast — A Nondisease? New England Journal of Medicine 307: 1010—1014.
Magarey, C. J., P. Todd, and P. Blizard
  1977 Psycho-Social Factors Influencing Delay and Breast Self-Examination in Women with Symptoms of Breast Cancer. Social Science and Medicine 11: 229—232.
Marmot, M.
  1976 Facts, Opinions and Affaires Du Coeur. American Journal of Epidemiology 103: 519—526.
Mathews J. et al.
  1984 The Protection of Workers' Health and Safety: Vol. 1: Report of the Occupational Safety, Health and Welfare Steering Committee. Presented to the South Australian Ministers of Labour and of Health, May 1984.
McCarty, et al.
  1981 Selecting Patients with Fibrocystic Disease for Subcutaneous Mastectomy. Resident Staff Physician, March: 34—47.
McGehee, H., J. Bordley III, and J. A. Barondess
  1979 Differential Diagnosis: The Interpretation of Clinical Evidence. 3rd. ed. Philadelphia: W. B. Saunders Co.
Mulvihill, J. J. et al.
  1982 Prevention in Familial Breast Cancer: Counseling and Prohylactic Mastectomy. Preventive Medicine 11: 500—511
Najman, J. M.
  1980 Theories of Disease Causation and the Concept of General Susceptibility: A Review. Social Science and Medicine 14A: 231—237.
O'Neill, J.
  1982 Essaying Illness. In V. Kestenbam (ed.), The Humanity of the Ill: Phenomenological Perspectives. Knoxville: The University of Tennesse Press, pp. 125—141.
Ratcliffe, J. et al.
  1984 Perspectives on Prevention: Health Promotion vs. Health Protection. In J. De

Kervasdoue, J. R. Kimberly and V. Rodwin (eds.), The End of An Illusion: The Future of Health Policy in Western Industrial Nations. Berkeley: Univesity of California Press, pp. 56—84.

Rawlinson, M. C.
    1982 Medicine's Discourse and the Practice of Medicine. *In* V. Kestenbaum, (ed.), The Humanity of the Ill: Phenomenological Perspectives. Knoxville: The University of Tennessee Press, pp. 69—85.

Rosenkrantz, B. G.
    1976 Causal Thinking in Erewhon and Elsewhere. Journal of Medicine and Philosophy 1: 372—384.

Sartwell, P. E.
    1960 On Methodology of Investigations of Etiologic Factors in Chronic Diseases: Further Comments. Journal of Chronic Disease 11: 61—63.

Scalon, E. F.
    1981 The Early Diagnosis of Breast Cancer. Cancer 48: 523—6

Schutz, A.
    1967 The Phenomenology of the Social World. Northwestern University Press.

Schwartz, G. F.
    1982 Risk Factors in Breast Cancer: A Clinical Approach. Breast 8: 26—29.

SEER
    1984 Cancer Incidence and Mortality in the United States. U.S. Department of Health and Human Services.

Susser, M.
    1973 Causal Thinking in the Health Sciences: Concepts and Strategies in Epidemiology. New York: Oxford University Press.

Toulmin, S.
    1975 Concepts of Function and Mechanism in Medicine and Medical Science. *In* H. T. Engelhardt and S. F. Spicker (eds.), Evaluation and Explanation in the Biomedical Sciences. Dordrecht-Holland: Reidel Publishing Company, pp. 51—66.
    1976 On the Nature of the Physician's Understanding. Journal of Medicine and Philosophy 1: 32—50.

Treacher, A. and P. Wright
    1982 The Problems of Medical Knowledge. Edinburgh: Edinburgh University Press.

Yerushalmy, J. and C. E. Palmer
    1959 On Methodology of Investigations of Etiologic Factors in Chronic Disease. Journal of Chronic Disease 10: 27—40.

Young, A.
    1978 Mode of Production of Medical Knowledge. Medical Anthropology 2(2): 97—124.

SECTION IV

PSYCHO-SOCIAL CONDITIONS

JOHN D. O'NEIL

COLONIAL STRESS IN THE CANADIAN ARCTIC: AN ETHNOGRAPHY OF YOUNG ADULTS CHANGING

INTRODUCTION

The "stress of change" is one of the most studied phenomena in the social and health sciences. Variously described as acculturation, urbanization, migration, modernization, or Westernization, rapid sociocultural change has become a daily fact of life for all but the most isolated of the world's populations. A large and multidisciplinary literature has generally argued that the health consequences of rapid sociocultural change are higher levels of morbidity and mortality along both physical and psychological dimensions. The prevailing view has been that rapid sociocultural change brings about social disorganization and cultural disruption which is in turn responsible for role confusion, cultural identity conflicts and feelings of alienation and anomie. This psychosocial "stress" is then implicated etiologically in the development of a variety of health problems including alcohol abuse, suicide, schizophrenia, hypertension, diabetes and, increasingly, other chronic illnesses including cancer (Dressler 1982; Appell 1980; Antonovsky 1979; Carstairs and Kapur 1976; Dohrenwend and Dohrenwend 1981; Graves and Graves 1979; Marmot and Syme 1976; Reed et al. 1970).

The study of the "stress of change" is particularly appropriate in this volume because there has already been a long history of collaboration and exchange of ideas between epidemiologists and anthropologists (Scotch 1963; Cassel 1974; Leighton 1959; Murphy 1973; Ness 1977). However, our basic understanding of the relationship of social and cultural change to health status remains clouded by inconsistencies and contradictions. Although most research suggests that change is inherently stressful, there is growing evidence which argues that we need to look at other contributing factors. For example, Beiser and colleagues (1978: 86—87) argued for an analysis of the broader sociopolitical context in a study of rural Senegalese who had migrated to Dakar:

Thus, in revising our too simplistic theories about the effect of social change, we must take care to distinguish between situations of change which confer subordinate status, powerlessness, joblessness and frustration upon people, from those which offer openness and real opportunity.

Therefore, we must continue to ask ourselves: Is change itself stressful, or are there other factors relevant to particular situations that are responsible for these high rates of stress and illness that people sometimes experience in changing contexts?

Craig R. Janes et al. (eds.), Anthropology and Epidemiology, 249—274.
© 1986 *by D. Reidel Publishing Company.*

This controversy is significant on other than theoretical grounds. Socio-cultural change is ubiquitous. If we accept that sociocultural change is the primary independent explanatory variable in determining changes in health status, we must also conclude that the best way to improve people's well-being is to act conservatively on both macro and micro levels. Either society must resist innovation and heterogeneity, or people must learn to adjust and accommodate themselves to the majority perspective.

Although both of these conservative arguments may now prevail in both scientific and popular ideologies, there is an equally compelling alternative argument.[1] The sources of distress that presently affect many of the world's acculturating, migrating, urbanizing or modernizing populations have less to do with change per se and more to do with the political and economic structures which constrain individual and community attempts to construct meaningful and rewarding social environments. Conservative concepts such as adaptation, adjustment or accommodation which imply an acceptance of stressful life situations should be discarded and replaced with a more progressive set of conceptual tools designed to examine the relationship of health to the construction of new social realities. In other words, change should be regarded as a solution to, rather than a cause of, stressful life situations and associated morbidity and mortality.

This chapter will address this issue by examining the impact of *colonial stress* on Inuit youth in the Canadian Arctic.[2] I will argue that epidemio-logical studies of change-related stress suffer from a failure to evaluate critically underlying theoretical assumptions about social structure and process, and the relationship of persons to these phenomena. The first portion of the paper will be a theoretical discussion of different models for the analysis of change and stress. I will provide first of all a rationale for selecting "internal colonialism" rather than "acculturation" as an analytical framework for understanding change-related stress in situations where one ethnic group is surrounded and dominated by another. I will then argue that a processual and interactionist approach to the analysis of social change must replace the structural-functional bias that prevails in most epidemiological and medical anthropological studies. Finally, I will discuss the role that human agency plays in the social change process.

The second portion of the paper will illustrate these arguments with reference to the everyday lives of young Inuit in the Canadian Arctic. There is presently an "epidemic" of suicides in this young adult population which can be interpreted as an indicator of extraordinary stress. This discussion will introduce the concept of "participatory stress" and describe a series of case studies which illustrate the way in which stress arises from a person's involvement in the construction of their social worlds. In this context, reality construction, and its attendant stress, occurs as people attempt to redefine the nature of the invidious social contract that characterizes their internal colonial relationship with the wider society.

ACCULTURATION OR INTERNAL COLONIALISM IN THE CANADIAN ARCTIC

Inuit in northern Canada are often cited as a classic example of acculturation. During the 1950s and 1960s, the literature on northern Canada emphasized the adaptive accommodations that Inuit were making to southern industrial society. Several prominent anthropologists argued that Inuit represented a case of successful assimilation because many communities seemed to be making the transition with a minimum of stress-related problems (Chance 1965; Honigmann 1965). Where problems existed, it was suggested they were due primarily to the failure of individuals or communities to accommodate themselves to modern orientations. Psychodynamic explanations were often offered for problems associated with modernization. Traditional Inuit socialization and personality structure was thought to be inappropriate for the exigencies of the modern world (Lubart 1969; Parker 1962)!

The most current expression of this approach appears in the work of Berry, a cross-cultural psychologist, and his colleagues, who have carried out a ten year prospective study in northern Quebec on the Cree Indians' capacity to cope with the stresses of culture change (1970, 1976, 1981, 1984). Berry's "acculturative stress" model proposes that when modern community standards and expectations are at greatest variance from traditional culture, the prevalence of acculturative stress will be high.

Significantly, Berry (1981) has recently introduced a political dimension to his work which suggests that when communities have achieved a certain level of self-determination, individuals experience less identity confusion and acculturative stress. For the Cree Indians in northern Quebec, this means that the political autonomy generated by the land claims settlement surrounding the James Bay Hydroelectric Project has resulted in a marked decrease in stress-related problems, particularly among youth.

This latest finding is significant in light of the broader analysis of northern Canada as an internal colony (Dacks 1981; Brody 1975; Paine 1977; Graburn 1981). Internal colonialism describes the political and economic relationship of hinterland or frontier regions to the metropolis in nation-states. It refers to situations where the original inhabitants of remote regions have been disenfranchised economically and politically by the nation states which surround them (Hechter 1975). Commodities are valued according to national and international economic priorities which have little to do with economic conditions in hinterland regions. Populations are maintained as cheap and mobile labor forces for the shifting priorities of resource extraction industries. The dominant (and usually White) minority also allocates social roles and thereby creates a cultural division of labor where indigenous peoples occupy the lower rungs of institutional ladders (Graburn 1981).

Ethnic identification in internal colonies generally emerges in the form of nationalistic efforts to regain control over local affairs from the dominant minority. Whereas the acculturative stress model suggests that assimilation into the dominant society is most likely to reduce the "stress of change", the internal colonial model argues that assimilation into the values and ideas of the dominant society will not necessarily bring about changes in the political and economic conditions which are stressing members of minority communities. The nationalistic movements which are increasingly characteristic of internal colonies are usually fundamentally opposed to assimilation and committed to restructuring the political and economic environment. This process of restructuring, by definition, requires further sociocultural change and varies in expression from violent revolution in contexts such as Northern Ireland and Central America to the more peaceful negotiation of the constitutional rights of indigenous peoples such as is occurring in northern Canada (Wolf 1983).

ANTHROPOLOGICAL APPROACHES TO SOCIAL STRUCTURE AND PROCESS

The use of an internal colonial model in this analysis also suggests that we reassess our concepts of social and cultural change. Too often, anthropologists or anthropologically-oriented health scientists, studying the health consequences of social change, fail to review their use of models and concepts critically in light of current anthropological theory regarding social structure and process. Since the publication of Barth's (1967) essay on social change, and later publication of the monograph on ethnic groups and boundaries (1969), anthropological models for the study of social change have undergone considerable revision. Barth's work was critical of the structural-functional bias in the then prevailing approach to the study of social change (e.g., acculturation theory) which tended to focus on the effect that changing institutional forms had on people's ideas and behaviour. Barth (1967) argued that social institutions were the product of people's interactions and the proper locus of study should be on how people's actions affect the structure and content of institutions.

This approach has been adopted particularly in political and economic anthropology and has also become the basis for the study of the strategic construction of ethnic identity in complex and plural societies (Barth 1983; Hicks and Leis 1977). A "processual" and "interactionist" analysis of sociocultural change draws attention to the way in which individual entrepreneurs, brokers and other "decision-makers" manipulate resources and symbols to *construct* a social reality that both protects their communities from external exploitation and simultaneously enhances their own position in that community (Braroe 1975; Despres 1975; Hannerz 1980; Isaacs 1975).

Some anthropologists have argued that the "social constructionist" model which informs much of the research on social change and ethnicity derives from a fundamentally different epistemology than the structural-functional paradigm which has previously dominated anthropological reasoning:

Thus, the division is not simply about whether or not research takes into account society on the one hand and people's activities on the other. It is basically about the autonomy of agency: if society, or structure, is an objective reality to whose demands people respond in specific ways, then it is an autonomous agency and the individual people are its agents, and the only acceptable explanation is in terms of the functioning of the system. If on the other hand, society or structure emerges from, and is maintained or changed only by what people do, then individuals are autonomous agents and systems are consequences of their actions and, in the last instance, explicable by them. (Holy and Stuchlik 1983: 2)

Although the processual/interactionist model has been widely adopted for analysing changing social systems in most other branches of anthropology, much of medical anthropology still clings tenaciously to the structural-functional model and related concepts of equilibrium, adjustment, disorganization and disintegration. Rather than considering people as "actors", and looking at the way in which their everyday activity brings about changes in beliefs, values, social institutions, resource allocation and power structures, medical anthropology and allied health disciplines continue to view people as reacting to changes in the world around them. This structural-functional approach assumes that people "cope" with these changes through continual adjustment and adaptation, and those identified as "at risk" are those whose attempts at adjustment or adaptation have failed. If medical anthropology is to grow theoretically and make a meaningful contribution to the epidemiology of sickness associated with sociocultural change, these contrasting epistemologies must be critically examined and reconciled.

Despite its obvious structural bias, the internal colonial model is compatible with an actor-centered approach because it is essentially a conflict model. It does not rely on an organic analogy to argue for a prototypical social structure but suggests instead that the maintenance of a colonial structure is a product of elite manipulation of power to ensure the domination of one group's interests over others'. This perspective shifts analysis to actions taken by individuals to restructure inequities and create new social arrangements. Stress arises from the tensions that prevail in a conflict model of society. Stress is also inherent in social activity directed to reconstruct the social context (Berreman 1981; Wolf 1983).

HUMAN AGENCY IN THE ANALYSIS OF STRESS AND COPING

Although the concepts of stress and coping have been utilized primarily in conjunction with the structural-functional model that I have critiqued above, they remain valuable tools for a processual/interactionist analysis with some clarification and revision. I will not attempt to review the history and changing definitions of these concepts here. Excellent reviews are already available elsewhere in this volume and in Dressler (1982).

These reviews identify one theme that is central to this analysis. There is a serious debate in this literature regarding the extent to which stress should be considered in 'meaningful' terms. More empirically-minded scholars have argued that stress can be measured objectively and its health consequences are not significantly affected by the way in which people interpret events and the world around them (Selye 1956; Holmes and Rahe 1967). A better definition of stress and coping adopts the phenomenological approach of Lazarus (1981) and his colleagues, with some fundamental revisions. Stressors are objective features of the environment such as extreme cold, limited opportunities for employment, political domination, family pressure to complete school or various life events such as death of a parent, which are of little predictive power analytically except at the most descriptive level. Stress derives from the meaning associated with the experience of various stressors in terms of their challenge to the individual. The meaning of stressors, however, is inextricably a product of social and cultural participation and should not be attributed individually.

Coping should be considered the more important analytical focus for predicting health outcomes of certain behaviours (Lazarus, ibid). Coping, however, involves more than the marshalling of cognitive, social and material resources to defend against appraised threats, a definition couched in the conservative notions of adjustment or adaptation to external demands on an organism. Coping must be defined in "activist" terms:

> With moral agency as its starting point, a humanistic theory of coping would investigate the person in his social and moral settings, his construction of such settings, *the role of power in the imposition and resistance to such constructions,* and the ways in which cultures, societies and political economies serve as resources and constraints . . . . In such a theory, coping would be understood as the *capacity for culture creation* . . . coping involves *competence in symbolic construction* . . . coping is not merely a matter of job satisfaction or personal adjustment. Instead it is a question of *potency in creating meaning and form.* (Brown 1980: 43, 45, emphasis added)

Coping behavior occurs in a competitive context, structured to some extent by age-related interests. Given prevailing assumptions about appropriate social action that are supported by the larger society, each successive cohort must generate a version of reality which accommodates age-related interests and priorities (Keith 1980). Given particular historical conditions such as internal colonialism, these constructions may be more or less ambiguous and/or variant from prevailing understandings about social roles and action. Increased ambiguity within cohorts often results in contrasting or competing definitional ideas where individuals or sub-groups attempt to dominate the construction of new social realities. Clearly, this competitive process can entail stressful experiential aspects of a chronic quality which should be fundamental to any explanation of links between sociocultural stress and illness. It should also be noted that this model directs equal attention to both the structure of the political economic context which sets limits on possible constructive social action *and* to the transactional situation where change is generated.

Since in this paper we are addressing specifically the situation of young adults, a further clarification is necessary. Young adulthood is a particularly "creative" period in the sense that young people must not only begin to participate in the general selection of strategies to improve the local community's situation with respect to the larger society but they are also faced with the task of gaining access to already occupied productive roles and statuses in the community's social structure. In the words of Eric Erikson (1968: 23):

We cannot separate personal growth and communal change nor can we separate ... the identity crisis in individual life and contemporary crisis in historical development because the two help to define each other.

Thus, it is essential that our model distinguishes between stress arising out of life-cycle changes and stress arising out of general participation in social change. While this distinction is generally relevant to society as a whole, it is particularly significant for young adults. Young adulthood is a period characterized by strong ties of identification to a narrowly defined cohort of peers. In traditional societies, where young people were expected (and were able) to assume previously defined roles in the larger society, cohort identification may not have been as strong or important. However, in situations where innovation is the key to constructing new social realities successfully, young people are under considerable pressure to construct sub-cultures which give them an edge on exploiting new resources or greater access to resources previously allocated. In situations of rapid social change, successive cohorts have not only experienced history differently but they confront different structural constraints and resources as they adopt adult roles (Foner 1984).

For example, *teenage* Inuit were born after the epidemics of infectious diseases that had forced their parents to resettle around trading posts and missions. They had also come through adolescence in the period following alcohol prohibition. These experiences were quite distinct from the *early twenties* cohort, who had been teenagers during a period of excessive alcohol-related social unrest in the community; and different as well from the *late twenties* cohort, who had largely spent the first ten years of their lives in nomadic hunting camps. Furthermore, each cohort came of age when different economic opportunities were available. As a result, each cohort perceives the world differently and has developed distinctive coping styles (O'Neil 1984; 1985).

DEVELOPMENT OF THE RESEARCH PROJECT

The research was designed to address a problem of grave significance in the contemporary Canadian North. Young Inuit and Indians (particularly young men between the ages of 15 and 25) have been committing suicide at epidemic rates far above the expected levels of non-Natives in Canadian society generally. In 1971, the suicide rate in the Northwest Territories was below or near the Canadian average of 10 per 100,000.[3] By 1978, the incidence rate had risen to 35 per 100,000. Indeed, there have been periods where rates have been as high as 170 per 100,000. Psychiatrists have painted the following portrait of a high-risk individual: he is a young man in his late teens, recently returned from high school, often the firstborn son and usually the family favorite, and regarded by peers as a leader and potentially successful in the White world. Further, the suicide often occurs in the context of romantic problems and alcohol use (Rodgers 1982; Seltzer 1980; Atcheson and Malcolmson 1976). These suicide outbreaks also appear to have a contagious quality. In several instances, the suicide of one young man appears to have triggered the self-destruction of five or six of his friends within a few short weeks. For a community of five or six hundred people consisting of 10 to 15 extended families, the social and psychological impact of these deaths has been devastating.[4]

In response to requests from elders in an Inuit community which had experienced several tragic incidents, I developed a research program to identify the coping strategies young Inuit had developed. The analytical task was to correlate health status indicators with coping strategies and thereby identify behavioural risk factors that indicated a significantly stressful life-style. Although this research design would not identify risk factors explicitly linked to suicidal outcomes, it would provide a framework for community workers to identify young people whose life circumstances left them at risk. This broader approach was also necessary in order to validate the theoretical argument that an actor-centered model of participation in social change processes means that risk factors are different and will change for successive cohorts of young people as they age and change the society around them.

The initial research design combined a population survey of all young men in an Inuit community with in-depth life history interviews from a purposive, cohort-specific sample.[5] The survey questionnaire was designed to measure the nature of young peoples' participation in various sectors of community life and included both historical and structural dimensions. For example, one section of the questionnaire dealt with the degress of mobility experienced by the young person and his family and another section dealt with the family's economic and political status in the community.

The questionnaire also included a number of outcome measures to assess the past and present state of the respondents' health. Ten items were included from the Health Opinion Survey developed by the Leightons (1959) for the Stirling County Study. This instrument has been accepted generally as a reasonably valid cross-cultural indicator of psychiatric problems (Dohrenwend and Dohrenwend 1981; Macmillan 1957). Questionnaire items also asked respondents to indicate the extent of their alcohol and drug use and whether they had ever been in trouble with local authorities. Lastly, respondents were asked for their written consent for me to review various institutional records, including medical records, police records and educational records. With one exception, permission was universally given.

Inuit communities are relatively "captive" in the sense that all their health care is provided through the local, federally-funded health clinic. Thus, medical records represent a reasonably reliable measure of health care utilization since 1970 when the clinic was built. Variation in both recording techniques and personal recording style does occur, however, due to staff turnover and changing bureaucratic recording requirements. Utilization data must therefore be analyzed with some care. Indices were constructed which indicated: (1) overall frequency of utilization during different age stages (i.e., as children and as teenagers); and (2) proportion of visits at different age stages that could be considered stress-related (determined rather arbitrarily by subtracting obvious injuries, infectious diseases and/or chronic conditions — which left problems like headaches, nervous conditions, generalized aches and pains, skin inflamations, etc.). Blood pressures were not taken since the age of the respondents precluded any expectation that hypertension would be a significant indicator of stress. In the absence of hormone assays, or other empirical measures of stress, this holistic assessment of the individual's health along social, psychological and physiological dimensions was considered sufficient. It was also designed to assess diverse outcomes of stressful experiences which Dressler (1982: 134) has identified as an important area requiring further methodological development.

The population included fifty-seven young men between 15 and 30 years of age who indicated Sanctuary Bay as their "home town".[6] Eight of these young men were resident elsewhere and questionnaires were mailed to them for completion. Otherwise, I administered each questionnaire personally which took from one to three hours.

As a group, the study population clearly exhibits significant variation along most of the variables selected for analysis (see Table I). Some of these differences are developmental (e.g., higher income levels for older youth); others are related to changing historical circumstances (e.g., level of education completed, which is an indicator of changing educational opportunities); and others reflect age-specific stresses and coping strategies that change as the sociocultural context changes (e.g., age of first sexual experience). Determination of cohort boundaries was first suggested by ethnographic evidence that the community expected fundamental transitions to occur at ages 20 and 24; and was further substantiated by significant correlations between age and selected social variables.[7]

From this population of fifty-seven young men, I selected a sample of twelve individuals for intensive case-study analysis. Wherever possible, I participated in the lives of these informants fully. In some cases, I lived in

TABLE I
Variation among young adult cohorts

	Junior team (20)	Polar bear hunters (17)	Managers (14)	
Historical/Biographical Factors				
1. Born in or near Sanctuary Bay	60	41	36	a
2. Lived in Sanctuary Bay entire life	50	35	14	b
3. Lived part of life outside Kitikmeot region	20	24	64	b
4. Related to Whites by descent or marriage	30	41	36	N.S.
5. Had experience with Boarding School as a child	0	18	36	b
6. Parents encouraged education	75	41	21	b
7. Have no secondary education	10	6	57	b
8. Completed secondary education	5	6	14	b
9. Able to work as a translator	10	18	21	N.S.
10. Prefer English to Inuktitut in everyday conversation	80	59	36	b
Domestic Context				
1. Majority of kindred lives in Sanctuary Bay	55	71	36	b
2. Currently residing with older relatives	90	76	14	b
3. Father still alive	80	88	43	b
4. Father is very active hunter/trapper	45	53	21	b
5. Father has full-time employment	30	24	29	N.S.
6. Had first sexual experience younger than fifteen	20	41	21	b
7. Marriage was arranged by parents	N/A	29	43	N.S.
8. Wife is from another village	N/A	41	36	N.S.
9. Child(ren) adopted by older relative	N/A	41	50	N.S.
Contemporary Coping Behavior				
1. Only travel is to nearby villages by snow-mobile	20	41	21	b
2. Have travelled out of Kitikmeot in past two years	80	59	79	N.S.
3. Have visited at least four different villages in past two years	75	41	36	b
4. Go onto the land at least twice per month	55	71	57	N.S.
5. Never attend church	55	59	43	N.S.
6. Earned more than $10,000 in 1981	0	47	57	b
7. Had a full-time job in 1981	15	41	57	b
8. Enjoy indoor jobs the most	30	12	36	b
9. Worked only in indoor jobs in 1981	45	12	36	b
10. Earned more than $250 carving in 1981	10	24	43	b
11. Have been elected to political office	N/A	47	29	a
12. Watch television news almost every night	45	24	36	a
13. Go to the gym almost every night	75	24	21	b
14. Go to almost every dance	75	47	64	a

Table I (Continued)

	Junior team (20)	Polar bear hunters (17)	Managers (14)	
Health Behavior				
1. Started smoking cigarettes younger than fourteen	70	35	7	b
2. Smoke at least half package of cigarettes per day	85	71	86	N.S.
3. Do not drink any alcohol	70	41	36	b
4. Occasionally use alcohol illegally	5	12	22	b
5. HOS score higher than 30 (at risk for psychiatric problems)	55	12	21	b
6. Frequent visitor to Nursing Station as a teenager	25	47	43	a
7. More than 1/3 of visits to Nursing Station in past two years are stress-related	5	12	29	b
8. More than 1/2 of visits to Nursing Station in past two years are minor injuries	40	12	0	b

All numbers expressed as percentage of total population of each cohort (indicated in brackets).
[a] — indicates x^2 statistic significant at $\alpha = 0.05$.
[b] — indicates x^2 statistic significant at $\alpha = 0.01$.
N.S. — not statistically significant.

their family households for periods of several months and, in most cases, I travelled extensively with them on hunting trips and/or trips to other villages.

COPING STYLES AND HEALTH

Data analysis for this study was difficult due to a number of epistemological and methodological problems. I had initially intended to analyse the survey data and find a number of empirically-based behavioural styles that correlated with evidence of stress-related health problems. For example, I expected to find that young people who participated infrequently in land activities and worked in a subordinate role for Whites would experience greater stress. Using multivariate regression techniques and factor analysis, I tested a broad range of similar hypotheses regarding empirically-defined behavioural styles and health status. The results were disappointing. Not only were the correlation statistics usually insignificant, those that were significant were generally too trivial to be meaningful in terms of my original objective to assist the community in developing programs to aid individuals at risk.

The analysis then shifted to a more qualitative approach. Based on insights from the case study material (which I had originally intended to use as illustrations of quantitatively identified stressful coping styles), I began to review each of the fifty-seven survey protocols for similar dynamic features.

I was able to identify five general coping styles that cross-cut actual behaviours in the different cohorts and were associated qualitatively with negative health consequences. For example, although the specific behavioural elements of the coping styles of a nineteen year old basketball player and a twenty-four year old polar bear hunter were distinctive, they could both be under stress if their respective coping styles were innovative attempts to create new cultural styles for the rest of their cohort. I have labelled this particular coping style the "stress of definition". This and other coping styles are listed here and described in detail below:

(1) The Stress of Definition
(2) The Stress of Isolation
(3) The Stress of Transition
(4) The Stress of Timing
(5) The Stress of Consolidation

1. *The Stress of Definition*

Those people who are most active in the construction of new social and cultural realities for groups confronting colonial constraints experience the stress of definition. In developmental terms, the stress of definition is experienced particularly by members of younger transitional cohorts who are negotiating entrance into a new social order (e.g., assuming adult roles) where access to resources defined as valuable by a dominant external elite is best facilitated by challenging those value definitions locally. Definitional copers must balance their own material and emotional needs with a vision of how their cohort will benefit most. The following case describes a definitional coper:

Case I: Tuvak Alooktook is 22 years old, married, with one child. He and his young family live with his wife's parents. He is seldom at home, however, preferring to spend most of his time alone on the land. He travels by snowmachine into unfamiliar areas in search of game and to satisfy his curiousity about the land of his ancestors. He wears skin clothing made for him by his wife and mother-in-law and presents a 'traditional' appearance in most social contexts. He expresses his commitment to hunting and the land as follows:

> Young people today have forgotten a lot of the survival skills of our ances-
> tors. In lots of places in the North, you can go out hunting and back in one day
> so young people don't have to learn how to camp. I always try to stay out for
> three or four days when I'm hunting. It seems like I never stay in town. I just go
> there to get more gasoline and other stuffs [amunition, food, oil, etc.] and then I
> go hunting again.
>   Sometimes you get homesick when you are hunting all the time. I really miss
> my little girl and my wife always worries when I'm out. But it seems like I can't
> stay in town either. It's so boring . . . it's like there's nothing to do even if you
> have a job. Hunting makes me feel like I'm an Inuk. It's never boring on the land
> even when you're travelling alone.

Tuvak's shift in focus in his early twenties to land activities, while consistent with a general shift in Inuit ethnicity towards "traditionalism", also meant that he was not fulfilling a major familial expectation to contribute wage income. Previously, young men in the contemporary Canadian North have achieved a degree of status within families by contributing wage income to the extended family's economic well-being. Older, uneducated and unilingual fathers, brothers and grandfathers are limited in the range of economic options open to them and already have the skills necessary to pursue hunting as their primary economic strategy. Although older men worry that young men are losing the ability to survive "in nature" — the symbolic hallmark of the Inummariit or "real people" — on balance they are more concerned that their families will lose the competitive edge in the wage economy. Cash has become essential for purchasing the expensive equipment (snowmobiles, gasoline, rifles, etc.) that is a key element in the modern hunting strategies of contemporary Inuit.

Tuvak has rejected the wage-oriented adaptation of the previous cohort and was instead trying to establish a coping style based on traditional subsistence activities. His wife works full-time in a clerical job where she is able to support his land activities by purchasing the necessary equipment, gasoline and supplies. He, in turn, contributes to the extended family's larder.

In the spring, Tuvak took his young family onto the land every weekend, often leading large parties of similar young couples to hunting areas he had explored during the winter. He was an innovator in designing a sled with a covered box where his wife could keep warm with their young child, wrapped in caribou and musk-ox skins.

Significantly, this coping style is emerging as the preferred pattern for other young couples in their early twenties as well. Tuvak is, however, the most aggressive and systematic in his pursuit of a hunter identity. While other young men engage in hunting activities between part-time jobs, Tuvak has turned down several well-paid job offers from construction crews. Despite recognized skills as a carpenter, he prefers to supplement his wife's earnings with money earned from selling furs — the most important of which is the polar bear.

In general, those who pursued a hunter's identity in Tuvak's cohort seemed to experience less stress than those with a town orientation. Also, members of both the older and younger cohorts appeared more stressed. HOS scores for the 20—24 year old cohort were significantly lower than either of the other cohorts, as was illegal alcohol consumption (see Table I). This would suggest that an active involvement in land-oriented activities creates less stress for people than a lifestyle based around the town.

However, Tuvak himself expressed many of the symptoms of a young person at risk. His HOS score was 31, which indicated the presence of psychopathology, and his medical record indicated frequent complaints for psychosomatic problems. Thus, had I relied simply on a measure such as "extent of land activities", I would probably have concluded that land activities mediated stresses that arose in other areas of community and family life. While this conclusion is generally valid in a cross-sectional and structural sense, it ignores the fact that a land-oriented lifestyle is a particular social construction related to specific historical circumstances and that those most involved in defining this adaptation may be "at risk" in an epidemiological sense.

The definitional nature of Tuvak's coping style is further evident if examined in historical perspective. As indicated, previous cohorts of young adults have generally created new roles for themselves in the White-dominated institutions that structure village life. These institutions reflect a colonial heritage through the persistence of a culturally-defined hierarchy within which Inuit continue to occupy subordinate positions. Despite both Inuit and White expectations that Tuvak and his cohort should follow in their older brother's footsteps and attempts to restructure these institutions, they have opted for a more 'traditional' lifestyle that inherently rejects wage-related economic success as meaningful.

Similar cases of definitional stress could also be cited for other young men in the older or younger cohort who were active in defining the prevailing understandings about social life meaningful to *their* peers. Despite significant differences in the empirical dimensions of their coping styles (i.e., a focus on recreational activities or administrative responsibilities) the underlying association of definitional stress remains significant.

2. *The Stress of Isolation*

When an age cohort is in the process of constructing a new social reality in which definitions of selves are embedded, some members of that cohort will find themselves alienated from the emergent definitions. Depending on the size of the interacting cohort, where interaction includes symbolic exchange through mass media as well as face-to-face transactions, those whose definitions of selves and society are different from the majority may experience the *stress of isolation*. In large interacting cohorts (i.e., American urban society) competing definitions may be of a "subcultural" nature and less stressful. However, in a small interacting cohort, such as an isolated village or a migrant community, competing constructions may be individually based. The following case illustrates the stress of isolation:

Case II: For most male teenagers in Sanctuary Bay, everyday life revolves around recreational activities in the school gymnasium each evening. Cut off from active participation in either wage-related or landbased economic activities for developmental and political reasons, male teenagers had constructed a social reality based on team sports. Their primary social identification was as a "player" and personal value flowed from athletic ability.

Joe Nanook is 18 years old, lives at home with his elderly grandparents and, although physically and intellectually the equal of his peers, rarely engages in sports or other recreational activities. Instead, he maintains his own trapline and hunts frequently in the company of older male kin. While most teenagers, at best, possess an old and broken-down snowmachine, Joe owns two well-maintained machines and most of the other equipment necessary to travel, hunt and camp on the land. While most other teenagers adopt a submissive and dependent role on the rare occasions when they do venture onto the land, Joe often left the hunting parties to travel alone, and older hunters were confident in his survival abilities.

Ironically, the respect he fostered among older hunters facilitated his election to the town's Recreation Committee which invested him with the responsibility to supervise teenage recreational activities. This meant he was expected to participate regularly in sports activities and teen dances. Since many of these activities occurred on weekends — a time when hunters are on the land — his public responsibilities and personal interests were in conflict.

Significantly, he was not marginal to his peers because of any imposed distance on their part. Other teenagers did not express negative sentiments about him, and indeed, expressed a begrudging respect for his competence on the land. His interactions with them were usually friendly, although without the warmth sometimes evident among teammates. His choice of coping style was clearly linked to wider societal definitions about appropriate "Inuit" be- haviour, but it could not be interpreted as a simple assumption of a previously defined role. His tendency to travel alone and his overall ability on the land were evidence for a particularly creative and unique coping style.

His HOS score was 32, indicative of psychological problems, and his medical record indicated frequent visits for colds, headaches, skin inflamations and generalized pains in the joints. He was reticent to discuss emotional issues (a typical traditional Inuit trait) but did indicate feelings of depression related to his alienation from his peers.

This case illustrates both the stress of isolation *and* the problem of assuming that universally-defined stresses have uniform meaning in the same social context. "Extent of land activities" clearly means something quite different to Joe Nanook than to Tuvak Alooktook's cohort described in Case I. If I had attempted to correlate a measure of "land attitudes and/or activities" with health problems, I would have missed the differential impact that changes in the meaning of a stressor may have on members of a seemingly homogeneous cultural group.

The case also illustrates that the stress of isolation should not be confused with "marginality" as it is usually defined in the social science literature (e.g., Velez-Ibanez 1983). In this case, the isolationist coping style was actively constructed by Joe Nanook, rather than thrust upon him. While the case material described here suggests that historical/biographical and structural factors probably contributed to the construction of the coping pattern (e.g., membership in a family with strong traditionalist tendencies), the specific features of the isolationist coping style are still unique to both the individuals involved and the cohorts they belong to.

3. The Stress of Transition

Young people of the same age within even a narrowly defined cohort experience the stress of transition as the cohort moves into another develop- mental age category. I must emphasize again the "constructive" nature of this transition. People do not simply exchange one set of roles, statuses and obligations for another set as they age. Instead, they discover that the cultural reality that has been previously successful no longer meets their social, economic and emotional needs. New coping strategies must be devised that result in the construction of an historically unique perspective and behav- ioural focus (Nydegger 1981).

To be more specific, as Inuit male teenagers move into their early twenties, it is unlikely they will universally adopt the land-oriented focus of their older brothers as described in Case I above. While this land-oriented focus is in part determined by general social expectations in Inuit society (i.e., all young men must learn to feed their families from the land), its particular early twenties manifestation is equally determined by historical/biographical factors and contemporary contextual opportunities and constraints. Since each of these other sources for social construction are different for teenagers (and, indeed, the general Inuit expectation to feed one's family from the land is also changing to meet new demands), their solutions to the problem will also be different.

Although optimum transitional ages are also subject to negotiation (i.e., transitions are delayed or advanced to meet changing needs), transitional stress for young Inuit presently occurs at nineteen and twenty-four. The principal determinants of these boundaries are familial obligations. At 19, young men are expected to initiate a marital relationship and start a family, and at 24 they are expected to reverse the support they have received from the extended family (particularly their in-laws) and establish an independent self-sufficient household. The following case will illustrate:

Case III: Pauloosie Kiviuk is nineteen years old and living in his grandparents' house with a young woman who is pregnant with their first child. Pauloosie was adopted by his grandparents as a child and, although his natural parents were alive, well and living in the same community, his principle obligations and emotional ties were to his grandparents. He is also their sole source of household-based economic support since all other children in the family are younger. His grandparents expected him to hunt regularly and, to this end, his grandfather had purchased a snowmachine for him out of savings from his pension cheques.

Pauloosie is also known as "Mr. Spike" to his peers, a reference to his exceptional skills on the volleyball court. He is captain of both the basketball and volleyball teams and participates on a regular basis in the evening sports activities. Most teenagers sleep during the day and socialize at night while the rest of the community is in bed; a pattern that concerns their parents because it precludes participation in either land-based or wage-related economic activities. Pauloosie's involvement and, indeed, leadership in this teenage lifestyle means that he experiences considerable stress in both his marital and familial relationships. His family is influential and able to arrange part-time work for him on local construction projects; work which limits him both in terms of energy and time for participation in sports activities. As a consequence, he frequently either quit or was fired from these jobs. The social activities of young, pregnant women living with their in-laws are severely restricted and his young wife was very jealous of Pauloosie's nightly socializing with other, unattached young men and women — activities which she was unable to join.

Pauloosie's HOS score was fairly high (27) but not indicative of psychopathology and about average for his peer group (who generally scored higher than other young adult cohorts). However, he was a frequent illegal drinker and, on several occasions, became violent when drunk. In conversations, he indicated he experienced broad shifts in mood with occasional periods of despair.

During the period when Pauloosie and his cohort were negotiating their transition into early twenties young adulthood, older members of the community were beginning to place considerable emphasis on formal education and training for the teenage cohort. Various locally supported programs emphasized trades apprenticeships in areas previously monopolized by transient Whites; trades such as plumbers, electricians, mechanics, etc. These trades require more career committment (in terms of attending courses away from the community and pursuing one job for long periods) than part-time construction work (the favoured wage activity of Tuvak Alooktook and his early twenties cohort described in Case I). Opportunities for developing land skills are therefore more restricted. Pauloosie and his cohort, at nineteen, had to select among three potential coping styles: (1) the attraction of continuing to play volleyball and basketball and delaying the assumption of young adult responsibilities, (2) the difficult but previously defined orientation to a hunter's lifestyle similar to Tuvak Alooktook's cohort or (3) the vague but emergent sense that participation in trades apprenticeships would become the new social and economic reality for young men in their early twenties.

Although a follow-up study would be necessary to determine which option Pauloosie and his cohort are likely to pursue, there were several indications that the tension is generated, again, from the colonial context in which these choices arise. In order to pursue the trades apprenticeship career option, young men must leave their villages for training during a developmental age stage when they should be maturing as independent hunters. Pauloosie's cohort are less likely to be successful in rejecting the wage-oriented option, because their cohort biography does not include the same degree of early childhood land experience as their older brothers. Due to the rapid development of centralized administrative facilities brought about by colonization in the North, Pauloosie's cohort have been almost entirely born and raised in villages, while Tuvak Alooktook's cohort generally lived in hunting camps for at least their infant years.

In summary, Pauloosie's case illustrates the stress of transition for young men involved in redefining their relationship with their society as they mature. Old solutions to social stresses, successfully constructed by older cohorts, may offer some features to be incorporated into the transitional cohort's coping repertoire but, in most cases, political and economic circumstances will have changed sufficiently to require new solutions.

This initial socialization experience has also had long term implications in the extent to which Tuvak's cohort has participated, as children, in their fathers' hunting activities. As a result, they are better prepared than Pauloosie and his peers for achieving young adult status as independent hunters.[8]

4. The Stress of Timing

As cohorts age, transitional boundaries are negotiated as part of the social construction of new cultural realities (Keith 1980). Although changes in age cohort boundary definitions may be slow, competition over resources, political constraints and corresponding coping strategies related to social identification choices usually result in boundary flexibility. The classic example is, of course, the upward movement of the entry boundary into adulthood for members of the "baby boom" cohort in Western society.

The process of reaching consensus on boundary definition is a topic worthy of detailed investigation and beyond the scope of the present paper. Rather, the interest here is in the stress that is experienced by young adults who attempt to ignore transitional boundaries or whose efforts to renegotiate boundaries are unsuccessful.

These individuals often attempt to delay transitions by continuing to participate and define themselves in relation to the coping style of a younger cohort. In fact, however, their personal interpretation of the younger cohorts' coping style is often based on their *own* cohort's cultural constructions that they experienced when they were younger. The new, younger cohorts often define themselves quite differently (as argued above). As a result, off-timers find themselves alienated from both their own cohort, who have made a transition into a new social world, *and* with the younger cohort who may appear to the off-timer to still offer an appropriate social reality but who, in fact, may see the world and themselves quite differently. The following case will illustrate:

Case IV: Joshua Ittinuaq is 26, is married to the favorite daughter of the village's most powerful spiritual elder and has three young children. His own extended family lives in another village three hundred miles to the south. He married his wife under conditions of extreme duress. She was promised to the son of another powerful elder in the village and her father strongly opposed her marriage. Joshua had come to Sanctuary Bay for a brief visit, but had become romantically involved with the young woman and had stayed with her, in spite of her father's objections. The father's dislike of him had erupted into violence on several occasions.

Joshua is the son of an Inuit Anglican minister. Joshua's involvement in alcohol-related illegality as a teenager had contributed to a serious estrangement from his father. His decision to move to Sanctuary Bay was in part motivated by a desire to escape his father's dominance.

Joshua was trained as a heavy equipment operator but was unable to obtain employment in Sanctuary Bay. Manual labor opportunities are controlled by the village's elders who sit on the various councils and associations which administer local municipal affairs. These men supported Joshua's father-in-law in his efforts to force Joshua to leave the community and refused to hire him. Without an independent source of income, or familial backing, Joshua was also unable to pursue a hunter's lifestyle and was forced to support his family on welfare and what little food his wife was able to beg from her family.

Joshua coped with these constraints by becoming heavily involved in the recreational activities of teenagers. Sleeping all day, playing basketball all evening and cards all night and organizing pop music dances whenever possible defined his everyday behaviour. His efforts in these areas surpassed a passive avoidance of other pursuits. He refereed and organized sports competitions, operated the sound equipment at dances and frequently hosted all-night poker parties. He dressed in the appropriate teenage uniform — wolf-trimmed bomber jacker, blue jeans and running shoes — and offered his house as a hang-out for young people who still lived with their parents.

However, the teenage cohort resented his involvement in their activities and attempted to exclude him whenever possible. Their attitude was not based on personal dislike but derived from a feeling that Joshua's participation in their social life further prejudiced older members of the community against what was generally perceived as an unproductive and socially disruptive coping pattern. Inuit feel strongly that personal economic productivity is an essential survival strategy; laziness and unproductive activity are considered as serious threats to the community's future. Teenage recreational activities were tolerated as long as no one indicated this pattern might continue on into young adulthood and Joshua's presence threatened this as a distinct possibility.

Joshua expressed suicidal feelings on several occasions. His HOS score was extremely high and he was on medication for problems defined by the medical staff in strictly psychosomatic terms. He was a frequent illegal user of alcohol and had been arrested several times when drinking had led to violence.

Although it could be argued that Joshua's problems were psychodynamic or the product of stresses generated by his relationship with his family and in-laws, this case must also be understood in relation to other cases where young men were engaged in similar off-timed coping styles. Although these other cases also entailed a considerable degree of stress, the empirical dimensions of the cases were quite different (i.e., biographical data, relationships with families, spouses, etc.). The off-timeing coping strategy is generated instead in situations where colonially-produced economic and political factors force certain individuals to survive by creating a role for themselves in the social life of another cohort.

These cases also illustrate the chronic stress associated with attempts to delay or speed up transitional stages which are accepted by other members of one's cohort as legitimate. While transitional boundaries in situations of rapid sociocultural change are themselves the subjects of constant negotiation, changes are nonetheless gradual and usually require a degree of consensus from all groups on both sides of the boundary. For off-timers, participation in this process is definitional but it is also isolationist which compounds the experience of stress.

5. The Stress of Consolidation

This kind of stress occurs in situations of rapid social change where emerging adult cohorts construct identities and coping styles which are successful in mediating the stresses specific to their transition into adulthood at a particular point in history. As the cohort ages, these constructions are consolidated and further change is resisted. If the wider societal context continues to change rapidly, these consolidated coping strategies become somewhat anachronistic and people begin to experience stress in association with their attempts to defend definitions of selves and social reality. Particularly when coping styles are of themselves highly stressful, the stress of consolidation can have a particular impact.

In the Inuit context, several members of the Managerial cohort (24—29) are suffering considerably from the stress of consolidation. This cohort was the first thoroughly bilingual and literate cohort in the Village's history and, as a result, were well-qualified to assume the growing number of brokerage-type positions in the expanding institutional sectors of village life in the mid-seventies. Schools, stores, health services and other government agencies all required young people to work initially as translators. These roles quickly expanded to include other more administrative functions and the position of "Manager-Trainee" has become a fixture in almost all institutional sectors. Young people in these positions are expected to fulfill the symbolic requirement of local control over village affairs but at the same time remain accountable to usually White supervisors. In order to be successful, they must be able to perform well culturally in both the White and Inuit social realities but greater emphasis is placed on their "White" performance. As a consequence, they express a stronger assimilationist orientation and their behaviour manifests a recognizable identification with White symbolic structures such as nuclear family autonomy and middle-class consumerism.

If younger cohorts had continued to develop this adaptation, the stress of consolidation would not be as severe for the Managerial cohort. In fact, however, the opposite is occurring. Young men in their early twenties are not only avoiding jobs where White supervision is still a factor but they show little interest in office jobs or bookkeeping tasks generally. The new focus, as described earlier, is on part-time construction work or skilled trades and intensive land activities with a strong traditionalist orientation. This orientation manifests itself in such things as visiting patterns — where extended family solidarity and respect for elder's knowledge is emphasized; clothing styles — where the "trapper" look is the model rather than the briefcase and tie appearance of the Managerial cohort; and language use — where Inuktitut rather than English is increasingly the language of public discourse.

This new traditionalist emphasis of the early twenties cohort creates stress for the Managers because the Managers are no longer at the cutting edge of new cultural definitions and this loss of leadership in shaping a new society means that they are starting to lose control over economic resources that they were beginning to gain access to. In order to compete, some members of the Managerial cohort have become aggressively "traditional" in their public demeanor. Participation at drum dances, refusal to speak in English in private and avoidance of White coworkers and supervisors are indicative of their attempts to redefine the Managerial cultural style in a direction consistent with emergent cultural forms. For others, resistance to the threat of new definitions has taken the form of an entrenched rejection of Inuit identifications and a determined embracement of White cultural styles. Often this latter strategy involves an increase in social interaction with local Whites outside working hours and a concomitant increase in social distance with members of their own extended family.

SUMMARY AND DISCUSSION

In this paper I have presented a series of case studies which illustrate the variable nature of young people's relationships with their changing social world in a colonial context. These relationships are extremely complex and require more elaborate models for understanding the way in which people's activities entail stress and are detrimental to their physical and emotional health than are normally found in social and cultural epidemiological studies of change and health.

To summarize briefly, the paper has described the lives of young Inuit men between the ages of fifteen and thirty. It argues that rapid social change and age-related developmental differences are responsible for the emergence of three narrowly defined cohorts which have been heuristically identified as the Junior Team (15—19); Polar Bear Hunters (20—24); and Managers (25—30). Members of these cohorts are actively engaged in coping with the constraints implicit in an internal colonial context by struggling to construct meaningful social realities which simultaneously facilitate a tolerable everyday life *and* contribute to Inuit societal efforts to restructure or survive in the political economy in which they live.

This struggle, unavoidably, entails the experience of stress, which for some young adults puts them at risk for suicidal outcomes among other destructive illness behaviours. This risk is understood as a dynamic component of creative and participatory coping styles rather than as fixed behavioural or cognitive traits.

Typically, the empirical bias in the epidemiological approach, with its emphasis on the measurement of social variables along a continuum (i.e., people have more or less of a particular social commodity such as kin support) produces a static and synchronic understanding of behavioural risk factors. Even when diachronic or 'prospective' epidemiological studies attempt to measure changing levels of social and cultural variables over time, the analysis is still limited by a reliance on predefined variables that may not reflect the changing nature of people's construction of their social worlds (Savishinsky 1974).

This paper argues that our understanding of people's participation in their changing social world must be cast in an *active* multidimensional mode and that the *meaning* of that participation must be understood in the particular context where the behaviour occurs. Sociocultural change must be understood as the *product* of, as well as the stimulus for human activity. Stress arises from a variety of participatory styles not all of which can be cast as failing to cope effectively. Often, those most involved in defining new social realities experience as much or more stress as those who become marginal or alienated from the process.

This paper has also argued that our understanding of different participatory styles, and the context-embedded meaning of that participation to the actors, can only be understood within a political economic framework. Social participation is more than simply a *meaningful* activity, it is a *competitive* series of events where ideological and material resources are marshalled and deployed to protect and enhance the interests of individuals and groups in plural (or, in this case, colonial) societies structured by inequality and injustice. The social constructions of Inuit youth must be understood in context but our understanding of context must be more than a set of culturally-defined symbols and ideas. It must be based on a dynamic understanding of the relationship between history and biography. This understanding places greater emphasis on the nature of structured access to symbols and ideas, as well as food and guns, and emphasizes the role of elites in the maintenance of ideologies which are used to justify the limitations and constraints that people struggle to deconstruct (Young 1980; Gellner 1979).

Finally, this paper contributes to our understanding of the nature of people's participation in the social change process and the potential health consequences that can accrue. It will be more difficult to develop a methodology that is suitable for adapting the model to broader population-based epidemiological research. The issue is more than simply designing epidemiological instruments that are sensitive to cultural factors; it may require a fundamental re-thinking of the positivist and empirical epistemological bias in epidemiological research if future research is to fully understand the meaning of change-related stress in people's lives.

ACKNOWLEDGEMENTS

Fieldwork for this paper was supported in 1977—78 and 1981—82 by a National Health Research and Development Pre-Doctoral Fellowship from Health and Welfare, Canada and in 1981—82 by a research grant from the Arctic Institute of North America with assistance from the Firestone Foundation. Preparation of the manuscript was made possible by a Post-Doctoral Fellowship from the National Health Research and Development Program, Health and Welfare, Canada. I am indebted to the people of Sanctuary Bay, and particularly their young people, who must remain anonymous for purposes of confidentiality. Fred Dunn, Nelson Graburn, Gerald Berreman, Corinne Nydegger, Fredrik Barth and Richard Lazarus have personally influenced the development of ideas contained in this paper and I am grateful. I would also like to thank Craig Janes, Ron Stall and Sandra Gifford for their helpful editorial comments during the preparation of this manuscript, and Charlene Ball and Jackie Linklater for their editorial assistance.

NOTES

1. Allan Young (1980) has written a provocative critique of stress ideology which he argues is asociological and ahistorical in its analysis of sickness and social life. While Young rejects stress theory on the basis that it reinforces the status quo, I argue here that the basic theoretical framework can be valuable if a political economic perspective is introduced.
2. *Inuit* means "The People" and has replaced the term Eskimo (with its derogatory "primitive" connotations) in standard scientific and popular usage in Canada. It is the preferred self-referent of the indigenous people living North of the treeline.
3. The Northwest Territories (NWT) is a vast region of approximately three million square miles in northern Canada of which nearly two million lie north of the treeline. Of the

approximately 45,000 people who live in the NWT, 15,000 are Inuit, 20,000 are White and 10,000 are Indian or Metis. North of the treeline, 85% of the population is Inuit.
4. McElroy (1975) has described the situation of Inuit women in similar terms as this paper discusses young men. While young women also seem to be at risk because of colonial stress, there are fewer cases of completed suicides. A full analysis of both men and women was not possible for methodological reasons.
5. The sample was selected on the basis of an initial assessment from the survey of stress indicators for each person. I selected six people from each of the three age cohorts with two individuals representing low, medium and high stress indicator scores.
6. Sanctuary Bay is a pseudonym as are the names provided for the case studies to follow.
7. For ease of reference I have somewhat arbitrarily assigned descriptive labels to each cohort: (1) Junior Team (15—19); (2) Polar Bear Hunters (20—24); and (3) Managers (25—30). Each of these labels does, however, capture the behavioural focus of each cohort.
8. It is also interesting to note that the boarding school experience of young men in their late twenties (which Tuvak's cohort were spared) has had a similar kind of differential socialization impact on the oldest young adult cohort.

REFERENCES

Appell, G. N.
   1980 The Health Consequences of Social change: A Set of Postulates for Developing General Adaptation Theory. *In* L. Stark and T. Macdonald (eds.), Amazonia: Extinction or Survival: The Impact of National Development on the Native Peoples of Tropical South America. Madison: University of Wisconsin Press.
Antonovsky, A.
   1979 Health, Stress and Coping. San Francisco, CA: Jossey-Bass.
Atcheson, J. D. and S. A. Malcolmson
   1976 Psychiatric Consultation to the Eastern Canadian Arctic Communities. *In* R. J. Shepard and S. Itoh (eds.), Circumpolar Health, Toronto: University of Toronto Press, pp. 539—542.
Barth, F.
   1967 On the Study of Social Change. American Anthropologist, 69: 661—669.
   1969 Ethnic Groups and Boundaries. Boston: Little, Brown.
   1983 Sohar: Culture and Society in an Omani Town. Baltimore: Johns Hopkins University Press.
Beiser, M. et al.
   1978 Author's abstract. Transcultural Psychiatric Research Review, 15: 86—87.
Berreman, G. (ed.)
   1981 Social Inequality. New York: Academic Press.
Berry, J. W.
   1970 Marginality, Stress and Ethnic Identification in an Acculturated Aboriginal Community. Journal of Cross-Cultural Psychology, 3: 239—52.
   1976 Acculturative Stress in Northern Canada: Ecological, Cultural and Psychological Factors. *In* R. J. Shepard and S. Itoh (eds.), Circumpolar Health. Toronto: University of Toronto Press, pp. 490—497.
   1984 Acculturative Stress in Northern Quebec. Paper presented at International Symposium on Circumpolar Health, Anchorage, Alaska.
Berry, J. W., R. M. Wintrob, P. S. Sindell, and T. Mawbinney
   1981 Culture Change and Psychological Adaptation Among the James Bay Cree. *In* B. Harvald and J. P. Hart-Hansen (eds.), Circumpolar Health 81. Nordic Council on Arctic Medical Research Report, Series 33.

Blauner, R.
1972 Racial Oppression in America. New York: Harper and Row.
Braroe, N. W.
1975 Indian and White: Self-Image and Interaction in a Canadian Plains Community. Stanford: Stanford University Press.
Brody, H.
1975 The People's Land: Eskimos and Whites in the Eastern Arctic. Middlesex: Penguin Books Ltd.
Brown, H.
1980 Identity, Politics and Planning: On Some Uses of Knowledge in Coping with Social Change. In G. V. Coelho and P. I. Ahmed (eds.), Uprooting and Development: Dilemmas of Coping with Modernization. New York: Plenun Press, pp. 41—66.
Carstairs, G. M. and R. L. Kapur
1976 The Great Universe of Kota: Stress, Change and Mental Disorder in an Indian Village. Berkeley: University of California Press.
Cassel, J.
1974 Psychosocial Processes and Stress: Theoretical Formulations. International Journal of Health Services 4: 471—482.
Chance, N.
1965 Acculturation, Self-Identification and Personality Adjustment. American Anthropologist, 67: 372—373.
Dacks, Gurston
1981 A Choice of Futures: Politics in the Canadian North. Toronto: Methuen.
Despres, L. A. (ed.)
1975 Ethnicity and Resource Competition in Plural Societies. The Hague: Mouton.
Dohrenwend, B. S. and B. P. Dohrenwend
1981 Stressful Life Events and Their Contexts. New York: Prodist.
Dressler, W.
1982 Hypertension and Culture Change: Acculturation and Disease in the West Indies. South Salem, N.Y.: Redgrave Publishing Co.
Erikson, E. H.
1968 Identity: Youth and Crisis. New York: W. W. Norton and Co. Inc.
Foner, N.
1984 Ages in Conflict: A Cross-Cultural Perspective on Inequality Between Old and Young. New York: Columbia University Press.
Gellner, E.
1979 Spectacles and Predicaments. Cambridge: Cambridge University Press.
Graburn, N. H. H.
1978 Inuit Pivalliajut: The Cultural and Identity Consequences of the Commercialization of Canadian Inuit Art. In L. Muller-Wille et al. (eds.), Consequences of Economic Change in Circumpolar Regions. Boreal Institute for Northern Studies. Occasional Publication #14, pp. 185—200.
1981 1, 2, 3, 4 . . . Anthropology and the Fourth World. Culture, 1(1): 66—70.
Graves, T. D. and N. B. Graves
1979 Stress and Health: Modernization in a Traditional Polynesian Society. Medical Anthropology 3: 23—59.
Hannerz, U.
1980 Exploring the City. New York: Columbia University Press.
Hechter, Michael
1975 Internal Colonialism: The Celtic Fringe in British National Development, 1536—1966, London. Routledge and Kegan Paul.
Hicks, G. L. and P. E. Leis (eds.)
1977 Ethnic Ecounters: Identities and Contexts. North Scituate, Mass.: Duxbury Press.

Holmes, T. H. and R. Rahe
  1967 The Social Readjustment Rating Scale. Journal of Psychosomatic Medicine 11: 213—218.
Holy, L. and M. Stuchlik
  1983 Actions, Norms and Representations: Foundations for an Anthropological Inquiry. Cambridge: Cambridge University Press.
Honigmann, J. J.
  1965 Eskimo Townsmen. Ottawa: Canadian Research Centre for Anthropology.
Isaacs, H. R.
  1975 Idols of the Tribe: Group Identity and Political Change. New York: Harper and Row.
Keith, Jennie
  1980 The Best is Yet To Be: Toward an Anthropology of Age. Annual Review of Anthropology 9: 339—64.
Lazurus, R. S.
  1981 The Stress and Coping Paradigm. In C. Eisdorfer et al. (eds.), Models for Clinical Psychopathology. New York: Spectrum Publications.
Leighton, A. H.
  1959 My Name is Legion: Foundations for a Theory of Man in Relation to Culture (Stirling Country Study of Psychiatric Disorder and Sociocultural Environment, 1). New York: Basic Books.
Lubart, J. M.
  1969 Psychodynamic Problems of Adaptation — MacKenzie Delta Eskimos. Ottawa: Department of Indian Affairs and Northern Development.
Macmillan, A. M.
  1957 The Health Opinion Survey: Technique for Estimating Prevalence of Psychoneurotic and Related types of Disorder in Communities. Psychological Reports 3: 325—339.
Marmot, M., and Syme, S. L.
  1976 Acculturation and Coronary Heart Disease in Japanese-Americans. American Journal of Epidemiology 104: 225—247.
McElroy, A.
  1975 Canadian Arctic Modernization and Change in Female Inuit Role Identification. American Ethnologist 2—4: 662—686.
Murphy, J. M.
  1973 Sociocultural Change and Psychiatric Disorder Among Rural Yorubas in Nigeria. Ethos 1: 239—262.
Ness, R.
  1977 Modernization and Illness in a Newfoundland Community. Medical Anthropology 1(4): 25—53.
Nydegger, C.
  1981 On Being Caught Up in Time. Human Development 24(11): 1—13.
O'Neil, J. D.
  1984 Is it Cool to be an Eskimo?: A Study of Stress, Identity, Coping and Health Among Canadian Inuit Young Adult Men. Ph.D. thesis, University of California (San Francisco/Berkeley).
  1985 Self-Determination and Inuit Youth: Coping with Stress in the Canadian North. In R. Fortuine (ed.), Circumpolar Health '84. Seattle: University of Washington Press.
Paine, R. (ed.)
  1977 The White Arctic: Anthropological Essays on Tutelage and Ethnicity. Newfoundland Social and Economic Papers No. 7. Toronto: University of Toronto Press.
Parker, S.
  1962 Eskimo Psychopathology in the Context of Eskimo Personality and Culture. Ameri-

can Anthropologist 64: 76—95.

Reed, D., D. Labarthe, and R. Stallone
1970 Health Effects of Westernization and Migration Among Chamorroo. American
      Journal of Epidemiology 92: 94—112.

Rodgers, D. D.
1982 Suicide in the Canadian Northwest Territories, 1970—1980. *In* B. Harvald and J. P.
      Hart-Hansen (eds.), Circumpolar Health 81, Nordic Council for Arctic Medical
      Research Report, Series 33.

Savishinsky, J. S.
1974 The Trail of the Hare: Life and Stress in an Arctic Community. New York: Gordon
      and Breach.

Scotch, N. A.
1963 Sociocultural Factors in the Epidemiology of Zulu Health. American Journal of
      Public Health, 53: 1205—1213.

Seltzer, Allan
1980 Acculturation and Mental Disorder in the Inuit. Canadian Journal of Psychiatry
      25(2): 173—81.

Selye, H.
1956 Stress of Life. New York: McGraw-Hill.

Tyroler, H. A. and J. Cassell
1974 Health Consequences of Culture Change II: The Effect of Urbanization on Coro-
      nary Heart Disease in Rural Residents. Journal of Chronic Disease 17: 167.

Velez-Ibanez, C. E.
1983 Rituals of Marginality: Politics, Process and Culture Change in Urban Central
      Mexico, 1969—1974. Berkeley: University of California Press.

Wolf, E.
1983 Europe and the People Without History. Berkeley: University of Califonira Press.

Young, Allan
1980 The Discourse on Stress and the Reproduction of Conventional Knowledge. Social
      Science and Medicine 14B: 133—146.

RON STALL

RESPONDENT-IDENTIFIED REASONS FOR CHANGE AND STABILITY IN ALCOHOL CONSUMPTION AS A CONCOMITANT OF THE AGING PROCESS

INTRODUCTION

It has become commonplace to point out that the proportion and raw numbers of the elderly in the United States will continue to increase until the midpoint of the next century (e.g., Hauser 1976). Current experience suggests that future senior citizens will demand a proportion of health care expenditures far in excess of their actual percentage of the population, thus creating a formidable socio-medical problem (Shanas and Maddox 1976). In order to continue to provide an adequate level of health care for America's aged of the 21st century, health care strategies designed specifically to meet the needs of the elderly — including effective preventive health components — must be developed and implemented.

The efforts to design effective preventive health care strategies are complicated by the fact that behavioral factors have been implicated in the etiologies of the diseases expected to be most prevalent among the future elderly. Certain behavioral factors important to the etiologies of serious disease states (e.g. smoking) have proven to be intractable in the face of intervention efforts and, as of yet, the most effective strategies for the prevention of such behaviors are poorly understood.

One behavioral risk factor implicated in disease causation among the elderly is that of alcohol use. It is a well-known fact that heavy alcohol use has been implicated as a risk factor for tuberculosis, a range of cardiovascular problems, trauma, suicide, lung cancer, oesophageal varices, alcoholic cirrhosis, and brain cancer (e.g. Brenner 1967; Schmidt and de Lint 1972; Costello 1974; Schmidt and Popham 1975; Robinette, Hrubel, and Fraumeni 1978), not to mention the severe psychological and socio-economic problems which often accompany heavy levels of alcohol use by an older person. However, it is less widely recognized that a body of cross-sectional alcohol use studies among non-institutionalized American samples have provided consistent evidence suggesting that a significant decrease in alcohol consumption, alcohol-related problems and alcoholism occurs after middle age. This consistent finding may suggest that a "maturational" or "remission" process is at work among aging drinkers. If remission of alcohol-related problems is typical of many aging Americans, interesting epidemiological and health policy questions emerge. These questions include: What factors contribute to a decrease in alcohol consumption and alcohol-related problems after late middle age? Once such "natural" factors for decrease in alcohol use with aging are identified, could intervention efforts be designed to take advantage

275

Craig R. Janes et al. (eds.), Anthropology and Epidemiology, 275—301.
© 1986 *by D. Reidel Publishing Company.*

of "natural" factors for decrease among aging heavy drinkers who continue to drink problematically in later life? How powerful of an effect do decreases in alcohol consumption during later life have on decreasing the burden of disease among the elderly?

This chapter is principally concerned with respondent-identified reasons for change in alcohol-related behaviors during the second half of the life course. This topic is addressed in relation to the analysis of a 19-year prospective study of change and stability in alcohol use. The prospective data generated by this research project were useful in determining proportionate change (or stability) in alcohol consumption, but could not be used to determine the reasons behind such change or stability. Since the small sample size at follow-up precluded multivariate prediction of drinking outcomes, it was decided to consider respondents' own explanations for change or stability. Combined with the prospective findings, the analysis of respondent-identified reasons for change provides a rich source of data from which exploratory hypotheses concerning alcohol-related behaviors during the second half of life might be developed. It is hoped that future research concerning alcohol use patterns during the latter half of life (based in part of the testing of hypotheses suggested here) will allow the construction of informed health policy and prevention guidelines concerning alcohol use among aging populations.

Parenthetically, long-term prospective alcohol use research designs can be usefully employed to provide further insights concerning processes of social aging. In particular, this focus is amenable to the study of changes that occur in recreational or "time out" behavior over the second half of the life course (e.g. MacAndrew and Edgerton 1969: 83—99). Alcohol use is generally relevant to many dimensions of an individual's life: a behavior expressive of relaxed intimacy, a seal for a new social bond, a ritualized courtesy denoting a cordial business relationship, a means of announcing celebration, or a tonic to salve a one's own or a friend's troubles. The study of alcohol use over the life course can thus contribute to the construction of a portrait of an informant's social networks, how the respondent has built a social identity, occupational life, and the quality and forms of social relationships. How such issues change or stay the same as individuals experience the aging process is of great interest in the further construction of aging theory. That is, the study of changing alcohol use contexts can perhaps tell us a great deal about the processes of social aging as well as of the processes of changing alcohol use patterns. Although a literature has emerged within the field of gerontology which addresses such issues (e.g. particularly in regard to the controversies surrounding the "activity" and "disengagement" theories), this literature might be augmented through the use of a relatively unique "window", such as might be obtained through the study of alcohol use patterns over time, on how the social lives of persons change in the face of the aging process. Thus, the study of change and stability in alcohol use patterns over long periods of time is of interest to both the social and health sciences.

ALCOHOL USE AND AGING: A REVIEW

Despite the etiological importance of alcohol use in the distribution of health and disease patterns among the aged, alcohol use among American elderly is an understudied topic. Furthermore, the retrospective, cross-sectional and prospective designs used to study alcohol use and aging have generated relatively divergent pictures of age-related alcohol use changes. Yet, a careful consideration and integration of findings from these three research designs is necessary if we are to further our understandings of the natural history of alcohol use and abuse across the life course.

Retrospective designs have been used to generate a typology of the elderly who manifest problems in their consumption of alcohol, i.e. the early-onset and late-onset geriatric problem drinker (Droller 1964; Glatt and Rosin 1964; Bahr 1969; Glatt 1978). Each of the projects cited share similiar design shortcomings, i.e. an exclusive reliance on clinical or atypical drinking populations, a heavy reliance on informant or significant-other retrospective reports, and (with the exception of the Bahr 1969 report) the use of opportunistic or convenience sampling techniques. The documentation of significant differences along psychological and social measures between early-and late-onset elderly problem drinkers has also been replicated in research which has employed retrospective designs among more typical populations of the elderly (e.g., Abelson and van der Spuy 1978; Foulds and Hassall 1969). Further, Zimberg (1974) reports that the early and late-onset problem drinking dichotomy is of use in intervention efforts designed to modify the alcohol consumption of elderly drinkers. An important implication of this literature, however, is that significant numbers of elderly first experience drinking problems in later life and that these problems may be related to the special circumstances of the aged.

The vast majority of the research relevant to considerations of alcohol use across the life course has adopted a cross-sectional research design. This body of literature allows the estimation of the prevalence of varying levels of alcohol use and alcohol-related problems across age strata, and these rates are customarily reported. In the way of a general summary statement, cross-sectional or prevalence surveys among the non-institutionalized elderly have generated comparatively low prevalence rates of problem drinking or alcoholism. A key word in the previous sentence is "comparatively", for the problem drinking or alcoholism prevalence rates for those persons past the age of 65 appear to be significantly lower than the rates generated for younger cohorts.

Three classic studies are of particular interest to the alcohol use and aging literature. These research projects have served to independently replicate each other, despite the use of inconsistent measurement and sampling techniques and application of these divergent methodologies to distinct populations. For example, Knupfer and Room (1964) reported the results of a survey of a sample of 1,268 San Francisco adults interviewed in 1962. By decades of age, the prevalence of heavy drinking steadily decreased from 39% among males aged 21—19 to 19% for those men 60 years of age and older. Conversely, the proportion of abstainers increased from 13% of the men aged 21—29 to 32% of the older men. Cohort effects (both for the older and younger cohorts), decreased stress for the aged, attenuated social networks, and increase in health concerns for the elderly were suggested by Knupfer and Room as important to this decreasing pattern of alcohol consumption with aging.

Johnson (1974) measured the frequency of drinking occasions of persons aged 65 in a multi-ethnic and lower-class district of Manhattan. Johnson's research is unusual in that she reported factors associated with alcohol use along with measures of the social and psychological realms of the informant's lives. Based on a random household survey of 169 elderly in this district, Johnson found that approximately half of the informants were abstainers. The prevalence of heavy drinking was quite low, approximately 1.2%. Poor health, being a woman, and being a Spanish-speaker were associated with lighter and less frequent drinking patterns.

Barnes' (1979) description of the drinking habits of a stratified random sample ($n = 1041$) of Buffalo, New York adults is notable in that she attempted to test specific hypotheses concerning the relationships between processes of social aging and drinking habits. Consistent with other research reported here, Barnes found a general decrease in quantity/frequency drinking scores and a concomitant increase in abstention with increasing age (for example, heavy drinkers amount to 24% of men aged 50—59, 10% aged 60—69, and 4% above the age of 70). The notion that bereavement — especially that associated with widowhood — is a significant factor for high alcohol consumption in old age was tested by Barnes. She found that heavy drinking was actually more prevalent among the married (3% widowed, 10% married). Elderly male widowers and married men did not differ significantly in heavy drinking rates (17% married, 14% widowers). A test of the "retirement hypothesis" — that the cessation (or "disengagement from") a career predisposes to heavy alcohol use among men also yielded results which contradicted commonly-held perceptions concerning alcohol use and aging. Among the men over 60, heavy drinkers were twice as likely to be found among the employed (12%) than the unemployed/retired (6%). Interestingly, for the men aged 50—59, of whom those not working were generally unemployed and not voluntarily retired, the reverse pattern obtained (heavy drinking among the unemployed 71%; heavy drinking among the employed males, 36%). Sex differences in drinking habit distributions were pronounced, females exhibiting the same general time trends as the males, but for whom heavy drinking was so rare as to virtually disappear after the age of 60. A series of national random household probablity samples taken during the 1960s (i.e. Cahalan et al. 1969; Cahalan 1970; Cahalan and Room 1974) have largely replicated the findings concerning alcohol use and aging from the cross-sectional studies described above.

Despite the importance of long-term prospective research to the study of aging and alcohol-related problems, few such projects have been attempted. The bulk of the prospective research projects (e.g., Cahalan 1970; Clark and Cahalan 1976; Orford and Edwards 1977; and Polich et al. 1981) are of such short time frames that they are of limited use in understanding the relationship between alcohol use and aging processes. Longer-term prospective studies have been primarily concerned with change in alcohol use patterns from youth to middle age (e.g., Fillmore et al. 1979) and so cannot be generalized to processes of aging and alcohol use. Other long-term panel studies of possible relevance to the study of alcohol use and aging report data from populations whose lifestyle is a wide variance to populations of elders living in the U.S. (e.g., Öjesjö 1980; 1981). The Glynn et al. (1983) report documented considerable stability in quantity of alcohol use among older men over time, but also noted that if men over the age of 59 changed alcohol use patterns they were significantly more likely to decrease use than increase use. One report (Schuckit et al. 1980) has attempted to analyze three year prospective data from institutionalized repondents in such a way as to provide estimates of the incidence of alcohol-related problems in old age (5% for a 3 year period).

In summary, cross-sectional surveys of general, non-institutionalized elderly yield much lower prevalence rates of alcohol-related problems than those generated for younger age levels. Retrospective data, however, suggest that a sizable percentage of geriatric problem drinkers first experience alcohol-related problems in old age. One prospective report which describes a non-institutionalized sample found considerable stability in quantity of use over time among aging drinkers, but also supported the cross-sectional findings in that if men changed alcohol consumption over time they were likely to decrease use. The weight of evidence from this literature, then, can be interpreted to suggest that important decreases in heavy alcohol consumption and related problems occur in conjunction with the aging process among American populations. Despite the considerable health policy and theoretical implications of the study of decreases in alcohol consumption and related-problems, no research has been attempted which explores the reasons reported by aging drinkers, themselves, for any increased or decrease in alcohol use as a concomitant of the aging process.

METHODOLOGY

The primary focus of this chapter is on retrospective data concerning the reasons given by respondents for change in their alcohol use habits over time. These retrospective data were collected as part of a larger 19 year prospective study of change in alcohol use habits. In order to investigate such changes, a sample of San Francisco adult white males aged 30—69 interviewed in 1964 ($n = 246$) was selected for reinterviewing. Follow-up of this sample occurred during the summer and fall of 1983 — a 19 year period during which members of the sample moved towards "old" age.

Upon follow-up, 85 of the 246 respondents first contacted in 1964 were successfully reinterviewed.[1] To test for the possibility of loss to follow-up bias in this research, the 1983 respondents were compared to the 1964 sample of white males between 30—69 along the variables of age, number of reasons for drinking, income, education, religion, and a series of alcohol consumption measures (including quantity, frequency and a quantity-frequency measure). Of these only the distributions of age (due to the loss of the older respondents to death) and education (due to the inordinate loss to follow-up of men with less than a high school education) were significantly different between the 85 reinterviewed men and the entire sub-sample.

Age distributions for the sub-sample were between 30—69 in 1964 and thus these men were aged 49—88 in 1983. The modal age range from the sample in 1983 was between 59—68, with the majority of the sample (67%) in their sixties or older.

Respondents at both waves were asked a series of items which measured typical frequency and quantity of drinking. That is, respondents were asked how often they typically drank as well as the typical number of drinks that they took when they did drink. These measures were multiplied to generate an estimate of the previous year's number of drinks, which was divided by 365 for an estimate of the typical daily number of drinks. These data are presented in categories (e.g., 2.01 to 3 drinks per day) to summarize how alcohol consumption changed or stayed the same over a 19 year period of time in Table I and II. The chi square tests reported here were performed on the categorized data; the matched t-test on the uncollapsed continuous data.

The respondents for the 1983 wave of interview were also asked a set of open-ended retrospective questions regarding reasons for change or stability in alcohol consumption from 1964 to 1983. First, men were asked whether they thought that their alcohol use had changed at all. If the response was positive, then they were asked whether they had increased or decreased drinking. Finally, these men were asked why they thought their alcohol use had changed. If an informant felt that his alcohol use had been stable over the years, he was also asked a set of open-ended questions which elicited his reasons for stability. The attempt was made to elicit four reasons for change or stability over time; some respondents were able to identify four such reasons while most (58%) were not.

The respondents' reasons for change and stability were coded according to their own categories, which were later grouped according to a set of larger categories imposed by the author (e.g., "social", "health", "stress", etc. reasons for change). Both the respondents' and the author's categories are given in Table III—V, the author's categories being italicized.

Originally it was thought possible to compare statistically the men who decreased, were stable, or increased alcohol consumption according to the larger categories imposed by the author. However, an examination of the content of the respondents' reasons for stability and change makes it clear that such tests are not possible. That is, even in the case where a larger category is present for both the increasers and decreasers (e.g. social reasons), the specific social factors that prompted an increase in use are so different from those that prompted a decrease that comparison of proportions of the larger categories is clearly not appropriate. Description and analysis of the reasons that these men gave for change and stability in alcohol use will therefore proceed independently according to whether they increased, decreased or were stable over time. In the discussion of individual cases, professional affiliations and other identifying characteristics have been altered to protect respondents' anonymity.

FINDINGS

Prospective Analysis of Change and Stability in Mean Number of Drinks Per Day

Analysis of change and stability in mean number of drinks per day will focus on the aggregrate (presented in Table I) and individual (presented in Table II) levels. The aggregate analysis will compare the prevalences of varying levels of mean number of daily drinks in 1964 and 1983. For this analysis it is important to clarify the differences between the "two" 1964 samples. The 1964a sample ($n = 246$) consists of all the white males interviewed in 1964 between the ages of 30 and 69; the 1964b sample ($n = 85$) reports Time I data drawn from the men interviewed in 1964 and 1983. Comparison of the 1964a and 1964b samples allows consideration of the possible effects of loss the follow-up bias. Comparison of the 1964b and 1983 samples allows the consideration of change in alcohol consumption over time. The 1964b and 1983 samples will be referred to collectively as the "follow-up" or "longitudinal" samples. The individual analysis will examine patterns in individual drinking outcomes and the incidence, remission and chronicity in daily drinking levels.

Table I presents the frequency distributions for mean daily number of drinks for 1964 and 1983. When specific frequency levels for mean daily number of drinks are collapsed, only small diferences are apparent between the 1964a and 1964b samples. The frequency distributions for mean daily number of drinks were collapsed into three categories: 3.01 or more drinks

TABLE I

Mean daily number of drinks; 1964 and 1983 frequency distributions; by absolute frequency and percentages

	1964a	1964b	1983
8.01 or more drinks	4.5% (11)	2.4% (2)	0% (0)
4.01—8 drinks	8.1% (20)	4.7% (4)	10.6% (9)
3.01—4 drinks	11.4% (28)	14.1% (12)	9.4% (8)
3.01 or more drinks	*24.0% (59)*	*21.2% (18)*	*20.0% (17)*
2.01—3 drinks	3.7% (9)	3.5% (3)	2.4% (2)
1.51—2 drinks	14.6% (36)	10.6% (9)	18.8% (16)
1.01—1.5 drinks	8.1% (20)	10.6% (9)	5.9% (5)
1 to 3 drinks	*26.4% (65)*	*24.7% (21)*	*27.1% (23)*
0.51 to 1 drink	9.8% (24)	9.4% (8)	10.6% (9)
0.01 to 0.5 drink	30.5% (75)	35.3% (30)	21.2% (18)
Abstainer or no drinks during the past year	9.3% (23)	9.4% (8)	21.2% (18)
0 to 1 drink	*49.6% (122)*	*54.1% (46)*	*53.0% (45)*
Total	100% (246)	100% (85)	100.1% (85)

per day, the "heavy" drinkers; 1.01 to 3 drinks per day, the "moderate" drinkers; and 1 or less drinks per day, the "light" drinkers. These categories will also be employed in the presentation of individual change over time. The lack of difference between the 1964a and 1964b samples indicates that loss to follow-up bias is not an important consideration in the analysis of this variable. A chi-square test of independence between the 1964a and 1964b samples was insignificant.

A comparison the collapsed mean daily drinking levels reveals very little change in the longitudinal sample. The ratios of each of the collapsed drinking categories in the longitudinal sample approach 1, indicating a high degree of stability in aggregate alcohol consumption among these men over time. The one level of drinking where important changes appear to have occurred was among the abstainers: the men in this sample were 2.3 times more likely to be abstainers in 1983 as in 1964.

The exploration of individual change over time within the longitudinal sample is summarized in Table II. This analysis employs the same collapsed levels of mean daily drinks as were defined in Table I. Table II distinguished those individuals who have exhibited change from those who showed no change at follow-up. The underlined diagonal row of three cells contains the individuals who have been stable in their alcohol use over the years. The three cells in the bottom left corner contain information concerning those

TABLE II

Change in mean daily number of drinks; longitudinal sample; absolute frequencies and row percentages

	1983 Mean number of daily drinks			
	Light	Moderate	Heavy	Total
1964b Mean				
Light	<u>32</u> 69.6%	8 17.4%	6 13.0%	46 100%
Moderate	7 33.3%	<u>9</u> 42.9%	5 23.8%	21 100%
Heavy	6 33.3%	6 33.3%	<u>6</u> 33.3%	18 99.9%
Total				85 100%

individuals who have increased daily mean number of drinks at Time 2; similarly the three top right hand corner cells describe those individuals who decreased alcohol consumption over time. The top line of each cell gives the absolute frequency for each cell, the second line the percentage figure of the row total (a measure of continuity and change from the Time I drinking level). The marginal figures give the combined absolute frequencies and row totals.

It can be seen that general stability in the number of mean daily drinks, as indicated by the underlined figures in Table II, is the dominant pattern over time. 55.3% (47) of the men in this sample fall into this category. However, it should also be pointed out that of the men who were stable across time the majority (68%) were at the lowest drinking level. Of the men who changed alcohol consumption over time, equal numbers of men increased as decreased use. A paired T-test conducted within the longitudinal sample proved to be insignificant.

Continuity of drinking (as measured by the row percentages) was greatest among the light drinkers. That is, nearly 70% of the light drinkers remained at that level at follow-up, while only a third of the heavy drinkers continued drinking at that level. The Time 2 level of drinking was most difficult to predict among the moderate drinkers — approximately a third of the moderate drinkers decreased use, 43% stayed the same, and 24% increased use. The Time 1 heavy drinkers were very likely to decrease consumption over the follow-up period — 2/3rds of the original heavy drinkers decreased consumption by Time 2.

By way of a summary statement, dramatic changes were noted in neither the aggregrate nor the individual prospective analysis of mean daily number of drinks. Collapsed categories of the aggregate data yielded ratios approximating I within the longitudinal sample. Similarly, the dominant pattern of alcohol use over time, as measured at the individual level, was one of stability. Continuity of drinking was greatest among the light drinkers, the heavy drinkers being highly likely to decreased mean number of daily drinks over time. It should be emphasized, however, that when quantity of consumption and frequency of consumption are analysed separately, significant decreases are found in quantity of use. It appears that when summary measures are employed to explore change over time, stability of frequency of use masks important changes in quantity of use (Stall 1986).

It should also be stressed that the documentation of general stability in mean daily number of drinks is largely due to the continuity of the light drinkers. Two-thirds of the heavy drinkers cut back consumption over the years — a finding which replicates the consistent cross-sectional finding of decreases in heavy consumption at the older age levels.

The general impressions to be gained from the prospective analysis are, however, in some contrast to the respondents' retrospective impressions of their patterns of alcohol use over time.[2] That is, as shown below, approximately 18% of the men claimed an increase in consumption, 27% claimed stability, and 55% claimed a decrease in alcohol consumption over the years. In short, it would appear that the retrospective measures of change exaggerate decrease at the expense of stability, at least according to the impression derived from the prospective measures. Since the majority of the men who were stable were drawn from the ranks of light and moderate drinkers, one working assumption might be that this overstatement of declining use occured among the lighter, stable drinkers. These men may have been inclined to perceive themselves as moderating their alcohol use over the years, while, in fact remaining relatively stable. An equally compelling explanation of this dissonance, however, would be that agreement between the prospective and retrospective mesures could be achieved were a summary score which incorporates quantity, frequency, most quantity and number of alcohol-related problems employed in a test of agreement. Clearly, both hypotheses are of great methodological interest, but are beyond the definitional bounds of this chapter.

Regardless of the agreement between the cross-sectional, prospective and retrospective findings, it is clear that some men in the longitudinal sample increased consumption over time, most of the men were generally stable in their use of alcohol, and some men decreased use. These important differences in drinking outcomes are of great theoretical and treatment interest, yet the small sample size precludes the use of sophisticated statistical techniques to determine the social and psychological predictors of these three distinct outcomes. Furthermore, few hypotheses have been proposed to explain differential drinking outcomes in later life and so hypothesis generation would have to proceed within a theoretical vacuum. Given the limitations of the available prospective data bases as well as the scientific literature concerning alcohol use and aging, the understandings held by these men for the reasons behind their change and stability in drinking over the years are thus quite valuable. The perceptions formed by these men for the reasons why their alcohol use changed or stayed that same can serve as important clues to initial hypothesis generation and contribute to theory building. The balance of this chapter is an analysis of the reasons, given by these men themselves, for change and stability in alcohol use as a concomitant of the aging process.

Retrospective Reasons Given for Increase in Drinking over Time

Table III summarizes the 42 reasons given by 15 men for why they thought their alcohol use increased from 1964 to 1983.

The men who claimed an increase in use of alcohol gave an average of about three reasons for their change in consumption. That is, although most of the following discussion is in terms of specific reasons for increased drinking, most of these men had more than one reason for increasing use. This fact also explains respondent-indentified reasons for increase which are not entirely exclusive. For example, one of the retired respondents has increased frequency of alcohol use to include lunchtime drinking since he no longer has to be on the job in the afternoon. He also mentioned that since he retired he has a great deal more leisure time, part of which he spends in long poker games which includes some alcohol use. Further, since his children are all now self-supporting he has more money and time for activities that include drinking. So this informant has increased his drinking due to a combination of increased leisure time, a reaction to retirement, maturation of the nuclear family, and finances.

Although most of the social reasons for increased drinking are straight-forward, some of these reasons merit further discussion. The first of these concerns increased drinking within respondent's social networks. For example, one of the respondents became romantically linked with "an alcoholic" about ten years ago. He became intensely involved before he realized that his friend drank at a dangerous level. To his alarm, he has become increasingly aware that, over the years, he has approximated his friend's alcohol consumption rather than serving as a moderating effect on his friend's drinking. They socialize with another, rather wealthy couple, and he admitted that it was not uncommon for the four of them to be forcibly evicted from restaurants. One of the group recently lost his driver's license due to driving while intoxicated and another a job due to drinking. The respondent recently decided that he has become an alcoholic and is in the process of trying to get his friend to quit drinking as well. This is a delicate procedure for the respondent. Although he highly values the relationship he feels that the

TABLE III

Respondents' reasons for increased use of alcohol from 1964 to 1983, frequency distributions

Social

1. Financial situation	4
2. Increased drinking within social networks	7
3. Maturation of nuclear family	5
4. Increased use part of job	2
5. Reaction to retirement	2
6. More leisure time	6
Total	26 (62%)

Stress

7. Increased psychological stress	3
Total	3 (7%)

Health

8. Health concerns, M.D. Orders to drink more	2
9. Reaction to chronic pain	2
10. Incapacitated in 1964, now can drink	2
Total	6 (14%)

Change in style of drinking

11. Change in type of alcohol, e.g. wine to vodka	1
12. Increase to daily use	4
13. Has become alcoholic	2
Total	7 (17%)
TOTAL RESPONSES	42 (100%)

relationship will not survive the shock of both of them ceasing to drink. Does he give up a 10-year relationship or keep drinking at a level he presumes to be dangerous to his health? As a contingency he has taken to only drinking white wine during the week, and then keeping up with his friend's vodka consumption during the weekends. He also said that he plans to get professional help to cut down on his drinking in the near future. Other, less dramatic, examples of the influences of social network drinking patterns on respondents' drinking can also be found in this series of interviews.

A second process of interest to the increasing use of alcohol across the life span is the maturation of the nuclear family. One informant, currently a wealthy lawyer, exemplifies this pattern. He mentioned that at the first interview he and his wife were quite preoccupied with raising their four children and were strapped financially, as are most families with young children. Even if they had the money to provide alcoholic beverages while entertaining, most of their friends were also just starting their families and finding the freedom to drink beyond strict moderation was difficult under these circumstances. Now, however, all of his children either are independent or in college, and the respondent and his wife have both the time and the money to engage in social activities that involve heavier drinking. A second informant also appears to have had his alcohol intake influenced over the years by the maturation of his family, but expressed this influence in terms of finances. Although not a wealthy man, he felt it best if he paid to have his children sent to parochial school instead of public school. This was an enormous drain on his budget and now that his children are independent he has money for luxuries such as alcohol.

The lawyer described above can also be cited as an example of another factor for increasing alcohol use over time. This is the increasing likelihood of having alcohol use become an important part of one's career as promotions occur. This man pointed out that when he was a junior partner he brought his lunch in a brown paper bag and ate while he worked. Now he is expected to entertain clients at posh private clubs as part of a typical business negotiation, and alcohol is invariably part of the meal. As a moderating factor he also mentioned that while he certainly enjoys drinking, he has to be careful in his position never to overdo it.

Another social process of interest to increasing alcohol use is that of adjustment to retirement. One man, formerly a high-level bank executive, has noticed a distinct increase in his alcohol use since retirement. He has taken informal steps to decrease his use, in part because of his wife's concerns. He feels that retirement has definitely increased the potential for alcohol use because he is socializing more, there is less pressure in his life and he has become more indulgent with himself. He mentioned that retired men are more prone to "enjoy themselves, kick back, and enjoy the fruits of their labor". Enjoying the rewards of retirement, for this man, includes alcohol use. Another informant feels that he is drinking more as a reaction to retirement since he has become completely bored since he quit working. As he put it, "Society pushes you aside. You are an old man, go away". His drinking, he claims, is due to the lack of a social life and of recreational activities rather than to any increase in leisure and social life.

On informant's experiences over the years illustrates how psychological stress and chronic pain can increase alcohol use. This man recently retired from the Navy, but spent much of the last 20 years in the Bay Area. He mentioned that his family had many problems during the 1960s and 1970s — one son became a drug addict and another was hospitalized numerous times over the years for a psychological problem. At one point this Navy officer and his family returned home to a stripped house — the furniture had been taken to pay for their son's drugs. During this period of heavy psychological stress for the respondent, he seriously injured his back which has placed him in continuous pain. He found that the pain medications didn't work particularly well unless combined with a few drinks. This effect, he discovered, soon wore off which necessitated the use of larger amounts of alcohol to cut his back pain. Over the years he has been able to sort out his family problems, but now has found that with retirement he has lost contact with old friends. He has found trying to construct a new social life for himself quite stressful. He is now worried about his alcohol intake and fears having nothing to do in his retirement. As he put it, "Guys who have more time and don't have anything to do, go down to a bar. They talk about baseball and soon they are real heavy alcoholics. They are just looking for companionship. Where else are they to go?".

Health concerns were also mentioned by another two men as a factor in their increased drinking. One informant was diagnosed as hypertensive shortly after he started a very stressful job. His physician suggested that when he arrived home after work, he lock himself in his study, mix himself a drink, lay on the floor and listen to music for 30 minutes as "relaxation therapy" for hypertension. Now, he mixes himself a drink or two before dinner, ". . . like Pavlov's dog, it has become a habit. It goes good with food." This respondent has since become quite interested in health matters and has continued to explore ways to fight stress in his life. He also jogs and takes vitamins. He did express some concern about his alcohol use, however. As he put it, "I've knocked off salt, caffeine, nicotine, and I'm almost ready to get rid of alcohol, too".

Retrospective Reasons Given for Stability in Drinking over Time

Table IV summarizes the 64 reasons why 23 men felt that their alcohol use had been stable from Time 1 to Time 2.

The men who claimed stability from 1964 to 1983 gave an average of approximately three reasons for their stability in alcohol use over time. As with the men who had increased use, although these reasons are discussed separately, the reader should keep in mind that these men were generally able to identify more than one reason for not changing over time. Respondent-identified reasons for stability may not always be mutually exclusive.

The most frequently stated explanation given by these men for stable consumption was that no reason had emerged over the years to force change. As one of the men put it, "I never drank so why should I start? That's not a good answer, but there are certain things in your life that you just don't change. Certain doctors have told me I'd be smart to take a drink with my wife, but I tell them I can't live forever. Also they told me to stop my coffee in the morning. I said that they can admit me to the hospital and that's when it will stop. The question is, do you drink or don't you drink? I don't." Another man expressed a similar opinion: "Why should it change? Nothing has happened. My pattern was set years ago. And I don't drink to cope with

TABLE IV

Respondents' reasons for stability in drinking from 1964 to 1983, frequency distributions

No reason to change	
1. No reason to change	23
2. Increase in use not enjoyable	7
Total	30 (47%)
Social	
3. "Significant other" intervention	2
4. Early socialization	4
5. No social pressure to drink	2
6. Religious beliefs	2
7. Structure of life prevents change	2
Total	12 (19%)
Fear of problems	
8. Health concerns	6
9. Strong dislike of alcohol-related problems	5
10. Former problem drinker, quit before 1964	1
Total	12 (19%)
Psychological	
11. Stable personality	7
12. Doesn't like taste of alcohol	1
Total	8 (13%)
Change in style, not intake	
13. Changed type of alcohol, not total intake	1
14. Eliminated spree drinking, increased daily use	1
Total	2 (3%)
TOTAL RESPONSES	64 (100%)

problems — when I have a problem I don't dwell on it. I don't take my problems to bed with me at night. Nothing has occurred to change it."

Of the social reasons for stability, two men mentioned that "significant other" support was important to their stability. By this they meant that individuals close to them would intervene if they began drinking at a dramatically heavier level. This was expressed succinctly by the man who exclaimed of heavy drinkers that his wife would "kill him" if he drank as much as they did.

Most of the men who cited early socialization experience as a factor in their stability were abstainers, and many of these men cited religious reasons for their abstinence. Many of these individuals had strong statements to make of their concerns of the "glamorization" of alcohol on television as well as in everyday business and social life.

A stable personality type and stable life structure were attributed by one individual as causal in his ability to keep his drinking patterns over the years. As he put it, "I'm a stable person. Around this office I'm known as 'Mr. Consistent' among my peers. While there are occasions where there is reason to drink, there is always the constant reminder that you have to keep your wits about you. The best CPA's are stable and that's the people with whom I live."

Another man indicated that he consciously structured his life so that he was not expected to drink to excess. He declined to go into business for himself because he did not want to have to entertain business clients on a regular basis. He said that he did not mind paying for clients' drinks when he put it on his employer's tab, but if he was expected to drink with his clients during lunch, then he was annoyed. He felt that having a drink was an inescapable part of being an independent businessman and so he was better suited to remain as an employee of a large business firm.

Six men indicated that they feared health problems if they drank at a higher level. Although these fears were rarely stated in specific terms, these men generally felt that alcohol use beyond light levels was not especially good for health. Five men indicated that they had strong feelings about individuals who drank problematically and were unwilling that they themselves should have such problems. For example, one man was reared in a family with a heavy drinking father. He explained that, ". . . seeing my dad coming home on weekends and taking it out on my mother is one of the reasons that I don't drink much." These early experiences kept this man from taking his first drink until he was in his 40's. Further, he has read a great deal concerning the health and social detriments of alcohol use and has purposely sought out friends who do not often drink.

Retrospective Reasons Given for Decrease in Drinking over Time

Table V summarizes the 144 reasons that 47 men gave for decreasing alcohol consumption over the years.

As with the men who claimed an increase or stability of use, the men who claimed that they decreased alcohol consumption over the years gave an average of approximately 3 reasons for decrease in use. As was the case with the increasers and the men who were stable, men experienced these reasons for decrease concurrently, although the discussion will treat reasons for decrease separately. Respondent-identified reasons for decrease may not always be mutually exclusive.

TABLE V

Respondents' reasons for declining alcohol consumption from 1964 to 1983, frequency distributions

Social

1. Financial situation	8
2. Job problems with drinking	4
3. Significant other intervention	5
4. Social networks decreased use	19
5. Has a demanding job	5
6. Maturation of the family	2
7. Less opportunity to drink	5
8. Religion	4
9. Reaction to retirement	8
Total	60 (42%)

Health

10. Health concerns	12
11. Physiological need less	6
12. Health problems	13
13. Weight control	3
Total	34 (24%)

Fear of problems

14. Growing distaste of alcohol-related problems	10
15. Fear of DWI arrest	1
16. Family problems (not the R's) with alcohol	1
17. Need to be a good example for R's children	1
Total	13 (9%)

Psychological

18. Maturation	11
19. Less stress in life	5
20. Significant accident	2
21. No longer cares for the taste	4
Total	22 (15%)

Change in style of drinking

22. Gradual, unplanned decrease	7
23. Joined AA, treatment for alcoholism	5
24. Changed type of alcohol, e.g. vodka to wine	3
Total	15 (10%)
TOTAL	144 (100%)

Among the social reasons for decreased alcohol use was an break in the respondents' social networks which precipitated a decrease in drinking. One man, currently a successful realtor, mentioned that his alcohol use decreased significantly after he divorced his wife. His wife was a heavy drinker and every day after work they had a few drinks before dinner. His wife also cultivated friendships with a "sophisticated" crowd and social events with these friends involved a fair amount of alcohol use. Now that he no longer lives with his wife and no longer sees his "sophisticated" friends (and he has searched out a new network of friends who hapen to drink less), his drinking has decreased significantly. Another man played in an orchestra at a dance hall. This man considered playing in the orchestra a hobby, an activity that was enjoyed with a group of musician friends. They often had to play until the early hours of the morning and during a typical evening the respondent drank as many as four beers. Beer was traditionally provided gratis to the musicians. Over the years, however, their music became less and less popular, and the dance halls that were willing to book the orchestra were farther and farther away from the Bay Area. Finally, this man had to give up playing in the orchestra since the commutes became too lengthy and he arrived home much too late at night. With the end of his musical career, the respondent's drinking decreased to mealtime consumption.

Some men mentioned that intervention from significant others, most generally spouses, was important in their decreases in alcohol use. One man said that, "My wife was against it. I was drinking too much. I was drinking on the job. That was bad. I got warnings about it and could have been fired. If I had been fired, then I would have lost my pension, too." His wife saw to it that he was "introduced" to her network of friends. These friends drank a good deal less than her husband's friends from work and having a social outlet with individuals who drank moderately helped this man to cut back on his alcohol consumption. This case can also be used as an example of the effect of job-related alcohol problems on declines in consumption.

A group of five men said that the demands of their jobs caused a decline in their alcohol consumption over the years. One man, a stock broker, said that he simply could not function if he were to arrive at work without a clear mind because he had been drinking the night before. He also expressed concern about many of his collegues who drank heavily as a means of dealing with the stress of working in the financial markets. Other men in this category expressed similar sentiments; e.g., that as they experienced advancements in their careers the demands of the new positions made immoderate alcohol use a dysfunctional behavior.

The men who mentioned "maturation of the family" as a reason for their decreased alcohol consumption felt that their children were now of an age where their alcohol use would be seen as an example. Whether this would still hold once the children left home remains an open question.

Some men felt that retirement was a factor in their decreased drinking.

Before retirement, one respondent ran a charitable foundation and had to do a great deal of socializing, which included a great deal of drinking. However, with retirement he did not have to socialize nearly as much and so had fewer occasions to drink. As he put it, "When you are working, whether you want to or not, you have to socialize. There's less opportunity to drink after retirement." Connected with retirement, he also found that he has been able to escape much of the stress in his life, which he feels has also contributed to a decline in drinking. Another man, a blue collar worker, also felt that retirement contributed to his lessening alcohol use. When he worked he used to stop off at a bar after work with his co-workers, an activity that would now be contrived at best, since he is no longer working.

Health concerns and health problems were the two more common reasons cited by these men for a decrease in alcohol use. As was the case with the men who were stable, many of the men who expressed concern about the health effects of alcohol use did so in general terms. These men felt that a certain amount of alcohol use was unhealthy, and decided to cut back on its use. As one man put it, "There are so many things that you don't have control over in your life, such as cancer, that to not take control over the things that you can is just ridiculous." Some men suffered health problems that made it difficult to drink. For example, one man, who had been a skilled tradesman, contracted arthritis and had to take medications which made drinking contraindicated. He mentioned specifically, however, that having to quit using alcohol had not affected his social life. He feels that his friends respect him even more for being able to quit. As he put it, "People don't realize that you can have a good time without drinking at parties. You can fit right in. But it's just like those cigarettes. I quit once for seven years just by making up my mind to quit. You can do it with the booze, too." Interestingly, some men stated that their desire for alcohol decreased as they aged. These statements were rarely specific in nature, but rather were assertions that the physiological need for alcohol lessens as one ages.

A group of men experienced a growing disdain for problem drinking as they aged. Many of these men had themselves been heavy drinkers and felt that they could no longer continue drinking problematically. One man, a self-identified alcoholic, felt that he and his wife could not continue drinking and expect to be able to take care of themselves in old age. He wanted, "a future life, my health, money in the bank. So we got together and decided to quit." With that decision, he and his wife managed to quit drinking. Of other problem drinkers the respondent said, "There, but for the grace of God, go I."

Some men felt that they had undergone a process of "maturation" over the 19 year period and that this process was important in their ability to lower their alcohol consumption. For example, a minister remembered that drinking was governed in his earlier years by, "the social mores of the period, peer pressure. Alcohol was more accepted. With more maturity you don't need

alcohol to have a good time. We've matured and the society has changed."
This statement also includes one of the rare references to a time period effect
on drinking behavior. Other men stated that as they aged they have become a
lot less receptive to being pressured into taking a drink.

A few men volunteered stories of "significant accidents" that were important in their ability to drink less. These sorts of accidents have been noted in
the "spontaneous remission" literature (Knupfer 1971; Stall 1983; Stall and
Biernacki 1986). The significance of these accidents is attributed by the
individual who experiences it, and serves to prompt a re-examination of the
drinker's view toward his alcohol consumption. One man, for example, had
an "alcoholic" friend who insisted that he take one drink too many. The
respondent felt that it would be rude not to accept the drink, and sure
enough, became inebriated. When he arrived home his daughter saw him in a
drunken condition and witnessed the next day's hangover, as well. Right then
and there he decided that he would never drink heavily again. As he put it,
"It's funny, but one little thing like that can embarrass you so much that you
say 'no more, never again' ".

Interestingly, a group of men were able to decrease their alcohol use over
this period although they had not consciously planned to do so. One of these
men said that, "Alcohol just doesn't do a thing for me, I never cared for the
taste anyhow. I even mix drinks for friends and not one for myself. It just
doesn't appeal to me anymore." Another man, when pressed on this point,
gave a remarkably similar quote, but added that since he never cared for
alcohol in the first place he felt that it was only natural that over the years his
drinking would decrease. Also, he pointed out that his friendships were never
based on drinking and this was another reason for him to stay away from
alcohol-soaked social circles. Another group of men changed the type of
alcohol that they consumed during the years 1964 to 1983, resulting in what
they felt was a total decrease in alcohol intake. Generally health reasons were
cited by these men, along with the belief that it has become less fashionable
to order "heavier" drinks.

Summary of Findings

The weight of the prospective data support the thesis that the dominant pattern of alcohol consumption in the face of aging is one of stability, although
sizeable proportions of these men increased or decreased use over time.
However, little has been published to indicate why these divergent outcomes
might occur in conjunction with the aging process. Given the importance of
alcohol use to the distribution of health and disease among elderly populations, furthering understandings of the reasons behind these divergent outcomes is warranted. Analysis of respondent-identified reasons for change and
stability is a valuable first step in the development of hypotheses suitable for
empirical testing concerning age-related decreases in alcohol consumption.

An inductive, qualitative analysis was conducted on the data concerning socio-cultural reasons identified by respondents for reasons as to why their alcohol use changed or stayed the same over time. Among the men who felt that their alcohol use had increased over the years, increased drinking within social networks, maturation of the nuclear family, alcohol use as an increasingly important part of one's professional life, and reactions to retirement were among the most frequent reasons mentioned as important factors in that increase. The men who felt that their alcohol use had been stable over the years cited most frequently not having a reason to change, as well as significant other intervention, general lifestyle preventing change, health concerns, and stable personality types as important to continuity in alcohol consumption over time. Reasons such as finances, decreased use of alcohol within social networks, significant other intervention, health concerns and problems, growing distaste of alcohol-related problems associated with aging, maturation, and a gradual unplanned decrease were given by the men who felt that they decreased over the years.

Discussion

The respondents for this study identified a number of reasons for change and stability in alcohol consumption as a concomitant of the aging process that are not directly relevant to socio-cultural forces (notably, current health status). However, since this book deals with the potential benefits of the integration of anthropology and epidemiology, the following comments will be restricted to a discussion of the socio-cultural reasons for change and stability over time. An interpretation of the meaning of such reasons within broader socio-cultural processes is an important consideration in the futher development of explanatory models concerning changes in drinking behaviors across the life course. The interpretations suggested here, although based on the inductive analysis, are suggested for further empirical testing.

For example, the mention of maturation of the family as important to changes in alcohol consumption is intriguing. What seems to be the crucial factor here is the search for new activities to take the place of those formerly associated with raising children. It appears that most typically men have expanded leisure activities as responsibilities for children declined. Some of these men, for reasons not now understood, expand their leisure activities in ways that include drinking. In contrast, while some men cited maturation of the family as important to declines in drinking behavior, these men were primarily concerned about the example that they were setting for their maturing children. Whether this would still be a factor once the children left home remains an open question.

A second reason for change and stability in alcohol use over time mentioned by these men included the influence of social networks. Whether men felt that their alcohol use increased, decreased or stayed the same, they felt that the pattern of alcohol consumption within their network of friends was an important consideration in their alcohol consumption over the years. Often this reason was expressed in terms of important relationships outside the family being, or not being, based on activities associated with alcohol use. It may be that, over time, men search out a group of friends with whom they feel most comfortable. Willingness to drink, and even the quantity of drinking, may play a part in this process of finding a group of friends with whom one can feel comfortable and who become, over time, important persons in these men's lives. This solidifying of social relationships over time, in which alcohol use plays a part, may be partly behind the modal response given by the men who did not change their alcohol use: that nothing occurred to make it change. That is, it would not be expected that these men would experience pressure to drink from their social networks unless most of friends began to drink more heavily or unless their social network relationships were severed. Yet little was said specifically about how social networks informally regulate drinking behaviors, that is, what the consequences within a social network might be if a member were suddenly to begin drinking too much or too little, within the informal bounds of that network. Certainly further inductive, observational research concerning the effects that social networks have on drinking behaviors is warranted.

Another reason cited for an increase in alcohol consumption was that of increases in consumption based on changes in career requirements as promotions occur. Specifically, it appears that for the upwardly mobile men in this sample, increasing situational pressure to drink was an important reason for increase in use. This pressure was most typically expressed in terms of business life, but it may be that as one climbs the class structure increasing pressure to consume alcohol as part of daily life increases. One counterbalancing factor, however, is that the men who felt that they were expected to drink more frequently than when they were starting their careers also said that they had to be careful not to drink too much. The dualistic nature of the effect of career trajectories on drinking is perhaps reflected by the fact that two men claimed this reason for an increase in use and another five men claimed this reason for a decrease in use. In any event, this change in alcohol consumption is based on differing expectations placed on the individual given certain socio-economic statuses.

Some men mentioned their reaction to retirement was important in their increases in consumption; others that this reaction was important in decreases in consumption. Why these men had such different reactions to ending their professional life is an intriguing question. Personality factors may certainly play a role in this variation, but it may also be that the construction of well-developed leisure skills, which do not involve alcohol use, may be implicated among the men whose alcohol use stayed the same or decreased after retirement.

Again, the effects of strong social network ties, not particularly grounded in alcohol-related activities, would seem to help these men weather the initial stress of retirement without a significant increase in alcohol consumption.

One puzzling aspect of the analysis of the respondent-identified reasons for change is that men who increased use sometimes identified the same factors as explanations for increase as did men who decreased use. Social networks and the experience of retirement were two such variables mentioned as causal of both increase and decrease in alcohol consumption. What seems to be the crucial factor in such cases is not the experience of certain, rather typical life events, but rather how such events are woven into the aging person's life history. That is, men who already had well-developed, non-drinking leisure skills and whose social identity was not entirely defined by the workplace seemed less likely to find retirement a shock that predisposed to increased alcohol use. Similarly, men whose social networks and corresponing social identity were less tied to alcohol-related activities were less likely to mention social networks as causal in increased use. In both of these cases, the influence of the aging person's social identity and drinking history are central to the definition of how typically-experienced life events shape alcohol use.

Thus, an inductive qualitative analysis of the reasons why these men, themselves, felt that their alcohol use had changed or stayed the same over time was useful in identifying a set of variables which help to explain changing patterns of alcohol use across the latter half of life. It is interesting to note that many of the reasons identified by these men (e.g., maturation of the nuclear family, drinking patterns within social networks, etc.) have heretofore been neglected in the alcohol use and aging literature as important explanatory variables. Further, is clear that the variables identified by these men are amenable to operationalization within future research strategies designed to explore changes in alcohol consumption as a concomitant of the aging process. For the time being, however, refinement of understanding concerning these processes would best be based on inductive, qualitative research strategies, since theory concerned with how these processes affect alcohol use is most tentative. This strategy would also possess the advantage of continuing to document the *style, context,* and *qualitative outcomes* of changes in drinking habits over time. These are crucial (although under-studied) aspects to the study of alcohol use and aging, and issues not readily addressed through the use of standard epidemiologic research designs. Stated most plainly, qualitative data collection techniques are necessary complements to quantitative methods if researchers wish to construct robust models which describe how changes in alcohol use occur across the life course.

The model for the integration of anthropology and epidemiology implicitly presented in this chapter also demonstrates the usefulness of the inductive identification of factors important to health-related behaviors. That is, one relevancy of medical anthropological research lies in the contributions that qualitative, inductive theory building has for a traditionally deductive, quantitative science such as epidemiology. These contributions are particularly likely to be valuable when, as is the case in the study of alcohol use and aging, little is understood of how socio-cultural forces shape health-related behaviors. A central task of epidemiology is the measurement of "suspected risk factors" in disease causation. In the construction of an etiological framework of disease, however, risk factors become "suspect" in a number of ways, deductive assertions of causation, "shoeleather epidemiology", and unorganized clinical impressions among them. Thus often the process of selecting risk factors to be measured in epidemiological surveys is to at least some degree a serendipitous process, and particularly so when the disease processes to be studied are poorly understood. Further, epidemiologists, sometimes lacking a sensitive *a priori* understanding of the risk factors to be studied, end up employing admittedly reductionistic or unreliable survey items, which tend to bias research findings in unknown ways. This is most likely to be the case when epidemiologists are called upon to create measures which need to be based on the careful conceptualization, observation, and measurement of socio-cultural variables. Inductive research, conducted before the process of survey instrument construction begins in full swing, can contribute to the process of the identification and measurement of risk factors. This contribution can be made through the creation of a preliminary working model of the organization of suspected risk factors in disease causation and through the refinement of risk factor measurement. The integration of careful inductive research as a part of the development of the research strategy would thus take the process of "shoeleather epidemiology" to a more organized, purposeful level.

In short, quantitative survey research methods (characteristic of epidemiological research) work best once specific and carefully conceptualized research hypotheses have been developed. Inductive, qualitative research designs can often serve a central role in the creation of such hypotheses, and may be particularly valuable when, as is the case in the study of changes in alcohol use across the life course, understandings of the processes of disease and health are tentative. The contributions of such efforts to the advancement of "theoretical epidemiology" (cf. Lilienfeld and Lilienfeld 1980) are obvious.

ACKNOWLEDGEMENTS

This chapter has benefited from critical comments and helpful suggestions from many sources, most notably Joan Ablon, Colleen Johnson and Corinne Nydegger of the Medical Anthropology Program, University of California, San Francisco; Robin Room of the Alcohol Research Group, Berkeley California; Patrick Biernacki of the Social Research Associates of San Francisco and my co-editors, Sandra Gifford and Craig Janes. This research was supported in part by two predoctorial training awards, one from National Institute on Alcohol Abuse and Alcoholism (AA 05173-01/02) and the second from the National Institute on Aging (AG 00045-07).

NOTES

1. A subsample of white San francisco males aged 30—69 and interviewed in 1964 ($n = 246$) was selected for reinterviewing. Follow-up of this sample occurred during the summer and fall of 1983 — a 19 year period during which member of the sample moved towards "old" age. The 1964 San Francisco study was itself in large part a reinteriew effort based on an earlier 1962 San Francisco study (reported in Knupfer and Room 1964). For the 1964 survey all of the heavy drinkers identified in 1962 were chosen for reinterview, plus all of the abstainers who had indicated that at some point in the past they had also been heavy drinkers. Further, half of all other respondents were reinterviewed in 1964, as well as all of the spouses of the 1962 respondents. The sampling procedures for the 1962 and 1964 studies have been described in greater detail elsewhere (Knupfer and Room 1964; Stall 1984). The fact that heavy drinkers were proportionately over-represented for the 1983 sampling frame constitutes the primary methodological variation from a typical community study of drinking habits.

   Upon follow-up, 85 (35%) of the 246 white male respondents aged 30—69 were successfully reinterviewed. Another 76 (31%) were deceased at Time 2 and 85 (35%) were either lost to follow-up or refused to be reinterviewed. To test for the possibility of loss to follow-up bias among the reinterviewed men, the 1983 respondents were compared to the 1964 sub-sample of white males between 30—69 along the variables of age, number of reasons for drinking, income, education, religion, as well as quantity, frequency and quantity-frequency of alcohol use. Of these, only the distributions for age (due to the loss of the older respondents to death) and education (due to the inordinate loss of men with less than a high school education) were significantly different between the 85 men who were successfully reinterviewed and the entire 1964 subsample. Age distributions for the sub-sample were betwee 30—69 in 1964 and so between 49—88 in 1983. The modal range from the sample in 1983 was between 59—68, with the majority of the sample (67%) in their sixties or older.

2. Since prospective data exist which measure patterns of alcohol consumption at Time 1 and Time 2, the question of how well the respondents' retrospective perceptions of their use of alcohol over time fit with the prospective measures should be raised. This issue is complicated by the form of the retrospective measure. That is, respondents were asked whether their alcohol use in general had changed over the past 19 years. As such the distributions reported here are not comparable to the prospective measures of quantity or frequency alone, or even a combined quantity-frequency measure. That is, respondents could have been referring to changes in quantity, frequency, most quantity of use during a specific occasion or even alcohol-related problems in their responses to the retrospective measure. Thus, an analysis which looked at agreement between the prospective and retrospective measures of change and stability according to only one of the measures of alcohol use would lack rigor, and it is difficult to determine how to construct a summary score which would adequately describe all of these aspects of alcohol use. Secondly, it is difficult to judge whether decrease in quantity but not in frequency of use should be counted as a pattern of decrease or stability. Thirdly, the troubling question of how closely the prospective measures must agree between Time 1 and 2 to constitute "stability" must be considered. That is, would an exact agreement on, say, the nine point frequency measure constitute "stability" or should a looser definition be used? Therefore, for the purposes of

this analysis which emphasizes respondent-identified reasons for change or stability, the broad outlines of the prospective measures have been described with an eye to judging approximate agreement with the respondents' reported impressions of how their alcohol use had stayed the same or changed over time.

REFERENCES

Abelson, D. S. and H. I. J. van der Spuy
    1978 The Age Variable in Alcoholism. Journal of Studies on Alcohol 39: 800—808.
Bahr, H. M.
    1969 Lifetime Affiliation Patterns of Early- and Late-Onset Drinkers on Skid Row. Quarterly Journal of Studies on Alcohol 30: 645—656.
Barnes, G. M.
    1969 Alcohol Use Among Older Persons: Findings from a Western New York State General Population Survey. Journal of the American Geriatrics Society 27: 244—250.
Brenner, B.
    1967 Alcoholism and Fatal Accidents. Quarterly Journal of Studies on Alcohol 28: 517—528.
Cahalan, D.
    1970 Problem Drinkers. San Francisco: Jossey-Bass, Inc.
Cahalan, D. and R. Room
    1974 Problem Drinking Among American Men. New Brunswick, N.J.: Rutgers Center of Alcohol Studies, Monograph # 7.
Cahalan, D., I. Cisin, and H. Crossley
    1969 American Drinking Practises: A National Study of Drinking Behavior and Attitudes. New Brunswick, N.J.: Rutgers Center of Alcohol Studies, Monograph # 6.
Droller, H.
    1964 Some Aspects of Alcoholism in the Elderly. Lancet 1964: 137—139.
Clark, W. B. and D. Cahalan
    1976 Changes in Problem Drinking Over a Four-Year Span. Addictive Behaviors 1: 251—259.
Costello, R. M.
    1974 Mortality in an Alcoholic Cohort. The International Journal of the Addictions 9: 355—363.
Fillmore, K. M., S. D. Bacon, and M. Hyman
    1979 The 27 Year Longitundinal Panel Study of Drinking by Students in College, 1949—1976. Final Report to NIAAA, Grant Contract # ADM 281-76-0015.
Foulds, G. A. and C. Hassall
    1969 The Significance of Age of Onset of Excessive Drinking in Male Alcoholics. British Journal of Psychiatry 115: 1027—1032.
Glatt, M. M.
    1978 Experiences with Elderly Alcoholics in England. Alcoholism 2: 23—26.
Glatt, M. M. and A. J. Rosin
    1964 Aspects of Alcoholism in the Elderly. Lancet 1964: 472—473.
Glynn, B., G. Bouchard, J. Locastro, and J. Hermos
    1983 Changes in Alcohol Consumption Behaviors Among Men in The Normative Aging Study. In Nature and Extent of Alcohol Problems Among the Elderly. NIAAA Research Monograph No. 14. Washington, D.C.: U.S. Dept. of Health and Human Services, pp. 101—116.
Hauser, P. M.
    1976 Aging and the World-Wide Population Change. In R. H. Binstock and E. Shanas

(eds.), Handbook of Aging and the Social Sciences. Pps. 58—86. New York: Van Nostrand-Reinhold Co.

Johnson, L. A.
  1974 Use of Alcohol by Persons 65 Years and Older, Upper-East Side of Manhattan. Final Report. Report to NIAAA, Grant Contract # HSM-43-73-38.

Knupfer, G.
  1971 Ex-Problem Drinkers. *In* M. Roff, L. N. Robins, and M. Pollack, (eds.), Life History Research in Psychotherapy, Vol. 2, pp. 256—282. Minneapolis: The University of Minnesota Press.

Knupfer, G. and R. Room
  1964 Age, Sex, and Social Class Factors in Amount of Drinking in a Metropolitan Community. Social Problems 12: 224—240.

Lilienfeld, A. and D. E. Lilienfeld
  1980 Foundations of Epidemiology. New York: Oxford University Press.

MacAndrew, C. and R. B. Edgerton
  1969 Drunken Comportment: A Social Explanation. Chicago: Aldine Publishing Co.

Ojesjo, L.
  1980 Prevalence of Known and Hidden Alcoholism in the Revisited Lundby Population. Social Psychiatry 15: 81—96.
  1981 Long-Term Outcome in Alcohol Abuse and Alcoholism Among Males in the Lundby General Population, Sweden. British Journal of Addiction 76: 391—400.

Orford, J. and G. Edwards,
  1977. Alcoholism. New York: Oxford University Press.

Polich, J. M., D. J. Armor, and H. B. Braiker
  1981 The Course of Alcoholism. New York: Wiley.

Robinette, C. D., Z. Hrubel, and J. Fraumeni
  1979 Chronic Alcoholism and Subsequent Mortality in World War II Veterans. American Journal of Epidemiology 109: 687—700.

Roizen, R.
  1981 The WHO Study of Community Responses to Alcohol-Related Problems: A Review of Cross-Cultural Findings. Report to NIAAA, Grant Contract # AA-05595-0324.

Schmidt, W. and J. De Lint
  1972 Causes of Death of Alcoholics. Quarterly Journal of Studies on Alcohol 33: 171—185.

Schmidt, W. and R. Popham
  1975 Heavy Alcohol Consumption and Physical Health Problems: A Review of the Epidemiological Evidence. Drug and Alcohol Dependence 1: 27—50.

Schuckit, M. A. *et al.*
  1980 Three-Year Follow-up of Elderly Alcoholics. Journal of Clinical Psychiatry 41: 412—416.

Shanas, E. and G. L. Maddox
  1976 Aging, Health and the Organization of Health Resources. *In* R. H. Binstock and E. Shanas (eds.), Handbook of Aging and the Social Sciences. Pp. 592—618. New York: Van Nostrand/Reinhold Co.

Smart, R. G. and C. B. Liban
  1981 Predictors of Problem Drinking Among Elderly, Middle-Aged and Youthful Drinkers. Journal of Psychoactive Drugs 13: 153—163.

Stall, R. D.
  1983 An Examination of Spontaneous Remission from Problem Drinking in the Blue-grass Region of Kentucky. Journal of Drug Issues 13: 191—206.
  1984 Alcohol Use and Aging: The Results of a 19 Year Prospective Study. Ph.D. Dissertation, Medical Anthropology Program, University of California, San Francisco and Berkeley.

1986   Change and Stability in Quantity and Frequency of Alcohol Use as a Concomitant
       of the Aging Process: a 19 Year Prospective Study. British Journal of Addiction 81:
       426—433.
Stall, R. D. and P. Biernacki
   1986   Spontaneous Remission from the Problematic Use of Substances: An Inductive
       Model Derived from a Comparative Analysis of the Alcohol, Opiate, Tobacco and
       Food/Obesity Literatures. International Journal of the Addictions 21: 1—23.
Zimberg, S.
   1974   Two Types of Problem Drinkers: Both Can be Managed. Geriatrics 29: 135—138.

ROBERT A. RUBINSTEIN AND JANET D. PERLOFF

IDENTIFYING PSYCHOSOCIAL DISORDERS IN CHILDREN: ON INTEGRATING EPIDEMIOLOGICAL AND ANTHROPOLOGICAL UNDERSTANDINGS

The development of a more satisfactory understanding of psychosocial disorders in children depends upon the successful combination of medical anthropological and epidemiological information. In this paper we describe one way this can be done. Our approach is to focus first on the level of the logic of inquiry, and only secondarily on the use of specific methods.

Questions of method become meaningful only after epidemiological and anthropological understandings have been used together to conceptualize a research project. Our approach therefore contrasts with some discussions in anthropology and in epidemiology which have been conducted as though problems of method can be considered alone. Some of these discussions have suggested that the methods of each discipline are complementary. Our view is that it is a serious mistake to focus discussions of the integration of anthropology and epidemiology primarily on the level of the methods or techniques of research. If the research question is set without the benefit of a conceptual integration of epidemiological and anthropological understandings, then a research program is unlikely to improve our understanding, no matter how sophisticated a combination of methods and techniques is used.

The success of researchers in integrating medical anthropology and epidemiology should not be evaluated by looking for the use of specific methods in particular ways. At times the conceptual integration may be successful yet the research question can be appropriately answered using methods from only one of the disciplines. In this paper we explore how better conceptual integration of these approaches, regardless of methods, can help to advance our understanding of psychosocial disorders in children. We seek to illustrate how taking up the concerns and asking the questions of one discipline can usefully inform work done using the methods of the other discipline.

We view this conceptual integration as important because often the focus on methods leads researchers to accept overly simple accounts of the phenomena they seek to understand. Too often the inadequacy of these accounts is discovered only after they have had harmful consequences (Rubinstein 1984; Simon 1983; Hall 1982). The principle reason for the failure of these understandings is that they have been developed using data from an artificially limited range of experience. Because of this observations are channeled toward particular normatively appropriate data, information anomalous to the model is discounted (Ward and Werner 1984; Argyris 1980; Rubinstein et al. 1984).

One way to avoid this is to insist that research keep theoretical models as

Craig R. Janes et al. (eds.), Anthropology and Epidemiology, 303–332.
© 1986 *by D. Reidel Publishing Company.*

open as possible to new information. To do this we must recognize that researchers interested in mental health and illness have recourse to a number of different "levels" of structure in their explanations of the behaviors they observe (e.g., genetic, cognitive, psychological, social structural, experiential, and the like). Frequently a single level is associated with the theoretical work of a single discipline. Yet each of these levels is comprised of organized subsystems (Whitehead 1960). Focusing on one level to the exclusion of others always leads to the confounding of scientific models rather than to their improvement (Quine 1964; Newell 1973).

Each level affects and is affected by adjoining levels. Because of this it is important to follow a "rule of minimal inclusion: any explanation of behavior must take into account any and all levels of systemic organization efficiently present in the interaction between the system operating and the environment of that system" (Rubinstein et al. 1984: 93). Precisely which systemic levels need to be considered varies with the research question asked.

It is additionally important to understand that (*both* basic and applied) scientific research is a continuing process alternating between inductive and deductive work (cf., Rubinstein 1984). Any research finding is a product of this process and is in a fundamental sense an artifact abstracted from ongoing activity. These research products can help to provide categories, such as nosological systems, through which useful judgements about the world can be made. But the value of such categories depends upon their providing information that is useful for particular purposes. It is, therefore, also important to be conscious that, fundamentally, categories are reifications of processes and do not exist independently of the purposes for which they are developed.

The evaluation of nosological categories in psychosocial work is one area in which it is possible to sketch a strategy for bridging between epidemiological and anthropological levels of analysis. We argue that this bridging can be accomplished, for example, by asking an essentially anthropological question about the nature, meaning and significance of a particular nosological category and answering that question using whatever methods turn out to be appropriate (whether quantitative, qualitative, or a combination of the two).[1] In this approach methodological decisions appropriately follow from theoretical judgements. Methodological decisions in turn allow the selection of methods; questions of technique are secondary to questions of logic. In the following sections of this paper we use the example of "hyperactivity" to illustrate how this approach can be used to further the integration of epidemiology and anthropology and ultimately the understanding of psychosocial disorders of children.

CHILDREN AND THE "NEW MORBIDITY"

During the past twenty-five years people interested in children's health in the

United States have become increasingly concerned with questions of mental health and illness. This shift in focus has several interdependent causes. Among these are the dramatic changes in patterns of childhood morbidity and mortality that took place prior to this time. During the first half of this century morbidity and mortality among children were due primarily to infectious diseases and acute illness. But, by the middle of the century, the development of antibiotics and public health programs which improved environmental conditions had virtually eliminated these as serious threats to children's health (Perloff et al. 1984).

As a result of these developments, patterns of practice changed among pediatricians and others involved with promoting child health (Pawluch 1983). These practitioners began to spend more time on "well-child" care than they had previously, and this led to an increasing concern with the behavioral, psychosocial problems of children (Haggerty 1983, 1982). Well-child care in part has come to be viewed as a way to prevent psychosocial problems in children (e.g., Green 1985, 1983; Green et al. 1982). Yet, despite such professional judgements and the faith of many in the value of well-child care, evaluations of the efficacy of well-child visits for preventing psychosocial problems yield results that are equivocal at best. At worst, such research suggests that well-child care does not help prevent psychosocial difficulties among children (Feldman 1984; Gilbert et al. 1984; Rogers et al. 1974).

Equally important in focusing attention on children's mental health and illness has been the perception that the incidence and prevalence of psychosocial difficulties among children have been increasing. In 1975 Haggerty and his associates identified this apparent trend as the "New Morbidity". The new morbidity is comprised of psychosocial, behavioral and other problems which involve processes outside of the "strictly medical" (or perhaps, traditionally medical) purview (Haggerty et al. 1975: 94). It includes "Learning difficulties, and school problems, behavioral disturbances, allergies, speech difficulties, visual problems, and the problems of adolescents in coping and adjusting . . . [and] family social problems and the management and handling of everyday life stresses" (Haggerty et al. 1975: 316). They noted the growing importance of these problems of children, and for their caretakers.

Reports from clinicians and researchers appear to confirm this judgement. Starfield et al. (1980: 159), for example, report that between 5% and 15% of all children seen at seven primary care facilities during 1977 were "recognized as having behavioral, educational, or social problems." More recently, Starfield reported that in a seven year longitudinal study of 2,591 children (from primarily white middle-class, two-parent homes), 25.1% were diagnosed as having "psychosocial morbidity" and 17.3% as having "psychosomatic morbidity" (Starfield et al. 1984: 825).

Several studies of mental health problems and the use of medical services by children in Monroe County, New York underscore this sense of a rising prevalence among children of psychosocial and behavioral problems. In a series of studies analyzing data from a cumulative psychiatric case register, Roghmann and his associates report that the treated prevalence of psychosocial problems among various categories of children ranges from 1% to 10%. They add that "as only about half of the children with such problems, as identified by pediatricians, are seen by psychiatric specialists, the total treated prevalence would be appreciably higher" (Roghmann et al. 1982). Their work thus suggests an identified prevalence of psychosocial problems among children of up of 20%, and leaves open the possibility that the true prevalence of such problems is in fact even higher.[2]

More detailed analyses of the cumulative psychiatric case register show increases in the treated incidence of situational disorders and behavioral disorders from 1960—1977. Roghmann et al. (1984: 789) suggest that this rise is due "partly to changes in diagnostic classification and partly due to changes in the availability of care". Although the observed rise in treated prevalence may be, in part, artifactual, they note that the "morbidity and mortality still encountered will increasingly be due to 'social causes' such as poverty or lack of care due to maldistribution of manpower and facilities" (Roghmann, et al. 1984: 372).

Despite such reports, it has turned out to be particularly difficult to identify cases of the new morbidity among children. This result is due to at least three factors. First, the new morbidity is comprised of a very heterogeneous set of difficulties. For instance, in a recent study Starfield, et al. (1980: 160), included;

psychoses, neuroses, personality disorders, behavioral and psychological problems, learning disabilities, educational problems, mental retardation, developmental problems, situational problems, social maladjustments, parent-child problems, syphills, gonorrhea, sexual problems, pregnancy, family planning, enuresis, urinary frequency, feeding problems, adverse effects of medicinal, chemical and environmental agents, and complications of medical care.

Second, each of the specific psychosocial disorders that make up the "new morbidity" is comprised not of a single distinguishing behavior but rather of a heterogeneous and sometimes overlapping complex of behaviors. Third, it has been observed that the "pathological behaviors" associated with some presumed psychosocial disorders show great context sensitivity. Some researchers have come to believe that many of the children classed as having psychosocial disorders suffer not from some deficit but from the "medicalization of deviance" (Conrad and Schneider 1980).

In some settings certain children behave in ways that are called "pathological", but in other settings these same children act "normally". Viewing this inconsistency these researchers conclude that the children's "sickness" is an artifact of social processes — that it is a socially constructed category — rather than an objective fact. The socially constructed nature of sickness categories, they say, is further demonstrated by the flexibility of the category boundaries. Frequently, they argue, the result of this flexibility has been that, as the authority of the medical profession has increased, behaviors or other characteristics previously thought of as odd, or curious, or handicapping have been redefined as sick; they have been medicalized. This medicalization, in turn, has the effect of narrowing the range of behaviors considered normal in a society and places many of these behaviors and attributes outside of the scope of things that lay-people can legitimately talk about (Conrad and Schneider 1980; Hufford 1982, 1983). In addition, the medicalization of deviance has been shown to lead to changes in the social roles (usually a narrowing) that are open to persons possessing the medicalized attribute (Penfold and Walker 1983; Scott 1969; Ablon 1984).

Kaplan (1983, see also Penfold and Walker 1983), for instance, shows how changes in psychiatric nosology have led to the linking of many feminine behaviors with specific psychiatric disorders (such as, "Hysterical Personality" or "Passive-Dependent Personality"). Conrad and Schneider (1980) show how this process has effected such diverse areas as alcoholism, opiate addiction, juvenile delinquency, child abuse, and homosexuality. Several researcher have argued that this same kind of social construction of sickness, and the increasing amount of behavior said to require medical rather than other kinds of attention, are illustrated by the case of "hyperactivity", which we discuss later in this paper.

Two research traditions have investigated the new morbidity. These two traditions can roughly be distinguished by their focus and research style. The first, grounded in epidemiological concerns, tends to seek patterns and to rely heavily on surveys and experimentation. The other, rather more anthropological in commitment, seeks to understand processes and favors the use of naturalistic observation and detailed behavioral description. Both traditions have produced interesting and important results. But, because they raise essentially different questions and use different logical rules of evidence and inference, each tradition has largely failed to take full account of the work of the other. Therefore, our understanding of the nature and significance of the new morbidity in children has not developed as fully as it could have.

COMBINING QUALITATIVE AND QUANTITATIVE APPROACHES

Coherently integrating qualitative and quantitative approaches is very difficult. Qualitative research, such a ethnographic descriptions of the context and meaning of particular behaviors, is often taken by survey researchers as interesting for its anecdotal value. But, because the results of this work are not generalizable to large populations and because the outcomes of ethnographic work may not be directly replicable, epidemiological researchers often value this anthropological research less than more traditional survey-style epidemiological research.[3] In their view, qualitative work is at best useful for preliminary studies associated with the subsequent validation of a survey instrument. For instance, a number of variables now generally considered important in psychosocial epidemiological studies — indices of social class, ethnicity, household patterning, social networks, and the like — were derived from anthropological understandings of particular communities (e.g., Hollingshead and Redlich 1958; Dunham 1959; Rapoport 1959; Srole et al. 1962; Leighton et al. 1966).

When viewed in this way, anthropological research is seen as valuable for two principle reasons. First, anthropological research can establish that some "things" previously unattended to should be taken into account. For instance, new "cultural" variables might be added to a survey questionnaire. Or, a traditional intervention (like psychotherapy) might be packaged differently for minority populations (e.g. Acosta et al. 1982). Second, the results of anthropological work undertaken early in a project can be built into sampling and questionnaire strategies. Such "preliminary" research may be seen as worth the investment of resources and time because it provides results that reused throughout the course of project can lead to improvements in research instruments.

Some qualitative researchers reject this conditional acceptance, claiming that it is mistaken for at least three reasons. First, they argue, it is wrong to assume that an anthropological understanding of a specific community can simply be transported to inform work in another, albeit demographically similar, community. They assert that survey instruments and questionnaire items can be developed which both assess social process in a community and reliably reflect the health care community's professional judgement of the nature of illness and disease in that community. Yet, when used in another community these questionnaires and surveys may not adequately reflect community definitions of illness and disease. Rating instruments, question- naire responses and the like, simply cannot be well understood without a thorough understanding of the specific context in which they are given (Adair and Deuschle 1970). Some epidemiological researchers have heeded this warning, but not always with results conforming to the spirit of the anthro- pological objection. For instance, cautions about the need to attend to social processes have often resulted in the definition of a new index (like, "ethnic group") rather than in a concern with the local meanings (of ethnicity, for example) and their impact on the research.

Campbell (1978) described some aspects of this situation when he noted that although,

rules regarding the use of qualitative knowing are clearly present in the quantitative methods books, they are rarely exercised. The researcher is apt to feel that presenting such content undermines the appearances of scientific certainly, or that weaknesses on these points are evidence of his own incompetence. The field experimenter's defensiveness vis-à-vis his labora- tory colleagues leads to further minimizing of this content and still more so when he is earning his living as a contractor in programme evaluation (Campbell 1978: 194).

Second, anthropologically-oriented researchers argue that because within a community the meanings and importance placed upon forms of behavior constantly undergo change, instruments appropriately used in a community at one time may at a later time be inappropriate. The anthropological understanding over time of even a single community requires ongoing qualitative research involvement (Ablon 1981, 1977; Foster et al. 1979). And, third, they argue that research structured around the use of preset questions excludes from consideration some types of important data (Argyris 1980; Rubinstein et al. 1984). The use of preset questions assumes a knowledge of the phenomenon being studied, often an inappropriate assumption. The structure hinders the revision of our knowledge in light of new information which might have been offered unsolicited.

For their part, anthropologically-oriented researchers have taken to heart some methodological lessons taught by epidemiological researchers, but not always in ways of which the latter would approve. Questions of sampling and the statistical treatment of data are now more widely used by anthropological researchers interested in health and behavior (Landy 1977; Brewer and Collins 1981; Schensul and Borrero 1982). Standardized interview schedules and survey questionnaires also sometimes comprise the major research focus in some areas of field work. However, the anthropological researcher's interest in these techniques often is not to make the research results generalizable but to deepen contextual understanding. For example, Estroff (1981) used the "Community Adaptation Schedule" with a convenience sample to gather texts that could then be analyzed in-depth, rather than only scored.

Despite the ambivalent attraction of anthropological researchers to epidemiological methods and of epidemiological researchers to anthropological information, attempts have been made at integrating the approaches. Yet, very little progress has been made. In part this is because attempts at integrating the two methods have most often really involved sanctioning under one administrative umbrella two parallel, but substantially separate, research programs, rather than the integration of them.

The results obtained by using either approach alone are incomplete and less robust than results obtained by successful integration of anthropological and epidemiological perspectives, employing a variety of methods and tools of inquiry (Campbell and Fiske 1959; Collins 1981; Wimsatt 1981). Even results of social research intended to provide information upon which interventions can be designed, if carried out within the canons of only one methodological approach, will be of limited use (Rubinstein 1984).

QUALITATIVE AND QUANTITATIVE UNDERSTANDINGS:
"HYPERACTIVITY"

The effect of the schism between anthropological and epidemiological researchers is extraordinarily clear in the case of "hyperactivity". As one of the most frequency diagnosed psychiatric disorders in children during the last two decades, "hyperactivity" serves as an exemplar of the new morbidity.[4]

Estimates of the prevalence of "hyperactivity" have varied widely (see, Table I). The generally accepted estimate is that "hyperactivity" affects between 3% and 5% of school-aged children (Barkley 1981). The prevalence of "hyperactivity" is thought to be higher in boys than in girls (around 6: 1), and in lower-income (or lower socio-economic) groups. Interestingly, however, based on analyses of teacher questionnaires or ratings, Trites (1979) classified as "hyperactive" 14.3% of a 14,083 sample of school children, and Lapouse and Monk (1958) estimated on the basis of teacher ratings that as many as 57% of boys and 42% of girls could be considered "hyperactive".

TABLE I

Some estimates of the prevalence of "hyperactivity" in children[a]

Source	Prevalence estimate
Huessy (1967; 1974)	10—20%
Hussy and Gendron (1970)	10—20%
Miller et al. (1973)	9.3% boys; 1.5% girls
Cantwell (1975)	5—20%
Wender (1971)	5—20%
Stewart et al. (1966)	4%
Renshaw (1974)	3%
Lambert et al. (1978)	1.19%
Barkley (1981)	3—5%
Trites (1979)	14.3%
Sprague et al. (1974)	9% boys; 2% girls

[a] After Bosco and Robin (1980).

Part of this great range in prevalence estimates is due to the fact that the behaviors thought characteristic of "hyperactive" children appear to be context sensitive. Thus, children may at one time display, and at other times not display, the diagnostically significant behaviors (Collins 1981; Douglas 1972; Sleator and Ullman 1981). In fact, Lambert et al. (1978) have shown that the diagnosis of "hyperactivity" varies depending upon whether the judgements of one or of a combination of parents', teachers', or physicians' determinations are accepted. They also argue that the diagnosis of "hyperactivity" varies as a result of the number of observers needed to agree on the diagnosis and the social position of these observers vis-à-vis the child.

Since the beginning of this century, the syndrome of behaviors that has been identified as hyperactivity have been classed under a series of changing diagnostic labels. Characteristically, children diagnosed as "hyperactive" are said to be more aggressive than non-hyperactive children, or to be "disruptive", because they often engage in "excessive vocal noises" that disrupt ongoing social activities. Risk-taking behavior of "hyperactive" children appears to exceed that of non-hyperactive children and is often associated with an increase in physical mishaps (like, scrapes and bruises, broken bones, and general accidents). Although generally not scoring significantly lower on intelligence tests (especially individually administered tests) than matched controls, "hyperactive" children are generally academic underachievers (Cantwell and Satterfield 1978; Douglas 1972), and their risk of school failure is 2—3 times greater than for non-hyperactive children.

In general, "hyperactive" children are thought to exhibit three types of problems which result in referral for treatment (Ross and Pelham 1981): (1) they tend to have problems in academic learning, resulting in school failure; (2) they seem to have trouble relating to their peers; and, (3) they have trouble complying with adult requests and commands (Safer and Allen 1976; Barkley and Cunningham 1979).

For some time researchers reasoned that since children who showed these troublesome behaviors acted very much like children with brain injuries, "hyperactive" children must also be neurologically impaired (Strauss and Lehtinen 1940). These children were therefore diagnosed as having Minimal Brain Damage (MBD). Much research effort went toward characterizing the differences between MBD and "normal" children and toward finding better ways to treat and manage troublesome MBD children. For the most part, this work proceeded using epidemiological research strategies such as various experimental designs and prevalence surveys among school-aged children. These efforts did not produce a convincing account of the etiology of MBD or effective treatments for these children.

In a recent review, Rutter (1978) noted that less than 5% of all children diagnosed as MBD show any evidence of structural brain damage, and that most children suffering brain damage did not develop the syndrome of behaviors used to define MBD children. Moreover, MBD children did not respond uniformly to pharmacologic treatment. This further indicated that it was unlikely that they suffered from some shared but unidentified organic disorder. MBD was replaced as a diagnostic category by the designation of "hyperactivity". This new diagnostic category was thought to have the advantage that it was descriptive of the "behavioral disorder" shown by this group of children.

When researchers working in qualitative traditions also became interested in the problem they noted that the group of children first diagnosed as MBD, and later as "hyperactive", was very heterogeneous. They relied mostly on naturalistic observation and pointed out that the behaviors of this group of children varied as to when, where and how troublesome they were. These researchers also noted that in everyday interaction many "hyperactive" children did not seem to be less bright than their peers. They therefore questioned whether the condition was really a disease entity. They offered a number of alternative explanations — labeling and the social control of deviance, for instance — to account for the difficulties faced by these children. Each account argued that these children did not have a disorder and hypothesized that the source of problems lies in their social environments (Conrad 1975).

Although the conclusion that hyperactivity was not a "disease entity" was objectionable to epidemiological researchers, their own work *also* suggested that children classified as "hyperactive" were a very heterogeneous group.[5] Continuing to rely heavily on the canons of epidemiological-experimental research, they too showed that although children diagnosed as "hyperactive" could be seen as different from other children on a number of measures of behavioral and cognitive activity, "hyperactive" children showed great variability in relation to all of these measures (e.g., Homatidis and Konstantreas 1981).

This turned out to be so, for example, for attention and impulse control (Douglas 1972; Brown and Quay 1977), for cognitive style (Sykes et al. 1973; Sprague et al. 1974), and for levels of motor activity (Whalen and Henker 1980). Variation in the characteristics of "hyperactive" children undoubtedly accounts in part for the wide range of estimates for the prevalence of "hyperactivity". This variation was troublesome to both clinicians and to researchers. And, in 1972 the epidemiological research community's attention was redirected when in an influential paper Douglas (1972: 260) argued that "hyperactivity is only one of a constellation of critical symptoms. [and that] it may be just as important to consider the quality of the hyperactive child's behavior as its quantity".

In addition to "over-activity", Douglas identified inability to sustain attention or to control impulsivity as important qualities of "hyperactive" children's behavior. It followed that disagreement about the etiology of these behaviors might be resolved (and appropriate interventions designed) if, rather than taking these children to form a single class whose behavior could be contrasted with other children's behavior, research efforts were directed at understanding the difficulties faced by smaller, better diagnosed and more homogeneous groups of children.

There were two possible responses to Douglas's suggestion. The first was to continue to view the global category of hyperactivity as consisting of a number of subtypes. Further research could then seek systematic contrasts between the global group of hyperactive children and other children, as well as to identify differences among subtypes of "hyperactive" children. This view depended upon interpretations of data that conformed to standards of experimental-epidemiological research.

An alternative response to Douglas's argument was to conclude that it was a mistake to cling to the global category of hyperactivity. This view would require that the global category be partitioned into a number of smaller categories; the adequacy of each as a diagnosis would then be evaluated.

Thus, through work with smaller well-described groups of children, a number of etiologies and syndromes might be defined or a portion of the children previously diagnosed as "hyperactive" (sick) would now be understood to be "normal". This conclusion would be congenial with that reached by the qualitative research community, who had already challenged the usefulness of the global category of hyperactivity.

The eventual response of the psychiatric community was to redefine the American Psychiatric Association's Diagnostic and Statistical Manual of Mental Disorders, Second Edition (DSM-II) diagnostic category of hyperactivity (properly, "Hyperkinetic Reaction of Childhood") as the DSM-III category of Attention Deficit Disorder. Included *within* Attention Deficit Disorder were two subtypes — "with hyperactivity" (ADDH) and "without hyperactivity" (ADD). This response expanded the earlier experimental-epidemiologically derived model of what is happening with these children, and required no change in the governing values of this clinical or research community.

EVALUATING NOSOLOGY: ANTHROPOLOGY AND EPIDEMIOLOGY COMBINED

The establishment of the nosological category of Attention Deficit Disorder with two subtypes appears to us to have pushed the results of the earlier experimental-epidemiological work to its limit. However, efforts have continued towards evaluating the new nosological category. To the extent that this empirical research shows that the category Attention Deficit Disorder fails to deal adequately with the earlier noted anomalies, it suggests the need for new models of research and practice.

There have been several evaluations of the reconceptualization of hyperactivity as an Attention Deficit Disorder. In each case the investigators have worked from only one theoretical level of analysis; be it psychological, sociological or clinical (Douglas 1972; Eysenck et al. 1983; Conrad and Schneider 1980; Russell et al. 1983; cf., Collins 1981). As a result these investigations each encompass only a single systemic level. They have, in effects, ignored the rule of minimal inclusion which would require that an explanation of "hyperactive" behavior in individuals take into account the other systemic levels interacting with and in the environment of the children (Rubinstein, et al. 1984: 93). Thus, this empirical work has resulted only in general disagreement about the nature and reality of "hyperactivity" and Attention Deficit Disorder.

Even in research reports that consider information from different disciplines, we find that the theoretical levels of analysis are separated while methodological debates are joined (Whalen and Henker 1980). This joining of questions of method, while expanding the methodological options for studying behavior, cannot hope to achieve the objective of expanding our fundamental understanding of behavior. Indeed, the latter is not possible unless our investigations encompass a broader range of systemic levels. As long as attention is focused on methodological issues, and the incorporation of conceptual materials from different levels is ignored, little progress toward better understanding this behavior should be expected (Rubinstein and Laughlin 1977; Argyris 1980).

A recent study undertaken to evaluate the diagnostic category of Attention Deficit Disorder (Rubinstein and Brown 1984) illustrates one way the bridging of levels might be achieved. In that study the investigators asked if the new nosological system presented in DSM-III served the joint diagnostic and research purposes for which it was developed. The strategy was to ask about the fundamental nature and role of the category of ADD/ADDH, much as anthropologists often ask about the nature and meaning of "folk" categories in everyday life. This essentially anthropological question might have been answered by detailed and intense observational study of children who had been diagnosed by clinicians and researchers as having ADD/ADDH. It turned out that the question could also be answered by using epidemiologic methods. The study serves to illustrate the point that the integration of different theoretical levels of analysis can provide results not obtained when efforts at integration are restricted to issues of method.

The heterogeneity of the group of children included in the category "Hyperkinetic Reaction of Childhood" provided an impetus for its redefinition as Attention Deficit Disorder with and without Hyperactivity. The psychological and epidemiological research in the area suggested that this difficulty could be dealt with if these children were sorted into two groups, one of which had more and the other of which had less severe problems. The qualitative research in contrast supposed that the heterogeneity of these children's behavior could be accounted for by seeing their difficulties as social, and therefore external to the children. The situation that results is a standoff: Qualitative researchers acknowledge the methodological rigor of psychological and epidemiological studies in the area but denigrate them for having reified social process; epidemiological and psychological researchers dismiss the qualitative results as unhelpful and hopelessly imprecise. The consequence for the research community in general is that both sets of heuristics and both sets of attendant biases are reinforced.

In order to avoid the methodological bickering that characterizes debates in this area, Rubinstein and Brown (1984) sought to evaluate the nosological category (in spirit a medical anthropological question) using a variant of a classic epidemiological research design, the retrospective case-control study.

Much epidemiological work takes place after some disease or disorder had affected a group. Because of this, epidemiologists interested in discovering the factors that increase an individual's risk of getting a disease or disorder must "work backward" from effect to cause. As epidemiology developed, a methodology for working with information about past exposures was articulated and refined. The result is the "case-control", or retrospective study, "probably the major contribution of epidemiologists and their predecessors to the general area of research methods" (Kleinbaum et al. 1982: 69). The *logic* of the case-control design requires that systematic, controlled comparisons be made between two groups, only one of which has the disorder or disease in question. Schlesselman (1982: 14) describes this research strategy:

The *case-control study,* also commonly called the *retrospective study,* follows a paradigm that proceeds from effect to cause. In a case-control study, individuals with a particular condition or disease (the *cases*) are selected for comparison with a series of individuals in whom the condition or disease is absent (the *controls*). Cases and controls are compared with respect to existing or past attributes or exposures thought to be relevant to the development of the condition or disease under study.

This kind of research is most straighforward when the conditions of interest are clearly bounded, identifiable entities. It is especially useful if these can be indexed by a specific test or syndrome. Even then retrospective data may be biased for a number of reasons, such as the refusal or the inability of study participants to respond to questions, lapses of memory, bias inadvertently introduced by the researcher, and the like. (See, Sackett 1979 for a review of these and other sources of bias.)

Assuming that cases are selected for clear reasons and that potential sources of bias in the retrospective data are guarded against, any case-control study is better or worse depending on the controls picked (Kleinbaum et al 1982: 67—70; Schlesslman 1982). In many studies controls have been selected from among healthy persons who otherwise are "matched" with the cases. But, this is a matter of tradition not of logic. Insisting that controls always be "normals" confuses issues of logic and design with questions of technique and strategy. Using normal controls can even result in a study's being less useful than it might be otherwise. There can be good reasons for choosing controls who share with the cases some general diagnosis (like, cancer) when trying to figure out what makes the different sub-diagnoses (like, breast, throat, lung, etc.) different.

One area for the potential integration of anthropological and epidemiological understandings is in the specification of appropriate controls. Anthropology's contribution can be made through better defining homogeneous groups through the proper identification of important demographic and other social characteristics. The Rubinstein and Brown study sought to assess to what degree children diagnosed as having Attention Deficit Disorder without Hyperactivity differ from children diagnosed as having Attention Deficit Disorder with Hyperactivity on a number of factors that previous research had shown to distinguish "normal" children from the general group of "hyperactive" children.

The specific objective of this research was to see whether a number of standard clinical measures and diagnostic measures available in program records could be used to successfully predict the diagnosis of children seen at a therapeutic research program for ADD/ADDH children during a single year. Upon entering the program children were classified as either ADD or ADDH, using the DSM-III criteria. The classifications were made using the independent judgements of two clinical members of the program staff. Clinical ratings were made without knowledge of each child's individual history. As a result of the classification, an ADD sample was identified ($N = 23$), an ADDH sample was identified ($N = 23$), and three cases for which the classification could not be decided were deleted from further study. A satisfactory level of interrater agreement was obtained. The samples were equivalent on a number of possibly confounding characteristics including age, sex, birth history, and intelligence test scores. In addition, before being treated at the clinic each child was given a thorough physical examination. If that examination showed evidence of gross neurological, sensory, or motor impairment, obvious physical defects, or major disease the child was refered elsewhere for treatment and not entered in to the clinic's program. Therefore, all 46 of the children included in the study showed no oganic basis for their diagnosis.[6]

Comparisons were made between the ADD and ADDH samples on number of variables that previous research had shown to distinguish normal children from "hyperactive" children. These factors are grouped in three sets of measures: attention and impulsivity measures; achievement tests; and rating scales of behavior. (These measures are described briefly in the Appendix to this Chapter, where the study means and standard deviations for each measure are also presented.)

Because the variable-to-subject ratio was too small to allow all of the variables to be used to estimate a discriminant function equation, a variable selection procedure was used. Three step-wise discriminant function procedures, using ADD/ADDH as the dependent variable, were carried out, one for each class of variables listed above (see, Table II). The objective was to select the measures that might be used in a fourth discriminant function analysis to best classify children as ADD or ADDH. Only one of the measures (Teacher Rating Scale of Impulsivity) had a level of significance sufficient for entry into the step-wise discriminant analysis.

Little success was achieved in sorting the children from each sample into ADD and ADDH categories on the basis of the discriminant function model containly only the TRSI (Wilk's lambda = 0.9153, $F(1, 38) = 3.517$, $p = 0.0684$). Using this model 54.5 percent of the children could be classified correctly as to diagnosis, only slighly more accurately than if the assignment had been made randomly (see, Table III).

Because hyperactivity is thought to increase the inability to control attention and impulsive behavior, ADDH children had been expected to score significantly lower on measures of achievement, attention, and impulse

TABLE II
Results of discriminant analyses

	R^2	F	P
Measure			
1. ATTENTION AND IMPULSIVITY			
Matching Familiar Figures Test			
Errors	0.0350	1.499	0.2278
Latency	0.0101	0.417	0.5221
Children's Checking Task			
Omissions	0.0089	0.368	0.5474
Commissions	0.0117	0.485	0.4899
Total	0.0160	0.667	0.4188
Embedded Figures Test	0.0000	0.000	0.9845
WISC-R Attention Concentration			
Arithmetic subtest	0.0202	0.846	0.3630
Coding subtest	0.0263	1.106	0.2992
Digit Span subtest	0.0022	0.089	0.7668
Total	0.0289	1.221	0.2765
2. ACHIEVEMENT			
Wide Range Achievement Test			
Arithmetic	0.0312	1.355	0.2510
Reading	0.0065	0.273	0.6043
Detroit Tests			
Related Words	0.0013	0.054	0.8177
Unrelated Words	0.0013	0.055	0.8154
Letters	0.0011	0.046	0.8308
Durrell Analysis	0.0022	0.007	0.9321
3. BEHAVIOR SCALES			
Conners Teacher Rating Scale	0.0024	0.093	0.7625
Conners Parent Rating Scale	0.0091	0.294	0.5914
Teacher Rating of Attention	0.0193	0.748	0.3924
Teacher Rating of Impulsivity	0.0847	3.517	0.0684[a]

[a] $p < 0.10$.

control, and on judgements of their behavior made by parents and teachers. The group means (presented in the Appendix, Table A1), which showed no significant differences between the two groups on the various measures, fail to support these expectations. The discriminant analyses presented in Table II and III, which yielded no significant ability to discriminate between the

TABLE III
Results of final discriminant analysis

| | Observations Classified into | | |
	ADD	ADDH	
	ADD (%)	ADDH (%)	Total (%)
Classified from			
ADD	12 (54.55)	10 (45.45)	22 (100)
ADDH	10 (45.45)	12 (54.55)	22 (100)
Total	22 (50.00)	22 (50.00)	44 (100)

two groups also failed to support these expectations. The diagnosis could not be predicted from these measures. Thus, a critical appraisal of this part of the psychiatric nosological system was achieved using methods from epidemiologic research.

Among the reasons for undertaking the work which lead to the DSM-III was a desire to improve the accuracy and reliability of psychiatric diagnostic assessment and so to improve its "clinical usefulness for making treatment and management decisions in varied clinical settings" (Spitzer 1980: 2). One of the goals involved in this was that the resulting nosological system be comprised of categories which were consistent with data from research evaluating the validity of those categories. The redefinition of the DSM-II category of Hyperkinetic Reaction of Childhood as comprised of ADD and ADDH is a change consistent with this goal.

The redefinition of the category respected the important and consistent research finding that those children diagnosed as displaying Hyperkinetic Reaction of Childhood actually constituted a very heterogeneous group. It respected too the research-based view that this class of children was comprised of two subclasses such that members of both displayed difficulty in controlling their attention and impulses, and that one group also showed overactive behavior, which was often variable with the context in which the child was observed. The partitioning of the diagnostic category into ADD and ADDH was motivated by the desire to have the diagnostic category be consistent with the research-based understanding of the group's heterogeneity. If diagnosis could be made in a system which allowed children to be referred to a category comprised of a more homogeneous group of children, then more effective treatment and management modalities might be developed.

Part of the heterogeneity characteristic of children who had been diagnosed as having Hyperkinetic Reaction Syndrome was great variation in the display of overactive behavior when these children were observed. The display of their hyperactivity was recognized as being context specific. Indeed, it was the context dependent nature of the display of hyperactivity that had lead some researchers to argue that, when there was no demonstrable organic basis for it, hyperactivity was in fact not a disease of the child.

In evaluating the independence of ADD and ADDH as psychiatric syndromes the underlying question is: does the partitioning of the diagnostic category into two subcategories account for the known heterogeneity of children diagnosed as "hyperactive"? The Rubinstein and Brown study suggests that this partitioning of the diagnostic category does not account adequately for the heterogeneity of behavior displayed by these children, whether for clinical or for research purposes. The clinical usefulness of the ADD/ADDH distinction is then doubtful.

In addition to showing that the distinction between ADD and ADDH does not adequately account for the heterogeneity of the behavior of hyperactive children, the results of the study may also be interpretated as supporting the view that hyperactivity is not a disease of the child. In fact, Rubinstein and Brown (1984: 412) concluded:

We interpret these results as supporting the view that many hyperactive children are not 'sick' in some medical sense but rather are involved in a complex process of social interaction, the meaning and significance of which we have yet to fully understand.

The results of this study bring into sharp focus two conflicting views of the nature of hyperactivity as a phenomenon. One view holds that hyperactivity is a real disease of the child, but one which must be conceptualized as having several distinct subtypes. The other holds that hyperactivity is not a disease of the child, but rather the reification of social processes which result in the labeling as sick of children who act badly.

Based on our reading of the literature in this area and on the results of the Rubinstein and Brown study we incline toward the latter view. The evaluation of the ADD/ADDH category serves to bring the two approaches into focus. This study is one step in an iterative process of research wherein our understanding of the phenomenon of "hyperactivity" is advanced by alternating attention between methodological concerns and conceptual levels. Neither the Rubinstein and Brown study nor other research can provide *the* clear result that can be used to arbitrate between the views of "hyperactivity" described above. For this, continuing research is needed.

This work can build on the basic anthropological insight that there is "such a vast variety of ways through which people conceive and interact with their environments and experiences that not even the most common objects or characteristics can be assumed by the researcher to have an invariant, objective existence outside of the context of some specified system of meanings" (Rubinstein 1984: 173). For the research community this means recognizing that problematic situations do not become problems until they are so defined (Schön 1983; Dumont 1984). One approach that the research and clinical communities can use to incorporate this recognition into their work is to seek nosological categories that explicitly tie diagnosis to context and social process, and always to consider these categories to be provisional in a fundamental sense.

Such research might be carried out using a combination of anthropological and epidemiological considerations. Anthropological understanding of hyperactivity can be used to stregnthen the design of studies that use epidemiological methods. One way this can be done is to use anthropological information to define the appropriate "case" and "control" groups. Thus, for instance, studies might be designed which incorporate widely used research and diagnostic measures and seek to predict on the basis of such instruments membership in *multiple* categories, rather than only in the two categories defined by ADD and ADDH.

This research process might begin by examining the *contexts* in which a child displayed behavior labeled as hyperactivity, as judged by multiple raters making multiple independent ratings. Then, the social processes through which children get diagnosed as "hyperactive in context 'X'" would be reported by researchers trained to make detailed descriptions of the interaction of children with their peers and with adults.

The literature on hyperactivity suggests that there are at least four contexts across which "hyperactive" children's behavior appears to vary: (1) home; (2) school; (3) clinician's office; and, (4) at play with peers. Since some children are reported to display hyperactive behavior in more than one of these contexts, categories need to be defined by the combination of these settings as well. An initial study might usefully examine hyperactive behavior in all of these four contexts, or that displayed in each of the four contexts, or at school, at home, and at play with peers, or only at home and at play with peers.

Work with appropriately specified groups of children would facilitate the exploration of questions of social process and meaning involved in the diagnosis of disorders like "hyperactivity". Beyond asking how a poorly defined group of children varies systematically from "normal" children, working with well-specified groups would allow the investigation of how the diagnosis of "hyperactivity" in specific contexts gains meaning from those contexts. It would also allow the exploration of the implications for the day-to-day lives of children diagnosed as disordered in those contexts.

Because they depart from earlier research which accepted the commitments of one or another tradition and incorporates some from each, such studies can properly be seen as indicating one way in which the understandings of psychosocial problems from different levels can be usefully incorporated into a coherent research program.

THE NONSPECIFICITY OF THE "NEW MORBIDITY"

The problems of reliability and validity confronting the diagnosis of psychosocial disorders in children are immense. Such difficulties are not unique to the category of Attention Deficit Disorder but must also be faced when determining that a child has behavioral, educational, social, or situational problems, or other of the many "disorders" that are taken to make up the "new morbidity" (e.g., Starfield et al. 1980: 160). In fact, the difficulties evident in the nosological treatment of childhood problems are also found in the professional categories used to deal with adults who have difficulties negotiating life (Dumont 1984).

Because the professional definitions of these disorders are said to be scientific and objective, and thus not culture dependent or culture specific in nature, anthropologically-oriented researchers object that this nosological system blurs the fact that all behavior is appropriate or inappropriate only in relation to specific contexts and in relation to the meanings that people give to those contexts. From this perspective what counts healthy or sick, or as desirable or nondesirable activities is socially constructed, and reflects the beliefs, values, and norms basic to an individual's society. This means that "folk" models of health and illness may vary substantially from professional models especially in the psychological and behavioral areas.

Examples of the disparity between professional and local models of health and illness are easily recognized in attempts to bring Western medicine to nonwestern settings (Foster and Anderson 1978). While there may be some resistance among health professionals to the idea that the Western medical and public health practices they champion are culturally situated, for the most part such cross-cultural work leads to an acknowledgement of and respect for the importance and reality of different culturally patterned ways of maintaining health and dealing with illness (Paul 1955, and compare Engleharht 1980 with Fox and Swazey 1984).

Qualitative researchers argue that in a plural society like the United States, it is equally important to pay attention to the different ways different groups of people socially construct health and illness. This claim is taken most seriously by health care workers when they deal with geographically or ethnically defined minority groups (e.g., Deuschle 1982; Harwood 1981).

Qualitative researchers extend this approach to the mainstream of our own society. They argue that in psychosocial work it is particularly important to recognize that there are many coexisting constructs of health and illness. Behavior deemed appropriate by some groups of lay-people may be defined as unhealthy both by professionals and by other groups of lay-people. Similarly health behavior, as professionally defined, may be seen as unhealthy by some nonprofessionals. This has led some researchers to claim that much of what is now called psychosocial disorder really reflects only culturally patterned variations of life style and social relations. The fact that health care providers see many of the psychosocial disorders as being most prevalent in poor and minority populations has reinforced this social and cultural interpretation, and led to the further argument that these phenomena are not really disorders.

Clinicians and epidemiological researchers find this proposal unacceptable, and in response they have redoubled their efforts to find and state precisely the characteristics of the various psychosocial disorders. The DSM-III is one such response, and renewed interest in demonstrating the efficacy of "well-child" visits to pediatricians is another. These researchers and clinicians respond that the children and adults they see *are* disturbed and deserve some help. This is a proper response. But further developing a model of these troubles as "mental disease", which has already been demonstrated to be by itself inadequate, moves us further away from being able to be really helpful (Eysenck et al. 1983).

Furthermore, the result "saves the appearance" of the wisdom of expert knowledge; it does not use the discovery of difficulties with this knowledge — anomalous data — to revise the model in ways that lead to conceptual advances.[7] This happens because each systematization directs attention toward specific characteristics of psychosocial problems, while also directing attention away from other aspects of those problems. Such selectivity makes it easier to make some useful judgements. But, directing attention away from some aspects of these problems also creates systematic biases in our research and clinical observations. If we are not self-conscious about this possibility, it may lead to over-simplification which hinders fuller understanding of psychosocial problems.

Unfortunately, neither anthropological nor epidemiological approaches escape this difficulty. After a point, the harder we strive to produce a picture of psychosocial problems consistent with either the basic concepts of the anthropological model alone or of the epidemiological model alone the less we put to good conceptual use data inconsistent with the framework from within which we work (Argyris 1980; Rubinstein et al. 1984).

Arguments over proper methodology and nomenclature further obscure our understanding of psychosocial problems. Giving voice to the difficulties this situation poses, Dumont (1984) provides the appropriate response of epidemiological researchers to extreme qualitative interpretations that deny the existence of psychosocial problems — "That the perceptions of a cloud are capricious and fleeting does not mean that a cloud is not there" (1984: 329). He also tells us how to reply to epidemiological researchers who would forge ahead insisting that their methodological strictures should always be used to measure the adequacy of research. Assuming that psychosocial problems have "objective" parameters permits "researchers and clinicians to draw meaningful inferences from statistical trends which, like the edges of any moving cloud tend to fulfill the fantasies of the beholder" (Dumont 1984: 328—329).

The role of the social environment and of social processes in the development of psychosocial difficulties is clearly significant, though poorly understood. It is therefore necessary to *understand* equally both how these problems develop, and how to form a useful set of nosological categories. Answers to these conjoined questions about the meaning, significance and nature of psychosocial problems for children, and for adults, clearly lie outside of the explanatory models of either anthropological or epidemiological research alone. They are also beyond the scope of traditional curative medical practice.

If we are to meet our desire to alleviate the suffering that psychosocial problems entail, we will need new forms of research collaboration, of theory, and of practice. To succeed these will need to include conceptual and social arrangements that are significantly different from those that now inform research and health care in the United States. These changes can most likely be brought about if emphasis is placed on the conceptual integration of different theoretical approaches rather than simply by attempting to coordinate separate, often inconsistent, methodological preferences.

APPENDIX

In the Rubinstein and Brown (1984) study, comparisons were made between the ADD and ADDH samples on a number of variables that previous research had shown to distinguish normal children from "hyperactive" children. These variables are assessed by three sets of measures: attention and impulsivity measures; achievement tests; and rating scale of behavior. This Appendix briefly describes these measures and presents the study means and standard deviations for each.

Measures of Attention and Impulsivity

Matching Familiar Figures Test (MFF). This test was developed to measure impulsivity. The MFF is a visual matching task in which a target figure and six alternatives are presented. The task is to choose from the six alternative figures the one that is identical to the target. Twelve target figures are presented during the test. Two measures are derived: (1) total number of errors in the choice of correct alternatives, and (2) the time in seconds between the presentation of the target and alternatives and the first response.

Children's Checking Task (CCT). The CCT was developed as a technique for measuring ability to sustain attention and effort to a task over time. During the CCT a child listens to a tape recording of a series of numbers. The child's task is to check off, in response to the tape recording, an almost identical series in a standard answer booklet. This checking task involves checking the recording against eighty 14-digit rows. Errors of omission are recorded.

TABLE A1

Means, standard deviations, and *t* tests for study measures

	ADD (N = 23)		ADDH (N = 23)		t^a
	X̄	SD	X̄	SD	
Measure					
Matching Familiar Figures Test					
Errors	13.25	7.51	16.17	7.73	1.30
Latency	126.83	50.09	135.39	89.09	0.40
Children's Checking Task					
Omissions	29.23	20.75	33.05	20.51	0.61
Commissions	10.77	15.75	15.76	29.47	0.69
Total	40.00	31.15	48.81	39.29	0.82
Embedded Figures Test	13.00	5.48	12.57	5.24	0.27
WISC-R Attention Concentration					
Arithmetic subtest	8.30	1.66	8.30	3.63	0.00
Coding subtest	35.43	11.68	37.61	15.43	0.54
Digit Span subtest	8.09	2.19	7.96	3.15	0.16
Total	51.83	12.93	53.81	19.46	0.42
Wide Range Achievement Test					
Arithmetic	27.62	6.06	25.22	7.47	1.16
Reading	54.62	16.68	51.96	17.65	0.52
Detroit Tests					
Related Words	34.55	7.90	34.73	10.30	0.07
Unrelated Words	43.41	15.13	43.26	15.73	0.03
Letters	10.54	0.86	10.04	1.00	0.38
Durrell Analysis	22.50	9.67	22.26	6.55	0.09
Conners Teacher Rating Scale	16.91	7.34	17.05	4.98	0.07
Conners Parent Rating Scale	19.18	4.97	20.65	4.31	0.06
Teacher Rating of Attention	52.68	12.26	55.90	11.28	0.86
Teacher Rating of Impulsivity	65.23	10.00	71.00	10.86	0.07

[a] Nonsignificant for all measures.

Embedded Figures Test (EFT). The EFT requires the discovery of a simple target figure in a complex background. It is a measure of the ability to focus attention and to organize a perceptual field. In the clinic's files scores for the EFT were recorded that indicated the number of correctly identified figures.

Attention-Concentration Factor of the WISC-R. This measure represents the scores of each child on three subtests of the WISC-R. These subtests are: (1) arithmetic subtest, which assesses the level at which a child can successfully carry out arithmetic computations; (2) coding scales, which provide an indication of how many target symbols a child can code to a corresponding space; and (3) digit span subtest, which indicates the number of increasingly large spans of digits a child can recall correctly.

Measures of Achievement

Wide Range Achievement Test (WRAT). The clinical assessment procedures of the clinic included the administration to each child of the reading and arithmetic subtests of the WRAT. These are widely used as indications of a child's ability and grade level.

Detroit Tests of Academic Achievement. Three subtests of the Detroit Tests of Academic Achievement were administered to each child in the program. Each of these assesses the recall of related words, of unrelated words, and of letters. Subtest scores have been shown to be related to achievement.

Durrell Analysis of Reading Difficulty. The Durrell subtests for oral reading, oral comprehension, listening comprehension, and spelling were administered to each child. Raw scores, on these subtests and scores convereted to grade level of achievement, were available in the clinic's files.

Rating Scales of Behavior

Conner's Rating Scales. Recorded for each child were the results of ratings by teachers (CTRS) and by parents (CPRS) on a ten item hyperactivity scale. Each teacher or parent rated the child on a four-point continuum (from "not at all" to "very much") for each of ten behaviors described on the scale. These included behaviors like, "restless and over active", and "sit and fidgets with small objects".

Teacher Ratings of Attention (TRSA). The attentional behavior of children who participated in the program was evaluated by their teacher using a scale that consisted of 19 descriptive statements that had been related to laboratory attention tasks. Teachers' judgements were made on a five-point scale ranging from "never describes this child" to "always describes this child".

Teacher Ratings of Impulsivity (TRSI). Each child's teacher completed a scale assessing impulsive behavior. It consists of twenty-one descriptive statements about impulse control that are responded to on a five point scale.

ACKNOWLEDGEMENTS

Portions of this paper were presented at the 1984 Annual Meeting of the American Public Health Association, November, Anaheim, California. Preparation of this paper was supported by United States Public Health Service grant MCJ-170486-01-0, to the American Academy of Pediatrics.

The views expressed in this paper are those of the authors and no official endorsement by the American Academy of Pediatrics is intended or should be inferred. We thank Mary LeCron Foster, David J. Hufford, Phil Kletke, Susan LeBailly, C. Timothy McKeown, James Orr, Sol Tax, and Jeffrey Ward for critical comments on an earlier draft of this paper.

NOTES

1. Although we refer to "qualitative" and "anthropological" methods interchangeably throughout this paper, it is important to note that traditional anthropological methods are only a subset of the qualitative approaches used in social research. Sociology, education, and other disciplines have also developed qualitative approaches to the study of social life. However, sometimes methodological terms shared by these approaches are given different meanings. For instance, traditionally anthropologists have used "ethnographic" to mean long term, participant-observation, while sociologists and education researchers use "ethnographic" to describe their observational methods (compare Estroff 1981; and Bluebond-Langner 1978 with Beuf 1979). Further contrasts among and between anthropological, sociological, education, and other approaches to qualitative research can be found by comparing Agar (1980), and Pelto and Pelto (1978) to Van Maanen (1983), and Miles and Huberman (1984); Spradley (1979) to Sudman and Bradburn (1982).
2. True prevalence refers to the number of people in a population who actually have a disease or disorder at a given point in time. Treated prevalence refers to the estimate of true prevalance based only on the number of people in a population who were under treatment for a disease of disorder at a given point in time. Similarly, true incidence measures the rate at which new cases of a disease or disorder occur during a specified period, and treated incidence is an estimate of true incidence based on the rate of new cases of a disease or disorder comming under treatment during a specified time. Because treated incidence and prevalence rates are based on a nonsystematic sampling of the population it is likely that they over- or underestimate the true incidence and prevalence rates of the disease or disorder.
3. Many of the epistemological issues that lead to the disjunction between qualitative and quantitative research are discussed by Rubinstein et al. (1984). The specifics of the clash between the foundational assumptions of psychosocial epidemiological research and anthropological research on mental health and illness are considered in detail by Rubinstein (1984).
4. There is considerable disagreement about the status of hyperactivity as a disease entity. For that reason, whenever we refer to hyperactivity as a diagnosis we enclose it in quotation marks.
5. Some epidemiologists would argue that, because what counts as a case is unclear, attempts at studying the epidemiology of psychosocial disorders are fundamentally misguided.
6. There are four general diagnostic possibilities. Children diagnosed as ADD could be: (1) true positives, that is there is a known organic basis for the diagnosis; (2) false positives, children incorrectly diagnosed as ADD; (3) children whose ADD diagnosis has an as yet undiscovered organic basis; and (4) children whose diagnosis has a social rather than organic basis. The study reported here examined only the latter three categories.
7. The general sociological reasons behind this "saving of appearances" by both qualitative and quantitative researchers is suggested by Merton's (1965) account of the "Hooke-Newton-Merton", or simply "kindle cole", principle of interaction among scientists: "when scientists report their differences in public, they are often moved to engage in polemical discourse designed to save their hypotheses (and so their faces) rather than to strive, quite disinterestedly, for Discovery of Truth" (Merton 1965: 29).

REFERENCES

Ablon, J.
    1984   Little People in America: The Social Dimensions of Dwarfism. New York: Praeger.
    1981   Urban Field Research in the United States: The Long Journey from the Exotic to the Mundane. Kroeber Papers 1981: 108—120.
    1977   Field Methods for Working with Middle Class Americans: New Issues of Values, Personality, and Reciprocity. Human Organization 36: 69—72.
Adair, J. and K. Deuschle
    1970   The People's Health: Medicine and Anthropology in a Navajo Community. New York: Appleton-Century-Crofts.
Acosta, F., J. Yamamoto, and L. Evens
    1982   Effective Psychotherapy for Low-Income and Minority Patients. New York: Plenum.
Agar, M.
    1980   The Professional Stranger: An Informal Introduction to Ethnography. New York: Academic Press.
Argyris, C.
    1980   Inner Contradictions of Rigorous Research. New York: Academic Press.
Barkley, R.
    1981   Hyperactive Children. New York: Guilford
Barkley and C. Cunningham
    1979   The Effects of Methylphenidate on the Mother-Child Interactions of Hyperactive Children. Archives of General Psychiatry 36: 201—211.
Beuf, A.
    1979   Biting off the Bracelet: A Study of Children in Hospitals. Philadelphia: University of Pennsylvania Press.
Bluebond-Langner, M.
    1978   The Private Worlds of Dying Children. Princeton, NJ: Princeton University Press.
Bosco, J. and S. Robin
    1980   Hyperkinesis: Prevalence and Treatment. In C. Whalen and B. Henker (eds.), Hyperactive Children, New York: Academic Press.
Brewer, M. and B. Collins (eds.)
    1981   Scientific Inquiry in the Social Sciences. San Francisco: Jossey-Bass.
Brown, R. and L. Quay
    1977   Reflection-Impulsivity in Normal and Behavior Disordered Children. Journal of Abnormal and Child Psychology 5: 457—462.
Campbell, D.
    1978   Qualitiative Knowing in Action Research. In M. Brenner, P. Marsh, and M. Brenner, (eds.), The Social Contexts of Method. New York: St. Martin's Press.
Campbell, D. and D. Fiske
    1959   Convergent and Discriminant Validation by the Multitrait-Multimethod Matrix. Psychological Bulletin 56: 81—105.
Cantwell, D. (ed.)
    1975   The Hyperactive Child: Diagnosis, Management, Current Research. New York: Spectrum.
Cantwell, D. and J. Satterfield
    1978   The Prevalence of Academic Under-achievement in Hyperactive Children. Journal of Pediatric Psychology 3: 168—171.
Collins, B.
    1981   Hyperactivity: Myth and Entity. In M. Brewer and B. Collins (eds.), Scientific Inquiry in the Social Sciences. San Francisco: Jossey-Bass.

Conrad, P.
    1975 The Discovery of Hyperkinesis: Notes on the Medicalization of Deviant Behavior.
          Social Problems 23: 12—21.
Conrad, P. and J. Schneider
    1980 Deviance and Medicalization: From Badness to Sickness. St. Louis: C. V. Mosby
          Co.
Deuschle, K.
    1982 Community-Oriented Primary Care: Lessons Learned in Three Decades. Journal of
          Community Health 8: 13—22.
Douglas, V.
    1972 Stop, Look and Listen: The Problem of Sustained Attention and Impulse Control in
          Hyperactive and Normal Children. Canadian Journal of Behavioral Science 4:
          261—281.
Dumont, M.
    1984 The Nonspecificity of Mental Illness. American Journal of Orthopsychiatry 54:
          326—334.
Dunham, W.
    1959 Sociological Theory and Mental Disorders. Detroit: Wayne State University Press.
Englehardt, H.
    1980 Bioethics in the People's Republic of China. Hastings Center Report 10: 7—10.
Estroff, S.
    1981 Making it Crazy: An Ethnography of Psychiatric Clients in an American Com-
          munity. Berkeley: University of California Press.
Eysenck, H., J. Wakefield, and A. Friedman
    1983 Diagnosis and Clinical Assessment: DSM-III. Annual Review of Psychology 34:
          167—193.
Foster, G. and B. Anderson
    1978 Medical Anthropology. New York: Wiley.
Foster, G., T. Scudder, E. Colson, and R. Kemper
    1979 Long-Term Field Research in Social Anthropology. New York: Academic Press.
Fox, R. C. and J. P. Swazay
    1984 Medical Morality is not Bioethics — Medical Ethics in China and the United States.
          Perspectives in Biology and Medicine 273: 336—360.
Gilbert, J. R., W. Feldman, L. Siegel, D. Mills, C. Dunnett, and G. Stoddart
    1984 How Many Well-Baby Visits are Necessary in the First 2 Years of Life?, Canadian
          Medical Association Journal 130: 857—861.
Green, M.
    1983 Coming of Age in General Pediatrics. Pediatrics 72: 275—282.
Green, M. (ed.)
    1985 The Psychosocial Aspects of the Family: The New Pediatrics. Lexington, MA:
          Lexington Books.
Green, M., T. Brazelton, D. Friedman, J. Reinhart, I. Schwartz, and P. Wallace
    1982 Pediatrics and the Psychosocial Aspects of Child and Family Health, Pediatrics 79:
          126—127.
Haggerty, R. J.
    1983 President's Report. William T. Grant Foundation 1983 Annual Report. New York:
          W. T. Grant Foundation.
    1982 Behavioral Pediatrics: Can it be Taught? Can it be Practiced?. Pediatric Clinics of
          North America 292: 391.
Haggerty, R. J., K. Roghmann, and I. Pless
    1975 Child Health and the Community. New York: John Wiley and Sons.
Hall, P.
    1982 Great Planning Disasters. Berkeley: University of California Press.

Harvard Child Health Project
   1977   Toward a Primary Medical Care System Responsive to Children's Needs. Volumes
           I—III. Cambridge, MA: Ballinger.
Harwood, A. (ed.)
   1981   Ethnicity and Medical Care. Cambridge, MA: Harvard University Press.
Hollingshead, A. B. and F. C. Redlich
   1958   Social Class and Mental Illness. New York: Wiley and Sons.
Homatidis, S. and M. Konstrantreas
   1981   Assessment of Hyperactivity: Isolating Measures of High Discriminant Ability.
           Journal of Consulting and Clinical Psychology 49: 533—541.
Huessy, H.
   1974   Hyperkinetic Problems Continue to Teens. Clinical Psychiatry News 2: 5.
   1967   Study of the Prevalence and Therapy of the Choreatiform Syndrome or Hyper-
           kinesis in Rural Vermont. Acta Paedopsychiatrica 34: 130—135
Huessy, H. and R. Gendron
   1970   Prevalence of the So-Called Hyperkinetic Syndrome in Public School Children of
           Vermont. Acta Paedopsychiatrica 37: 243—248.
Hufford, D. J.
   1983   The Supernatural and the Sociology of Knowledge: Explaining Academic Belief,
           New York Folklore Quarterly 9(1/2): 21—29.
   1982   The Terror that Comes in the Night: An Experience-Centered Study of Super-
           natural Assault Traditions. Philadelphia: University of Pennsylvania Press.
Kaplan, M.
   1983   A Woman's View of DSM-III. American Psychologist 38: 738—792.
Kleinbaum, D., L. Kupper, and H. Morgenstern
   1982   Epidemiologic Research: Principles and Quantitative Methods. Belmont, CA: Life-
           time Learning.
Lambert, N., J. Sandoval, and D. Sassone
   1978   Prevalence of Hyperactivity in Elementary School as a Function of Social System
           Definers. American Journal of Orthopsychiatry 48: 446—463.
Landy, D. (ed.)
   1977   Culture, Disease and Healing. New York: Macmillian.
Lapouse, R. and M. Monk
   1958   An Epidemiolgical Study of Behavior Characteristics in Children. American Journal
           of Public Health 48: 1134—1144.
Leighton, A., D. Leighton, and R. Danley
   1966   Validity in Mental Health Surveys. Canadian Psychiatric Association Journal 11:
           167—178.
Merton, R. K.
   1965   On the Shoulders of Giants: A Shandean Postscript. New York: Harcourt Brace
           Jovanovich.
Miles, M. and A. Huberman
   1984   Qualitative Data Analysis: A Sourcebook of New Methods. Beverly Hills, CA.: Sage
           Publications.
Miller, R., H. Palkes, and M. Stewart
   1973   Hyperactive Children in Suburban Elementary Schools. Child Psychiatry and
           Human Development 4: 121—127.
Naroll, R. and R. Cohen (eds.)
   1973   A Handbook of Method in Cultural Anthropology. New York: Columbia University
           Press.
Namir, S. and R. Weinstein
   1982   Children. In L. Snowden (ed.), Reaching the Underserved. Beverly Hills: Sage
           Publications.

Newell, A.
  1973 You Can't Play 20 Questions with Nature and Win. *In* R. Chase (ed.), Visual Information Processing, New York: Academic Press.
Paul, B. (ed.)
  1955 Health, Culture and Community. New York: Russell Sage Foundation.
Pawluch, Dorothy
  1983 Transitions in Pediatrics: A Segmental Analysis. Social Problems 30: 449—465.
Pelto, P. and G. Pelto
  1978 Anthropological Research: The Structure of Iquiry. Cambridge: Cambridge University Press.
Penfold, P. S. and G. Walker
  1983 Women and the Psychiatric Paradox. Montreal: Eden Press.
Perloff, J. D., S. A. LeBailly, P. R. Kletke, P. P. Budetti, and J. P. Connelly
  1984 Premature Death in the United States: Years of Life Lost and Health Priorities. Journal of Public Health Policy 5: 167—184.
Quine, W.
  1964 On Simple Theories of a Complex World. *In* Gregg and Harris (eds.), Form and Strategy in Science, Dordrecht: Reidel.
Rapoport, R. N.
  1959 Community as Doctor. London: Tavistock.
Renshaw, D.
  1974 The Hyperactive Child. Chicago: Nelson-Hall.
Rogers, K. D., R. Ernst, I. Shulman, and K. Reisinger
  1974 Effectiveness of Aggressive Follow-up on Navajo Infant Health and Medical Care. Pediatrics 53: 721—725.
Roghmann, K., H. Babigian, I. Goldberg, and T. Zastowny
  1982 The Increasing Number of Children Using Psychiatric Services: Analysis of a Cumulative Psychiatric Case Register. Pediatrics 70: 790—800.
Roghmann, K., R. Hoekelman, and T. McInerny
  1984 The Changing Pattern of Primary Pediatric Care: Update for One Community. Pediatrics 73: 363—374.
Roghmann, K., T. Zastowny, and H. Babigian
  1984 Mental Health Problems of Children: Analysis of a Cumulative Psychiatric Case Register. Pediatrics 73: 781—790.
Ross, A. and W. Pelham
  1981 Child Psychopathology. Annual Review of Psychology 32: 243—278.
Rubinstein, R. A.
  1986 Reflections on Action Anthropology: Some Developmental Dynamics of an Anthropological Tradition. Human Organization 45: in press.
  1984 Epidemiology and Anthropology: Notes on Science and Scientism. Communication and Cognition 17: 163—185.
  1983 Structuralism and the Study of Cognitive Process. *In* J. Oosten and A. de Ruijter (eds.), The Future of Structuralism, Gottingen: Edition Herodot.
Rubinstein, R. A. and R. T. Brown
  1984 An Evaluation of the Validity of the Diagnostic Category of Attention Deficit Disorder. American Journal of Orthopsychiatry 54: 398—414.
Rubinstein, R. A. and C. D. Laughlin
  1977 Bridging Levels of Systemic Organization. Current Anthropology 18: 459—481.
Rubinstein, R. A., C. D. Laughlin, and J. McManus
  1984 Science as Cognitive Process: Toward an Empirical Philosophy of Science. Philadelphia: University of Pennsylvania Press.
Russel, A., R. Mattison, and D. Cantwell
  1983 DSM-III in the Clinical Practice of Child Psychiatry. Journal of Clinical Psychiatry 44: 86—90.

Rutter, M.
   1978   Brain Damage Syndromes in Childhood: Concepts and Findings. Journal of Child
          Psychology and Psychiatry 18: 1—21.
Sackett, D.
   1979   Bias in Analytic Research. Journal of Chronic Diseases 32: 51—60.
Safer, D. and R. Allen
   1976   Hyperactive Children: Diagnosis and Management. Baltimore: University Park
          Press.
Schensul, S. and M. Borrero (eds.)
   1982   Action Research and Health Systems Change in an Inner-City Puerto Rican Com-
          munity. Special Issue of Urban Anthropology 11: 1—153.
Schlesselman, J.
   1982   Case-Control Studies: Design, Conduct, Analysis. New York: Oxford University
          Press.
Schön, D.
   1983   The Reflective Practioner. New York: Basic Books.
Scott, R.
   1969   The Making of Blind Men: A Study of Adult Socialization. New York: Russell Sage
          Foundation.
Simon, H. A.
   1983   Reason in Human Affairs. Stanford: Stanford University Press.
Sleator, E. and R. Ullman
   1981   Can the Physician Diagnose Hyperactivity in the Office? Pediatrics 67: 13—17.
Spitzer, R.
   1980   Introduction. In Diagnostic and Statistical Manual of Mental Disorders, Third
          Edition. Washington, D.C.: American Psychiatric Association.
Spradley, J. P.
   1979   The Ethnographic Interview. New York: Holt, Rinehart, and Winston.
Sprague, R., D. Christensen, and J. Werry
   1974   Experimental Psychology and Sitmulant Drugs. In C. Connors, (ed.), The Clinical
          Use of Stimulant Drugs in Children, New York: Elsevier.
Srole, L., T. Langer, S. Michael, M. Opler, and T. Rennie
   1962   Mental Health in the Metropolis: The Midtown Manhattan Study. New York.
          McGraw Hill.
Starfield, B., E. Gross, M. Wood, R. Pantell, C. Allen, I. B. Gordon, P. Moffatt, R. Drachman,
and H. Katz
   1980   Psychosocial and Psychosomatic Diagnoses in Primary Care of Children. Pediatrics
          66: 159—167.
Starfield, B., H. Katz, A Gabriel, G. Livingston, P. Benson, J. Hankin, S. Horn, and D.
Steinwachs
   1984   Morbidity in Childhood — A Longitudinal View. The New England Journal of
          Medicine 310: 824—829.
Stewart, M., F. Pitts, A. Craig, and W. Dieruf
   1966   The Hyperactive Child Syndrome. American Journal of Orthopsychiatry 36: 861—
          867.
Strauss, A. and L. Lehtinen
   1940   Psychopathology and Education in the Brain Injured Child. New York: Grune and
          Stratton.
Sudman, S. and N. Bradburn
   1982   Asking Questions: A Practical Guide to Questionnaire Design. San Francisco:
          Jossey-Bass.
Sykes, D., V. Douglas, and G. Morgenstern
   1973   Sustained Attention in Hyperactive Children. Journal of Child Psychology and
          Psychiatry 25: 262—274.

Trites, R.
   1979   Prevalence of Hyperactivity in Ottawa, Canada. *In* R. Trites (ed.), Hyperactivity in Children, Baltimore: University Park Press.
Van Maanen, J. (ed.)
   1983   Qualitative Methodology. Beverly Hills, CA.: Sage Publications.
Ward, J. and O. Werner
   1984   Difference and Dissonance in Ethnographic Data. *In* R. Rubinstein and R. Pinxten (eds.), Epistemology and Process: Anthropological Views, Ghent: Communication and Cognition Books.
Wender, P.
   1975   Minimal Brain Disfunction in Children. New York: Wiley.
Whalen, C. and B. Henker (eds.)
   1980   Hyperactive Children: The Social Etiology of Identification and Treatment. New York: Academic Press.
Whitehead, A. N.
   1960   Process and Reality. New York: Norton.
Wimsatt, W.
   1981   Robustness, Reliability, and Overdetermination. *In* Scientific Inquiry and the Social Sciences. San Francisco: Jossey-Bass.

LIST OF CONTRIBUTORS

Frederick L. Dunn, M.D., Ph.D., Department of Epidemiology and International Health, University of California, San Francisco, CA 94143.

Sandra M. Gifford, Ph.D., M.P.H., Health Department Victoria, Melbourne, Australia.

E. Michael Gorman, Ph.D., M.P.H., Center for Professional Development and Training, Centers for Disease Control, Atlanta, GA 30303.

Craig R. Janes, Ph.D., Department of Anthropology, University of Colorado, Denver, CO 80202.

Peter Kunstadter, Ph.D., Department of Epidemiology and International Health, University of California, San Francisco, CA 94143.

Marilyn K. Nations, Ph.D., Department of Internal Medicine, Division of Geographic Medicine, University of Virginia, Charlottesville, VA 22908.

John D. O'Neil, Ph.D., Department of Social and Behavioral Medicine, University of Manitoba, Winnipeg, Manitoba, R3E 0W3.

Janet D. Perloff, Ph.D., Center for Educational Development, Health Sciences Center, University of Illinois, Chicago, IL 60680.

Robert A. Rubinstein, Ph.D., M.S.P.H., Program in Ethnography and Public Policy, Department of Anthropology, Northwestern University, Evanston, IL 60201.

Ron Stall, Ph.D., M.P.H., Department of Urban Studies, Rutgers University, New Brunswick, NJ 08903.

James Trostle, M.A., M.P.H., Program in Medical Anthropolgy, University of California, San Francisco, CA 94143.

Craig R. Janes et al. (eds.), Anthropology and Epidemiology, 333.
© 1986 *by D. Reidel Publishing Company.*

INDEX OF NAMES

335

INDEX OF NAMES

INDEX OF SUBJECTS